Sudden Cardiac Death: Clinical Updates and Perspectives

Sudden Cardiac Death: Clinical Updates and Perspectives

Editors

Tobias Schupp
Michael Behnes

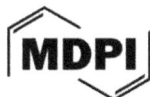

Basel • Beijing • Wuhan • Barcelona • Belgrade • Novi Sad • Cluj • Manchester

Editors

Tobias Schupp
University of Heidelberg
Mannheim, Germany

Michael Behnes
University of Heidelberg
Mannheim, Germany

Editorial Office
MDPI
St. Alban-Anlage 66
4052 Basel, Switzerland

This is a reprint of articles from the Special Issue published online in the open access journal *Journal of Clinical Medicine* (ISSN 2077-0383) (available at: https://www.mdpi.com/journal/jcm/special_issues/sudden_cardiac_death).

For citation purposes, cite each article independently as indicated on the article page online and as indicated below:

Lastname, A.A.; Lastname, B.B. Article Title. *Journal Name* **Year**, *Volume Number*, Page Range.

ISBN 978-3-0365-9198-8 (Hbk)
ISBN 978-3-0365-9199-5 (PDF)
doi.org/10.3390/books978-3-0365-9199-5

© 2023 by the authors. Articles in this book are Open Access and distributed under the Creative Commons Attribution (CC BY) license. The book as a whole is distributed by MDPI under the terms and conditions of the Creative Commons Attribution-NonCommercial-NoDerivs (CC BY-NC-ND) license.

Contents

Tobias Schupp, Ibrahim Akin and Michael Behnes
Special Issue: Sudden Cardiac Death: Clinical Updates and Perspectives
Reprinted from: *J. Clin. Med.* **2022**, *11*, 3120, doi:10.3390/jcm11113120 1

Tobias Schupp, Michael Behnes, Mohammad Abumayyaleh, Kathrin Weidner,
Kambis Mashayekhi, Thomas Bertsch and Ibrahim Akin
Angiotensin Converting Enzyme Inhibitors versus Receptor Blockers in Patients with Ventricular Tachyarrhythmias
Reprinted from: *J. Clin. Med.* **2022**, *11*, 1460 , doi:10.3390/jcm11051460 5

Yun Gi Kim, Kyungdo Han, Joo Hee Jeong, Seung-Young Roh, Yun Young Choi,
Kyongjin Min, et al.
Metabolic Syndrome, Gamma-Glutamyl Transferase, and Risk of Sudden Cardiac Death
Reprinted from: *J. Clin. Med.* **2022**, *11*, 1781, doi:10.3390/jcm11071781 17

Tsuyoshi Nojima, Hiromichi Naito, Takafumi Obara, Kohei Ageta, Hiromasa Yakushiji, Tetsuya Yumoto, et al.
Can Blood Ammonia Level, Prehospital Time, and Return of Spontaneous Circulation Predict Neurological Outcomes of Out-of-Hospital Cardiac Arrest Patients? A Nationwide, Retrospective Cohort Study
Reprinted from: *J. Clin. Med.* **2022**, *11*, 2566 , doi:10.3390/jcm11092566 29

Susanne Rysz, Malin Jonsson Fagerlund, Johan Lundberg, Mattias Ringh, Jacob Hollenberg, Marcus Lindgren, et al.
The Use of Levosimendan after Out-of-Hospital Cardiac Arrest and Its Association with Outcome—An Observational Study
Reprinted from: *J. Clin. Med.* **2022**, *11*, 2621 , doi:10.3390/jcm11092621 41

Ibrahim Akin, Michael Behnes, Julian Müller, Jan Forner, Mohammad Abumayyaleh, Kambis Mashayekhi, et al.
Prognostic Value of Cardiac Troponin I in Patients with Ventricular Tachyarrhythmias
Reprinted from: *J. Clin. Med.* **2022**, *11*, 2987 , doi:10.3390/jcm11112987 53

Quentin Delbaere, Myriam Akodad, François Roubille, Benoît Lattuca, Guillaume Cayla and Florence Leclercq
One-Year Follow-Up of Patients Admitted for Emergency Coronary Angiography after Resuscitated Cardiac Arrest
Reprinted from: *J. Clin. Med.* **2022**, *11*, 3738 , doi:10.3390/jcm11133738 73

Jakub Ratajczak, Stanisław Szczerbiński and Aldona Kubica
Occurrence and Temporal Variability of Out-of-Hospital Cardiac Arrest during COVID-19 Pandemic in Comparison to the Pre-Pandemic Period in Poland—Observational Analysis of OSCAR-POL Registry
Reprinted from: *J. Clin. Med.* **2022**, *11*, 4143 , doi:10.3390/jcm11144143 85

Miriam Renz, Leah Müllejans, Julian Riedel, Katja Mohnke, René Rissel,
Alexander Ziebart, et al.
High PEEP Levels during CPR Improve Ventilation without Deleterious Haemodynamic Effects in Pigs
Reprinted from: *J. Clin. Med.* **2022**, *11*, 4921 , doi:10.3390/jcm11164921 97

Hans van Schuppen, Kamil Wojciechowicz, Markus W. Hollmann and Benedikt Preckel
Tracheal Intubation during Advanced Life Support Using Direct Laryngoscopy versus Glidescope® Videolaryngoscopy by Clinicians with Limited Intubation Experience: A Systematic Review and Meta-Analysis
Reprinted from: *J. Clin. Med.* **2022**, *11*, 6291, doi:10.3390/jcm11216291 109

Jonathan Tjerkaski, Thomas Hermansson, Emelie Dillenbeck, Fabio Silvio Taccone, Anatolij Truhlar, Sune Forsberg, et al.
Strategies of Advanced Airway Management in Out-of-Hospital Cardiac Arrest during Intra-Arrest Hypothermia: Insights from the PRINCESS Trial
Reprinted from: *J. Clin. Med.* **2022**, *11*, 6370, doi:10.3390/jcm11216370 125

Piotr Duchnowski
Risk Factors of Sudden Cardiac Arrest during the Postoperative Period in Patient Undergoing Heart Valve Surgery
Reprinted from: *J. Clin. Med.* **2022**, *11*, 7098, doi:10.3390/jcm11237098 137

Manuel Obermaier, Stephan Katzenschlager, Othmar Kofler, Frank Weilbacher and Erik Popp
Advanced and Invasive Cardiopulmonary Resuscitation (CPR) Techniques as an Adjunct to Advanced Cardiac Life Support
Reprinted from: *J. Clin. Med.* **2022**, *11*, 7315, doi:10.3390/jcm11247315 145

Xuejie Dong, Liang Wang, Hanbing Xu, Yingfang Ye, Zhenxiang Zhou and Lin Zhang
Effect of a Targeted Ambulance Treatment Quality Improvement Programme on Outcomes from Out-of-Hospital Cardiac Arrest: A Metropolitan Citywide Intervention Study
Reprinted from: *J. Clin. Med.* **2023**, *12*, 163, doi:10.3390/jcm12010163 171

Yun Gi Kim, Kyung-Do Han, Seung-Young Roh, Joo Hee Jeong, Yun Young Choi, Kyongjin Min, et al.
Being Underweight Is Associated with Increased Risk of Sudden Cardiac Death in People with Diabetes Mellitus
Reprinted from: *J. Clin. Med.* **2023**, *12*, 1045, doi:10.3390/jcm12031045 185

Yun Gi Kim, Joo Hee Jeong, Seung-Young Roh, Kyung-Do Han, Yun Young Choi, Kyongjin Min, et al.
Obesity Is Indirectly Associated with Sudden Cardiac Arrest through Various Risk Factors
Reprinted from: *J. Clin. Med.* **2023**, *12*, 2068, doi:10.3390/jcm12052068 197

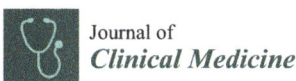

Editorial

Special Issue: Sudden Cardiac Death: Clinical Updates and Perspectives

Tobias Schupp, Ibrahim Akin and Michael Behnes *

First Department of Medicine, University Medical Centre Mannheim (UMM), Faculty of Medicine Mannheim, University of Heidelberg, 68167 Mannheim, Germany; tobias.schupp@umm.de (T.S.); ibrahim.akin@umm.de (I.A.)
* Correspondence: michael.behnes@umm.de; Tel.: +49-621-383-2512

Citation: Schupp, T.; Akin, I.; Behnes, M. Special Issue: Sudden Cardiac Death: Clinical Updates and Perspectives. *J. Clin. Med.* **2022**, *11*, 3120. https://doi.org/10.3390/jcm11113120

Received: 24 May 2022
Accepted: 29 May 2022
Published: 31 May 2022

Publisher's Note: MDPI stays neutral with regard to jurisdictional claims in published maps and institutional affiliations.

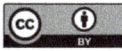

Copyright: © 2022 by the authors. Licensee MDPI, Basel, Switzerland. This article is an open access article distributed under the terms and conditions of the Creative Commons Attribution (CC BY) license (https://creativecommons.org/licenses/by/4.0/).

Sudden cardiac death (SCD) is defined as unexpected sudden death due to cardiac causes, occurring within one hour after the onset of symptoms [1]. In up to 50%, SCD occurs as initial manifestation of coronary artery disease (CAD) or other structural heart disease. The incidence of SCD has significantly decreased by 17% in men and 31% in women from 1997 to 2010 [2]. This may be related to the prognostic benefit of an implantable cardioverter-defibrillator (ICD), as well as important pharmacotherapies for the prevention of ventricular tachyarrhythmias (including beta-blockers, angiotensin converting enzyme inhibitors (ACEi), receptor blockers (ARB) and mineralocorticoid receptor antagonists (MRA)). Their prognostic impact has already been demonstrated within large randomized-controlled trials (RCT), leading to their implementation within current European guidelines with a class I indication and a level of evidence A [1,3]. By now, more than 38,000 articles on the topic "sudden cardiac death" are available on PubMed central. Due to the overall decreasing rates of SCD, the high evidence of guideline-recommended therapies and the overall increasing number of articles on the topic of SCD, one may therefore question whether updates on this "*old topic*" are necessary and worth a Special Issue?

Taking an in-depth view on the indication of pharmacological therapies reducing overall all-cause mortality and specifically SCD rates, it becomes apparent that most of the guideline relevant RCT—such as the "MERIT-HF", "CIBIS-II" and the "SOLVD" study—were published at the end of the last century [4–6]. For instance, the "CIBIS-II" study demonstrated decreased risk of all-cause mortality and SCD in 2647 heart failure (HF) patients with left ventricular ejection fraction (LVEF) of 35% or less treated with bisoprolol as compared to placebo at 1.3 years [4]. Although 96% of patients received concomitant treatment with an ACEi, the rate of digitalis treatment was 52%, which was shown not to improve cardiovascular mortality, leading to a significant decline of prescription rates over the past decade [7,8]. On the other hand, patients in the "CIBIS-II" study were median-aged 61 years, which may be partly related to exclusion criteria in RCT, but furthermore reflects the ongoing demographic changes and changes of patients' characteristics with cardiovascular diseases. Despite improvements of nationwide healthcare supply, adherence to international guideline recommendations and better coronary revascularization strategies have led to an older population of patients with cardiovascular diseases with an increased burden of comorbidities (such as atrial fibrillation, chronic kidney disease and severe HF) [9,10]. In line with this, the clinical presentation of SCD has also changed and far more patients present with an initial non-shockable rhythm, which reflects the improvements in diagnosis and treatment of structural heart disease [9]. However, only one RCT, the "PARADIGM-HF" trial, recently investigated the prognostic impact of pharmacotherapies regarding SCD. Thus, treatment with the angiotensin receptor–neprilysin inhibitor LCZ696 reduced the risk of SCD irrespective of the presence of an ICD despite optimal medical treatment [11,12]. Since the prognostic value of established pharmacotherapies remains questionable in the modern medicine era and no RCT are currently on the way to re-evaluating their prognostic impact, European guidelines demand the need for registry data [1]. Therefore, this Special Issue of the *Journal of Clinical Medicine* aims to provide insights on current research, focusing on the identification of patients at risk for SCD, as well as on the prognostic impact of diagnostic and therapeutic tools in patients with cardiac arrest or ventricular tachyarrhythmias, who are at highest risk of SCD. Currently, five studies have been published within the current Special Issue.

One study by Kim et al. investigated the prognostic impact of metabolic syndrome and gamma-glutamyl transferase (ɣ-GTP) on SCD. Including more than 4,000,000 patients undergoing nationwide health screenings in Korea, they demonstrated metabolic syndromes and elevated ɣ-GTP associated with increased SCD risk. It is of note that decreasing ɣ-GTP during follow-up has been shown to reduce the risk of SCD, which may be related to the effect of lifestyle modification [13]. These findings are important since risk stratification for SCD in clinical practice predominantly relies on LVEF. However, it was demonstrated that most SCD cases occur in patients with no evidence of depressed LVEF, who are considered as *"low risk"*, with no evidence of structural heart disease, which makes the identification of risk factors for SCD even more complicated [9]. Thus, especially in HF-related SCD, rates have improved due to ICD implantation and pharmacotherapies, whereas SCD decline was much lower in patients without depressed EF and without prior AMI [14]. Therefore, the study by Kim et al. is a relevant step to develop an improved SCD risk stratification tool within the general population at low risk of SCD.

Even fewer data are available that focus on diagnostic and therapeutic approaches in patients surviving aborted cardiac arrest (i.e., for the secondary prevention of SCD). Although these patients are at the highest risk of suffering from SCD, all RCT investigating prognosis of heart failure therapies included patients without HF or structural heart disease and without prior ventricular tachyarrhythmias (i.e., primary prevention of SCD) [4,5]. It is of note that only RCT demonstrating the prognostic superiority of an ICD included patients for secondary prevention of SCD [15]. Using a large registry of over 2400 patients, we recently identified age, sex, as well as important comorbidities (such as chronic kidney disease, LVEF, AMI, CAD) to predict outcomes following ventricular tachyarrhythmias [16–18]. Recently, biomarkers have gained more importance in predicting prognosis in patients with HF and AMI. In this Special Issue, we demonstrated that cardiac troponin I is a useful predictor of short-term mortality within 30 days following ventricular tachyarrhythmias, which was observed in both patients with and without CAD and AMI [19] This underlines the importance of cardiac troponins for the prediction of prognosis in high-risk patients despite their implementation in the diagnosis of AMI. With regard to pharmacotherapies, we were also able to demonstrate comparable benefit of ACEi as compared to ARB treatment following ventricular tachyarrhythmias, which is in line with prior studies including patients with AMI or HF [20–22]. ACEi and ARB were investigated in former studies including patients with AMI or HF, whereas again re-evaluation of "established" pharmacotherapies for the prevention of SCD within the current era of modern cardiovascular medicine is demanded in current European guidelines [1].

Within this Special Issue, two studies included patients with out-of-hospital cardiac arrests (OHCA). A study based on the "JAAM Out-Of-Hospital Cardiac Arrest registry" by Nojima et al. suggested blood ammonia levels at hospital arrival were useful to predict neurological outcomes following OHCA, taking into account whether the return of spontaneous circulation (ROSC) was achieved at hospital admission [23]. Given the overall poor prognosis of patients with OHCA, especially in the setting of refractory OHCA, these findings are important for the early identification of patients with presumably favorable outcomes. In line with this, Rysz et al. demonstrated within a propensity-score matched study of 940 OHCA patients from Sweden, that inotropic support with levosimendan was only used in 10% of OHCA patients and was not associated with favorable outcomes; however, a small subgroup of patients treated with levosimendan <6 h had improved mortality. Despite the overall limited data with regard to levosimendan use following cardiac arrest, further studies are warrened to identify patients that may benefit from levosimendan therapy [24]. Besides the prognostic impact of inotropic agents in patients with OHCA or cardiogenic shock, the use of mechanical circulatory support (MCS) devices may improve the in-hospital survival of these patients. Although the "ARREST" trial randomized only 30 patients to extracorporeal membrane oxygenation (ECMO) or standard treatment, improved survival until hospital discharge was shown in patients undergoing ECMO therapy [25]. On the contrary, the randomized controlled ECLS-shock trial (clinicaltrials.gov identifier: NCT03637205) is currently investigating the prognosis of ECMO therapy in patients presenting with cardiogenic shock. Considering the limited evidence from RCT, the investigation of both invasive strategies and pharmacological therapies in OHCA needs further investigation.

In conclusion, evidence regarding the prediction of SCD and treatment strategies of patients at high risk of SCD are scarce, despite the overall high number of studies in this field. This is related to ongoing demographic changes, improvements of HF and AMI therapies and the overall difficult scenario of developing appropriate SCD risk prediction models, which is related to the high absolute number of SCD occurring in patients with no evidence of structural heart disease or severe HF. However, the present Special Issue may provide further insights into SCD prevention and the treatment of OHCA/ventricular tachyarrhythmias in the current era of medicine.

As Guest Editors of this Special Issue, we would like to thank the authors for their valuable contributions and the *Journal of Clinical Medicine* Editorial Office for their continuous support.

Author Contributions: Conceptualization, T.S. and M.B.; project administration, M.B. and I.A.; data and writing, T.S.; original draft: preparation, T.S.; review and editing, I.A. and M.B.; supervision, I.A. and M.B. All authors have read and agreed to the published version of the manuscript.

Funding: This research received no external funding.

Conflicts of Interest: The authors declare no conflict of interest.

References

1. Priori, S.G.; Blomström-Lundqvist, C.; Mazzanti, A.; Blom, N.; Borggrefe, M.; Camm, J.; Elliott, P.M.; Fitzsimons, D.; Hatala, R.; Hindricks, G.; et al. 2015 ESC Guidelines for the management of patients with ventricular arrhythmias and the prevention of sudden cardiac death: The Task Force for the Management of Patients with Ventricular Arrhythmias and the Prevention of Sudden Cardiac Death of the European Society of Cardiology (ESC)Endorsed by: Association for European Paediatric and Congenital Cardiology (AEPC). *Eur. Heart J.* **2015**, *36*, 2793–2867. [CrossRef] [PubMed]
2. Feng, J.L.; Nedkoff, L.; Knuiman, M.; Semsarian, C.; Ingles, J.; Briffa, T.; Hickling, S. Temporal Trends in Sudden Cardiac Death From 1997 to 2010: A Data Linkage Study. *Heart Lung Circ.* **2017**, *26*, 808–816. [CrossRef] [PubMed]
3. Maggioni, A.P.; Anker, S.D.; Dahlström, U.; Filippatos, G.; Ponikowski, P.; Zannad, F.; Amir, O.; Chioncel, O.; Leiro, M.C.; Drozdz, J.; et al. Are hospitalized or ambulatory patients with heart failure treated in accordance with European Society of Cardiology guidelines? Evidence from 12,440 patients of the ESC Heart Failure Long-Term Registry. *Eur. J. Heart Fail.* **2013**, *15*, 1173–1184. [CrossRef] [PubMed]
4. The Cardiac Insufficiency Bisoprolol Study II (CIBIS-II): A randomised trial. *Lancet* **1999**, *353*, 9–13. [CrossRef]
5. Effect of metoprolol CR/XL in chronic heart failure: Metoprolol CR/XL Randomised Intervention Trial in Congestive Heart Failure (MERIT-HF). *Lancet* **1999**, *353*, 2001–2007. [CrossRef]
6. Yusuf, S.; Pitt, B.; Davis, C.E.; Hood, W.B.; Cohn, J.N. Effect of enalapril on survival in patients with reduced left ventricular ejection fractions and congestive heart failure. *N. Engl. J. Med.* **1991**, *325*, 293–302. [CrossRef]
7. The effect of digoxin on mortality and morbidity in patients with heart failure. *N. Engl. J. Med.* **1997**, *336*, 525–533. [CrossRef]
8. Lee, D.S.; Mamdani, M.M.; Austin, P.C.; Gong, Y.; Liu, P.P.; Rouleau, J.L.; Tu, J.V. Trends in heart failure outcomes and pharmacotherapy: 1992 to 2000. *Am. J. Med.* **2004**, *116*, 581–589. [CrossRef]
9. Al-Khatib, S.M.; Stevenson, W.G.; Ackerman, M.J.; Bryant, W.J.; Callans, D.J.; Curtis, A.B.; Deal, B.J.; Dickfeld, T.; Field, M.E.; Fonarow, G.C.; et al. 2017 AHA/ACC/HRS Guideline for Management of Patients With Ventricular Arrhythmias and the Prevention of Sudden Cardiac Death: A Report of the American College of Cardiology/American Heart Association Task Force on Clinical Practice Guidelines and the Heart Rhythm Society. *J. Am. Coll. Cardiol.* **2018**, *72*, e91–e220. [CrossRef]
10. Stathopoulos, I.; Jimenez, M.; Panagopoulos, G.; Kwak, E.J.; Losquadro, M.; Cohen, H.; Iyer, S.; Ruiz, C.; Roubin, G.; Garratt, K. The decline in PCI complication rate: 2003–2006 versus 1999–2002. *Hellenic. J. Cardiol.* **2009**, *50*, 379–387.

11. Rohde, L.E.; Chatterjee, N.A.; Vaduganathan, M.; Claggett, B.; Packer, M.; Desai, A.S.; Zile, M.; Rouleau, J.; Swedberg, K.; Lefkowitz, M.; et al. Sacubitril/Valsartan and Sudden Cardiac Death According to Implantable Cardioverter-Defibrillator Use and Heart Failure Cause: A PARADIGM-HF Analysis. *JACC Heart Fail.* **2020**, *8*, 844–855. [CrossRef] [PubMed]
12. McMurray, J.J.; Packer, M.; Desai, A.S.; Gong, J.; Lefkowitz, M.P.; Rizkala, A.R.; Rouleau, J.L.; Shi, V.C.; Solomon, S.D.; Swedberg, K.; et al. Angiotensin-neprilysin inhibition versus enalapril in heart failure. *N. Engl. J. Med.* **2014**, *371*, 993–1004. [CrossRef]
13. Kim, Y.G.; Han, K.; Jeong, J.H.; Roh, S.-Y.; Choi, Y.Y.; Min, K.; Shim, J.; Choi, J.-I.; Kim, Y.-H. Metabolic Syndrome, Gamma-Glutamyl Transferase, and Risk of Sudden Cardiac Death. *J. Clin. Med.* **2022**, *11*, 1781. [CrossRef] [PubMed]
14. Shuvy, M.; Qiu, F.; Lau, G.; Koh, M.; Dorian, P.; Geri, G.; Lin, S.; Ko, D.T. Temporal trends in sudden cardiac death in Ontario, Canada. *Resuscitation* **2019**, *136*, 1–7. [CrossRef]
15. Kuck, K.-H.; Cappato, R.; Siebels, J.; Rüppel, R. Randomized comparison of antiarrhythmic drug therapy with implantable defibrillators in patients resuscitated from cardiac arrest: The Cardiac Arrest Study Hamburg (CASH). *Circulation* **2000**, *102*, 748–754. [CrossRef]
16. Behnes, M.; Akin, I.; Kuche, P.; Schupp, T.; Reiser, L.; Bollow, A.; Taton, G.; Reichelt, T.; Ellguth, D.; Engelke, N.; et al. Coronary chronic total occlusions and mortality in patients with ventricular tachyarrhythmias. *EuroIntervention* **2020**, *15*, 1278–1285. [CrossRef]
17. Behnes, M.; Mashayekhi, K.; Weiß, C.; Nienaber, C.; Lang, S.; Reiser, L.; Bollow, A.; Taton, G.; Reichelt, T.; Ellguth, D.; et al. Prognostic Impact of Acute Myocardial Infarction in Patients Presenting With Ventricular Tachyarrhythmias and Aborted Cardiac Arrest. *J. Am. Heart Assoc.* **2018**, *7*, e010004. [CrossRef]
18. Weidner, K.; Behnes, M.; Schupp, T.; Rusnak, J.; Reiser, L.; Taton, G.; Reichelt, T.; Ellguth, D.; Engelke, N.; Bollow, A.; et al. Prognostic impact of chronic kidney disease and renal replacement therapy in ventricular tachyarrhythmias and aborted cardiac arrest. *Clin. Res. Cardiol.* **2019**, *108*, 669–682. [CrossRef]
19. Akin, I.; Behnes, M.; Müller, J.; Forner, J.; Abumayyaleh, M.; Mashayekhi, K.; Akin, M.; Bertsch, T.; Weidner, K.; Rusnak, J.; et al. Prognostic Value of Cardiac Troponin I in Patients with Ventricular Tachyarrhythmias. *J. Clin. Med.* **2022**, *11*, 2987. [CrossRef]
20. Schupp, T.; Behnes, M.; Weiß, C.; Nienaber, C.; Lang, S.; Reiser, L.; Bollow, A.; Taton, G.; Reichelt, T.; Ellguth, D.; et al. Beta-Blockers and ACE Inhibitors Are Associated with Improved Survival Secondary to Ventricular Tachyarrhythmia. *Cardiovasc. Drugs Ther.* **2018**, *32*, 353–363. [CrossRef] [PubMed]
21. Schupp, T.; Behnes, M.; Abumayyaleh, M.; Weidner, K.; Mashayekhi, K.; Bertsch, T.; Akin, I. Angiotensin Converting Enzyme Inhibitors versus Receptor Blockers in Patients with Ventricular Tachyarrhythmias. *J. Clin. Med.* **2022**, *11*, 1460. [CrossRef] [PubMed]
22. Ohtsubo, T.; Shibata, R.; Kai, H.; Okamoto, R.; Kumagai, E.; Kawano, H.; Fujiwara, A.; Kitazono, T.; Murohara, T.; Arima, H. Angiotensin-converting enzyme inhibitors versus angiotensin receptor blockers in hypertensive patients with myocardial infarction or heart failure: A systematic review and meta-analysis. *Hypertens. Res.* **2019**, *42*, 641–649. [CrossRef] [PubMed]
23. Nojima, T.; Naito, H.; Obara, T.; Ageta, K.; Yakushiji, H.; Yumoto, T.; Fujisaki, N.; Nakao, A. Can Blood Ammonia Level, Prehospital Time, and Return of Spontaneous Circulation Predict Neurological Outcomes of Out-of-Hospital Cardiac Arrest Patients? A Nationwide, Retrospective Cohort Study. *J. Clin. Med.* **2022**, *11*, 2566. [CrossRef]
24. Rysz, S.; Fagerlund, M.J.; Lundberg, J.; Ringh, M.; Hollenberg, J.; Lindgren, M.; Jonsson, M.; Djärv, T.; Nordberg, P. The Use of Levosimendan after Out-of-Hospital Cardiac Arrest and Its Association with Outcome—An Observational Study. *J. Clin. Med.* **2022**, *11*, 2621. [CrossRef] [PubMed]
25. Yannopoulos, D.; Bartos, J.; Raveendran, G.; Walser, E.; Connett, J.; Murray, T.A.; Collins, G.; Zhang, L.; Kalra, R.; Kosmopoulos, M.; et al. Advanced reperfusion strategies for patients with out-of-hospital cardiac arrest and refractory ventricular fibrillation (ARREST): A phase 2, single centre, open-label, randomised controlled trial. *Lancet* **2020**, *396*, 1807–1816. [CrossRef]

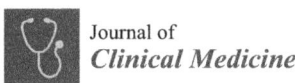

Article

Angiotensin Converting Enzyme Inhibitors versus Receptor Blockers in Patients with Ventricular Tachyarrhythmias

Tobias Schupp [1], Michael Behnes [1,*], Mohammad Abumayyaleh [1], Kathrin Weidner [1], Kambis Mashayekhi [2], Thomas Bertsch [3] and Ibrahim Akin [1]

[1] First Department of Medicine, University Medical Centre Mannheim (UMM), Faculty of Medicine Mannheim, University of Heidelberg, DZHK (German Center for Cardiovascular Research) Partner Site Heidelberg/Mannheim, Theodor-Kutzer-Ufer 1-3, 68167 Mannheim, Germany; tobias.schupp@umm.de (T.S.); mohammad.abumayyaleh@umm.de (M.A.); kathrin.weidner@umm.de (K.W.); ibrahim.akin@umm.de (I.A.)
[2] Department of Cardiology and Angiology II, University Heart Center Freiburg, 79189 Bad Krozingen, Germany; kambis.mashayekhi@universitaets-herzzentrum.de
[3] Institute of Clinical Chemistry, Laboratory Medicine and Transfusion Medicine, Nuremberg General Hospital, Paracelsus Medical University, 90419 Nuremberg, Germany; thomas.bertsch@klinikum-nuernberg.de
* Correspondence: michael.behnes@umm.de; Tel.: +49-621-383-6239

Abstract: Data investigating the prognostic value of treatment with angiotensin converting enzyme inhibitors (ACEi) and receptor blockers (ARB) usually focusses on patients presenting with heart failure (HF) or acute myocardial infarction (AMI). However, by preventing adverse cardiac remodeling, ACEi/ARB may also decrease the risk of ventricular tachyarrhythmias and sudden cardiac death (SCD). Although ventricular tachyarrhythmias are associated with significant mortality and morbidity, only limited data are available focusing on the prognostic role of ACEi/ARB, when prescribed for secondary prevention of SCD. Therefore, this study comprehensively investigates the role of ACEi versus ARB in patients with ventricular tachyarrhythmias. A large retrospective registry was used including consecutive patients with episodes of ventricular tachycardia (VT) or fibrillation (VF) from 2002 to 2015. The primary prognostic outcome was all-cause mortality at three years, secondary endpoints comprised a composite arrhythmic endpoint (i.e., recurrences of ventricular tachyarrhythmias, ICD therapies and sudden cardiac death) and cardiac rehospitalization. A total of 1236 patients were included (15% treated with ARB and 85% with ACEi) and followed for a median of 4.0 years. At three years, ACEi and ARB were associated with comparable long-term mortality (20% vs. 17%; log rank $p = 0.287$; HR = 0.965; 95% CI 0.689–1.351; $p = 0.835$) and comparable risk of the composite arrhythmic endpoint (HR = 1.227; 95% CI 0.841–1.790; $p = 0.288$). In contrast, ACEi was associated with a decreased risk of cardiac rehospitalization at three years (HR = 0.690; 95% CI 0.490–0.971; $p = 0.033$). Within the propensity score matched cohort (i.e., 158 patients with ACEi and ARB), ACEi and ARB were associated with comparable long-term outcomes at three years. In conclusion, ACEi and ARB are associated with comparable risk of long-term outcomes in patients presenting with ventricular tachyarrhythmias.

Keywords: ventricular tachycardia; ventricular fibrillation; mortality; ACE inhibitor; ARB; medical treatment; pharmacological drugs

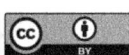

1. Introduction

Angiotensin converting enzyme inhibitors (ACEi) and receptor blockers (ARB) were shown to reduce all-cause mortality and risk of sudden cardiac death (SCD) in patients with acute myocardial infarction (AMI) and heart failure (HF) with reduced left ventricular ejection fraction (i.e., LVEF ≤ 40%) when prescribed for primary prevention of SCD [1–4]. By promoting transforming growth factor beta-1-synthesis, angiotensin II may stimulate the formation of fibrosis tissue, which increases the risk of arrhythmogenesis due to facilitation of re-entry, especially in patients with ischemic heart disease. Furthermore, angiotensin

II plays an important role as a vasoconstrictor. By increasing wall pressure and stretch, angiotensin II may also cause so-called electrical remodeling by prolonging conduction time and favoring conduction heterogeneity within cardiac myocytes. Moreover, angiotensin II was shown to have a direct effect on ion channels leading to increased calcium influx, which in turn favors the occurrence of atrial and ventricular tachyarrhythmias [5,6]. These pathophysiological aspects suggest decreased arrhythmic events in patients treated with ACEi/ARB. In line, decreased rates of SCD rates were observed within a large meta-analysis, including patients with AMI and HF [7]. However, Guideline recommendations for the prevention of ventricular tachyarrhythmias and SCD predominantly rely on patients treated with ACEi or ARB, who did not have prior episodes of ventricular tachyarrhythmias [6]. Therefore, within the current AHA/ACC/HRS Guidelines, ACEi/ARB have a class IA indication only in patients with LVEF $\leq 40\%$ [8]. Using a large retrospective registry, we recently demonstrated that prescription of ACEi/ARB is associated with decreased all-cause mortality at three years in patients surviving index episodes of ventricular tachyarrhythmias, when prescribed for secondary prevention of SCD as compared to patients not treated with ACEi/ARB. However, prognosis of patients treated with ACEi was not compared to patients with ARB [9].

Accordingly, the risk of ventricular tachyarrhythmias in the presence or absence of ACEi/ARB therapy was merely investigated within rather small registries [10,11]. The GRACE study is one of the largest trials that investigated the risk of appropriate ICD shocks in the presence or absence of ACEi/ARB in patients with systolic HF and LVEF $\leq 35\%$, demonstrating reduced risk of ICD shocks at five years of follow-up [12]. However, data directly comparing the prognosis of patients treated with ACEi versus ARB are limited [13–15]. Therefore, the present study investigates the prognosis for patients with ventricular tachyarrhythmias treated with ACEi as compared to ARB on the primary endpoint of all-cause mortality, as well as on secondary endpoints (composite arrhythmic endpoint (i.e., recurrence of ventricular tachyarrhythmias, appropriate ICD therapies, SCD) and cardiac rehospitalization) at three years.

2. Materials and Methods

2.1. Data Collection and Documentation

The present study retrospectively included all patients surviving index episodes of ventricular tachyarrhythmias (i.e., ventricular tachycardia (VT) and ventricular fibrillation (VF)) on admission from 2002 until 2016 at our institution as recently published [9]. The study is derived from an analysis of the "Registry of Malignant Arrhythmia and Sudden Cardiac Death—Influence of Diagnostics and Interventions (RACE-IT)", a single-center registry including consecutive patients presenting with ventricular tachyarrhythmias and aborted cardiac arrest being acutely admitted to the University Medical Center Mannheim (UMM), Germany, (clinicaltrials.gov identifier: NCT02982473) from 2002 until 2015. The study was carried out according to the principles of the Declaration of Helsinki and was approved by the medical ethics committee II of the Medical Faculty Mannheim, University of Heidelberg, Germany.

2.2. Inclusion and Exclusion Criteria

Consecutive patients with ventricular tachyarrhythmias were included [9]. The decision to treat patients with ACEi or ARB was based on the discretion of the cardiologists during routine care according to European guidelines [6,13–15]. Patients with death during index hospitalization, patients without ACEi or ARB treatment and patients with both ACEi plus ARB therapy were excluded from the present study. All other medical therapies apart from ACEi/ARB were allowed.

2.3. Primary and Secondary Endpoints

The follow-up period was set at three years for all outcomes. The primary prognostic endpoint was all-cause mortality. All-cause mortality was documented using our electronic hospital information system and by directly contacting state resident registration offices (Bureaux of Mortality Statistics) all across Germany. Identification of patients was verified by place of name, surname, day of birth and registered addresses. Secondary endpoints were a composite arrhythmic endpoint (i.e., recurrences of ventricular tachyarrhythmias, appropriate ICD therapies, sudden cardiac death) and cardiac rehospitalization. Cardiac rehospitalization comprised rehospitalization due to VT, VF, acute myocardial infarction (AMI), acute heart failure and inappropriate device therapy.

2.4. Statistical Methods

Quantitative data are presented as mean ± standard error of mean (SEM), median and interquartile range (IQR), and ranges depending on the distribution of the data and were compared using the Student's *t*-test for normally distributed data or the Mann–Whitney U test for nonparametric data. Deviations from a Gaussian distribution were tested by the Kolmogorov–Smirnov test. Spearman's rank correlation for nonparametric data was used to test univariate correlations. Qualitative data are presented as absolute and relative frequencies and compared using the Chi^2 test or the Fisher's exact test, as appropriate.

Firstly, the univariable Kaplan–Meier method was applied to evaluate prognostic differences within the entire cohort. Then, the impact of ACEi versus ARB was analyzed separated by LVEF $\geq$ 35% and <35%. Thereafter, multivariable Cox regression models were developed using the "forward selection" option, where only statistically significant variables ($p < 0.05$) were included and analyzed simultaneously. Predefined variables being used for multivariable Cox-regressions included: baseline parameters (age, gender), chronic diseases (chronic kidney disease, diabetes mellitus), coronary artery disease (CAD), acute myocardial infarction (AMI), LVEF < 35%, the presence of an ICD and ACEi versus ARB therapy.

Secondly, propensity score matching was applied retrieving data from the entire patient cohort. In RCTs, patients have a 50% chance of being treated with or without a specific medication (such as ACEi or ARB). Balanced measured and unmeasured baseline characteristics would then be expected. In an observational study recruiting real-life patients, the specific treatment is not randomized, resulting in varying chances between 0% and 100% to receive it, including imbalances in baseline characteristics. Consequently, differences of outcomes in specific treatment groups might be explained by heterogenous distribution of baseline characteristics. However, the consecutive all-comer study reflects a realistic picture of current health-care supply. Therefore, to reduce this selection bias, we used 1:1 propensity scores for the receipt of a specific discharge medication (i.e., ACEi versus ARB) to assemble a matched cohort in which patients receiving and not receiving the discharge medication would be well balanced on all measured baseline characteristics. Propensity scores were created according to the presence of the following independent variables: age, sex, diabetes, CAD, LVEF, in-hospital CPR, out-of-hospital CPR, index ventricular tachyarrhythmias (i.e., VT/VF), chronic kidney disease, and the presence or absence of an ICD. Based on the propensity score values counted by logistic regressions, for each patient, one patient in the control group with a similar propensity score value was found (accepted difference of propensity score values < 5%). Thereafter, univariable stratification was performed using the Kaplan–Meier method with comparisons between groups using univariable hazard ratios (HR) given together with 95% confidence intervals. Propensity score matching was calculated within the entire study cohort and then separated by LVEF $\geq$ 35% and <35%.

The result of a statistical test was considered significant for $p < 0.05$. SAS, release 9.4 (SAS Institute Inc., Cary, NC, USA) and SPSS (Version 25, IBM, Armonk, NY, USA) were used for statistics.

3. Results

3.1. Study Population

From a total of 2422 patients with ventricular tachyarrhythmias, 715 were excluded for in-hospital death, 477 for receiving neither ACEi nor ARB treatment and 24 patients for receiving both ACEi and ARB therapy (Figure 1; flow chart).

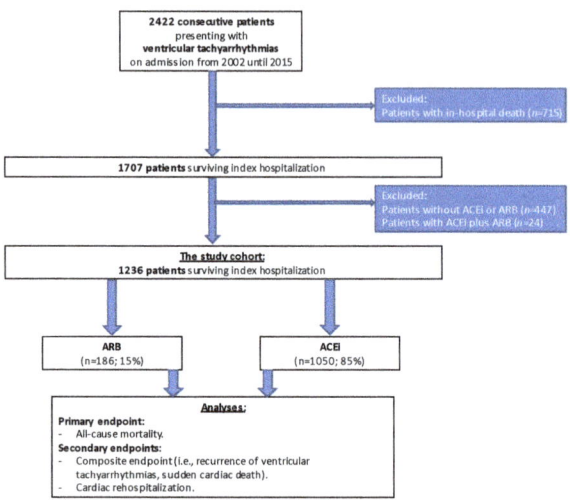

Figure 1. Flow chart of the study population.

The final study cohort comprised 1236 patients with ventricular tachyarrhythmias, 85% of whom were treated with ACEi and 15% were treated with ARB ($p = 0.001$). Within the ARB group, most patients were discharged on candesartan (53% with a mean daily dose of 15.3 mg $\pm$ 0.9 mg), followed by valsartan (19%; mean daily dose 121.0 mg $\pm$ 11.8 mg) (Table 1; study drugs). The most common type of ACEi was ramipril (71%; mean daily dose 5.4 mg $\pm$ 0.1 mg), whereas enalapril (19%; mean daily dose 12.3 mg $\pm$ 0.6 mg) and perindopril (5%; mean daily dose 3.5 mg $\pm$ 0.3 mg) were less common (Table 1).

Table 1. Study drugs.

Study Drugs; n (%); mg/day (Mean $\pm$ SEM)	ARB (n = 186; 15%)	ACEi (n = 1050; 85%)	p Value
Candesartan	99 (53)	-	-
	15.3 $\pm$ 0.9	-	-
Valsartan	36 (19)	-	-
	121.0 $\pm$ 11.8	-	-
Lorsartan	21 (11)	-	-
	53.8 $\pm$ 4.9	-	-
Other type of ARB	30 (16)	-	-
Ramipril	-	740 (71)	-
	-	5.4 $\pm$ 0.1	-
Enalapril	-	195 (19)	-
	-	12.3 $\pm$ 0.6	-
Perindopril	-	12 (5)	-
	-	3.5 $\pm$ 0.3	-
Other type of ACEi	-	103 (10)	-

ACEi, angiotensin converting enzyme inhibitor; ARB, angiotensin receptor blocker; SEM, standard error of mean.

As seen in Table 2 (left column), patients were median-aged at 69 years and most patients were males in both subgroups (75–77%). An index episode of VT was more common than VF in patients with ACEi and ARB treatment (66–73% vs. 27–34%; $p = 0.087$). In particular, the rates of arterial hypertension (79% vs. 65%; $p = 0.001$) and hyperlipidemia (42% vs. 34%; $p = 0.047$) were higher in patients treated with ARB. In contrast, rates of chronic kidney disease, prior heart failure and LVEF were equally distributed in both groups. Besides slightly higher rates of beta-blocker treatment in the ACEi group (89% vs. 83%; $p = 0.032$), no further differences regarding concomitant pharmacotherapies were observed.

Table 2. Baseline characteristics before and after propensity score matching.

Characteristic	Without Propensity Score Matching			With Propensity Score Matching		
	ARB (n = 186; 15%)	ACEi (n = 1050; 85%)	p Value	ARB (n = 158; 50%)	ACEi (n = 158; 50%)	p Value
Age, median (range)	68 (32–89)	67 (15–94)	0.001	68 (32–89)	68 (25–85)	0.239
Male gender, n (%)	139 (75)	810 (77)	0.473	119 (75)	126 (80)	0.345
Ventricular tachyarrhythmias at index, n (%)						
Ventricular tachycardia	135 (73)	695 (66)	0.087	112 (71)	110 (70)	0.806
Ventricular fibrillation	51 (27)	355 (34)		46 (29)	48 (30)	
Cardiovascular risk factors, n (%)						
Arterial hypertension	147 (79)	679 (65)	**0.001**	127 (80)	101 (64)	**0.001**
Diabetes mellitus	48 (26)	284 (27)	0.725	41 (26)	50 (32)	0.264
Hyperlipidemia	78 (42)	361 (34)	**0.047**	68 (43)	63 (40)	0.568
Smoking	46 (25)	365 (35)	**0.007**	39 (25)	62 (39)	**0.006**
Cardiac family history	20 (11)	118 (11)	0.846	17 (11)	17 (11)	1.000
Comorbidities at index stay, n (%)						
Prior myocardial infarction	61 (33)	291 (28)	0.157	53 (34)	56 (35)	0.723
Prior coronary artery disease	104 (56)	567 (45)	**0.004**	93 (59)	92 (58)	0.909
Prior heart failure	60 (32)	289 (28)	0.186	53 (34)	59 (37)	0.480
Atrial fibrillation	63 (34)	334 (32)	0.799	55 (35)	59 (37)	0.639
Non-ischemic cardiomyopathy	13 (7)	91 (9)	0.448	13 (8)	17 (11)	0.443
Cardiopulmonary resuscitation	35 (19)	346 (33)		27 (17)	40 (25)	
In hospital	18 (10)	129 (12)	**0.001**	14 (9)	29 (18)	**0.048**
Out of hospital	17 (9)	217 (21)		13 (8)	11 (7)	
Chronic kidney disease	84 (46)	428 (41)	0.254	76 (48)	67 (42)	0.309
COPD/asthma	18 (10)	83 (8)	0.416	13 (8)	15 (10)	0.692
Coronary angiography, n (%)	121 (65)	758 (72)	**0.048**	107 (68)	124 (79)	**0.031**
No evidence of CAD	40 (33)	177 (23)		34 (32)	28 (23)	
1-vessel disease	23 (19)	197 (26)	0.102	21 (20)	31 (25)	0.415
2-vessel disease	27 (22)	174 (23)		23 (22)	31 (25)	
3-vessel disease	31 (26)	210 (28)		29 (27)	34 (27)	
Chronic total occlusion	25 (21)	151 (20)	0.850	22 (21)	32 (26)	0.348
Presence of CABG	22 (18)	107 (14)	0.241	21 (20)	27 (22)	0.688
PCI	31 (26)	342 (45)	**0.001**	28 (26)	36 (29)	0.628
Acute myocardial infarction	22 (12)	326 (31)	**0.001**	19 (12)	31 (29)	0.064
STEMI	8 (4)	123 (12)	**0.002**	8 (5)	14 (9)	0.185
NSTEMI	14 (8)	203 (19)	**0.001**	11 (7)	17 (11)	0.235
LVEF, n (%)						
>55%	49 (31)	231 (26)		48 (30)	29 (18)	
54–45%	17 (11)	149 (16)	0.228	17 (11)	23 (15)	0.092
44–35%	33 (21)	184 (20)		32 (20)	37 (23)	
<35%	61 (38)	342 (38)		61 (39)	69 (44)	
No evidence of LVEF	26	144	-	-	-	-
Cardiac therapies at index, n (%)						
Electrophysiological examination	78 (42)	330 (31)	**0.005**	66 (42)	55 (35)	0.203
VT ablation therapy	20 (11)	61 (6)	**0.012**	15 (10)	8 (5)	0.130
Presence of an ICD, n (%)	109 (59)	560 (53)	0.184	100 (63)	105 (67)	0.556
Medication at discharge, n (%)						
Beta-blocker	155 (83)	933 (89)	**0.032**	136 (86)	144 (91)	0.157
Statin	126 (68)	752 (72)	0.283	108 (68)	117 (74)	0.264
Amiodarone	26 (14)	176 (17)	0.344	24 (15)	24 (15)	1.000
Digitalis	29 (16)	136 (13)	0.329	29 (18)	25 (16)	0.550
Aldosterone antagonist	29 (16)	128 (12)	0.199	32 (20)	17 (11)	**0.020**

ACE, angiotensin converting enzyme; ARB, angiotensin receptor blocker; CABG, coronary artery bypass grafting; CAD, coronary artery disease; COPD, chronic obstructive pulmonary disease; LVEF, left ventricular ejection fraction; NSTEMI, non-ST-segment myocardial infarction; PCI, percutaneous coronary intervention; SEM, standard error of mean; STEMI, ST-segment MI; VT, ventricular tachycardia. Bold type indicates $p < 0.05$.

3.2. Follow-Up Data, Primary and Secondary Endpoints within the Entire Study Cohort

Median follow-up time within the entire study cohort was 4.0 years (IQR 1.7–7.5 years). At three years of follow-up, the primary endpoint all-cause mortality occurred in 17% of the patients with ARB treatment and in 20% with ACEi. Accordingly, risk of all-cause mortality was not affected by treatment with ACEi versus ARB (log rank $p = 0.287$; HR = 0.965; 95% CI 0.689–1.351; $p = 0.835$) (Table 3 and Figure 2, left panel). Furthermore, risk of the composite endpoint was comparable in both groups (22% vs. 21%; HR = 1.227; 95% CI 0.841–1.790; $p = 0.288$). In contrast, ACEi was associated with a decreased risk of cardiac rehospitalization at three years (16% vs. 22%; log rank $p = 0.032$; HR = 0.690; 95% CI 0.490–0.971; $p = 0.033$) (Figure 2, middle and right panel).

Table 3. Endpoints and follow-up data before and after propensity score matching.

Characteristics	Without Propensity Score Matching					With Propensity Score Matching				
	ARB ($n = 186$; 15%)		ACEi ($n = 1050$; 85%)		p Value	ARB ($n = 158$; 50%)		ACEi ($n = 158$; 50%)		p Value
Primary endpoint, n (%)										
All cause-mortality, at 36 months	31	(17)	206	(20)	0.346	25	(16)	36	(23)	0.117
Secondary endpoints, n (%)										
Cardiac rehospitalization, at 36 months	41	(22)	165	(16)	**0.033**	38	(24)	35	(22)	0.689
Composite Endpoint (recurrence of ventricular tachyarrhythmias, sudden cardiac death), at 36 months	40	(22)	218	(21)	0.818	36	(23)	41	(26)	0.512
Follow up times, n (%)										
Hospitalization total; days (median (IQR))	9 (5–17)		14 (8–23)		0.069	10 (5–17)		13 (9–22)		**0.015**
ICU time; days (median (IQR))	1 (0–5)		3 (0–8)		**0.001**	2 (0–5)		2 (0–5)		**0.004**
Follow-up; days (mean; median (range))	1910; 1630 (68–4912)		1894; 1744 (15–5106)		0.399	1976; 1682 (68–4912)		1856; 1706 (18–5089)		0.418

ACE, angiotensin converting enzyme; ARB, angiotensin receptor blocker; ICU, intensive care unit; IQR, interquartile range. Level of significance $p \leq 0.05$. Bold type indicates $p \leq 0.05$.

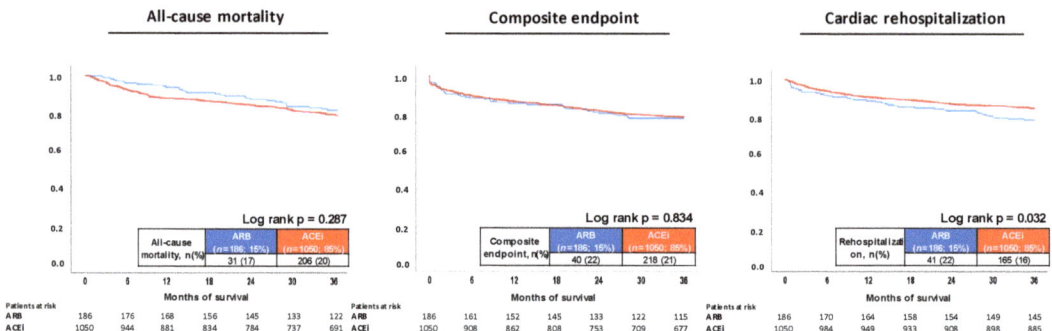

Figure 2. Prognostic impact of ACEi versus ARB treatment on all-cause mortality (**left panel**); risk of the composite arrhythmic endpoint (i.e., recurrence of ventricular tachyarrhythmias, sudden cardiac death) (**middle**); and cardiac rehospitalization (**right panel**) within the entire study.

3.3. Stratification by LVEF

Focusing on patients with LVEF $\geq 35\%$, no differences regarding all-cause mortality were observed in patients treated with ACEi or ARB (15% vs 11%; log rank $p = 0.255$; HR = 1.438; 95% CI 0.767–2.695; $p = 0.258$) (Figure 3, left panel). In line with those results, cardiac rehospitalization was not affected by ACEi or ARB (HR = 0.687; 95% CI 0.404–1.169; $p = 0.166$) (not shown).

In the presence of LVEF < 35%, similar mortality rates were observed at three years of follow-up (25% vs 25%; log rank $p = 0.909$; HR = 1.032; 95% CI 0.597–1.787; $p = 0.909$) (Figure 3, right panel), whereas a trend towards improved freedom from cardiac rehospitalization was seen in the ACEi group (HR = 0.624; 95% CI 0.385–1.012; $p = 0.056$) (not shown).

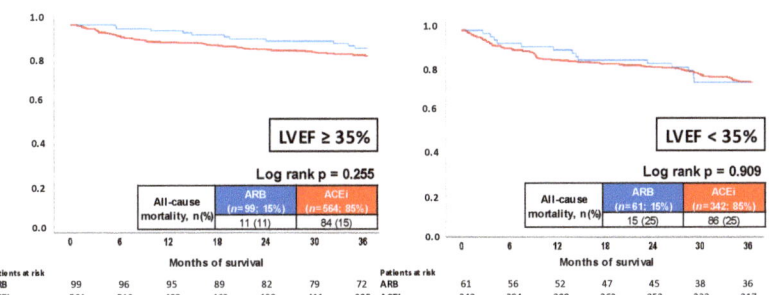

Figure 3. Prognostic impact of ACEi versus ARB treatment on all-cause mortality in patients with LVEF ≥ 35% (**left panel**) and LVEF < 35% (**right panel**).

3.4. Multivariable Cox Regression Models

After multivariable adjustment, ACEi was not associated with an increased risk of all-cause mortality at three years compared to ARB therapy (HR = 1.457; 95% CI 0.952–2.229; p = 0.083) (Table 4). In contrast, increasing age (HR = 1.057; p = 0.001), presence of diabetes mellitus (HR = 1.654; p = 0.001), chronic kidney disease (HR = 1.489; p = 0.007) and LVEF < 35% (HR = 1.909; p = 0.001) were associated with impaired prognosis, whereas an ICD was associated with decreased long-term mortality (HR = 0.462; p = 0.001). In line with these results, the risk of the composite endpoint (HR = 1.028; 95% CI 0.717–1.475; p = 0.880) was not affected by ACEi/ARB. Finally, ACEi was associated with improved freedom from cardiac rehospitalization compared to ARB after multivariable adjustment (HR = 0.688; 95% CI 0.478–0.990; p = 0.044) (Table 4).

3.5. Propensity-Score Matched Cohorts

To re-evaluate the prognostic impact of ACEi versus ARB therapy in a more homogenous subgroup of patients, additional propensity score matching was performed. The characteristics of patients with ACEi and ARB therapy after propensity score matching are presented within Table 2 (right column). Following propensity score matching, especially age, sex, LVEF, chronic kidney disease and distribution of coronary artery disease were equally distributed among patients with ACEi or ARB therapy (Table 2, right column). In contrast, CPR was more common in patients with ACEi (25% vs. 18%; p = 0.048).

After propensity score matching, ACEi and ARB were associated with comparable prognosis regarding the primary endpoint of all-cause mortality (HR = 1.496; 95% CI 0.898–2.493; p = 0.122), as well as the secondary composite arrhythmic endpoint (HR = 1.142; 95% CI 0.730–1.787; p = 0.560) and cardiac rehospitalization (HR = 0.902; 95% CI 0.570–1.428; p = 0.660) (Figure 4).

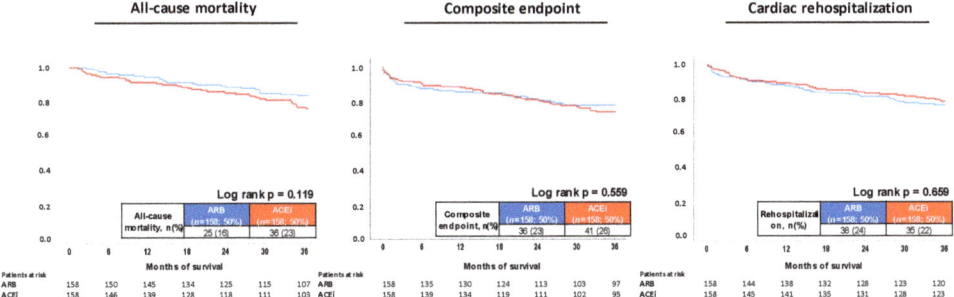

Figure 4. Prognostic impact of ACEi versus ARB treatment on all-cause mortality (**left panel**); risk of the composite endpoint (i.e., recurrence of ventricular tachyarrhythmias, sudden cardiac death) (**middle**); and cardiac rehospitalization (**right panel**) within the propensity-score matched cohort.

Table 4. Multivariable Cox regression analyses.

Endpoint	HR	95% CI	p Value
Mortality			
Age	1.057	1.040–1.073	**0.001**
Males	1.226	0.861–1.747	0.259
Diabetes	1.654	1.234–2.219	**0.001**
Chronic kidney disease	1.489	1.115–1.987	**0.007**
Acute myocardial infarction	0.628	0.424–0.932	**0.021**
Coronary artery disease	1.124	0.790–1.598	0.516
LVEF < 35%	1.909	1.407–2.590	**0.001**
Presence of ICD	0.462	0.336–0.636	**0.001**
ACEi versus ARB	1.457	0.952–2.229	0.083
Composite endpoint			
Age	1.006	0.994–1.019	0.310
Males	1.220	0.854–1.741	0.275
Diabetes	0.834	0.614–1.133	0.245
Chronic kidney disease	0.945	0.723–1.236	0.682
Acute myocardial infarction	0.961	0.647–1.428	0.843
Coronary artery disease	0.718	0.531–0.972	**0.032**
LVEF < 35%	1.142	0.870–1.499	0.338
Presence of ICD	7.752	4.829–12.445	**0.001**
ACEi versus ARB	1.028	0.717–1.475	0.880
Rehospitalization			
Age	1.006	0.992–1.020	0.423
Males	1.164	0.784–1.728	0.452
Diabetes	0.917	0.658–1.278	0.608
Chronic kidney disease	1.174	0.872–1.579	0.291
Acute myocardial infarction	1.246	0.841–1.845	0.273
Coronary artery disease	1.294	0.874–1.916	0.198
LVEF < 35%	1.442	1.058–1.965	**0.021**
Presence of ICD	3.057	2.045–4.571	**0.001**
ACEi versus ARB	0.688	0.478–0.990	**0.044**

ACE, angiotensin converting enzyme; ARB, angiotensin receptor blocker; CI; confidence interval; HR; hazard ratio; ICD; implantable cardioverter-defibrillator; LVEF, left ventricular ejection faction. Level of significance $p < 0.05$. Bold type indicates statistical significance.

Thereafter, propensity-score analyses were performed in the subgroups of patients with LVEF $\geq$ 35% and <35%, respectively. In patients with LVEF $\geq$ 35% (n = 97 patients with ACEi and ARB), comparable all-cause mortality at three years was observed (10% vs. 14%; log ran p = 0.319; HR = 1.507; 95% CI 0.669–3.393; p = 0.322) (Figure 5, left panel). In line, the composite arrhythmic endpoint (HR = 1.734; 95% CI 0.848–3.547; p = 0.132) and cardiac rehospitalization (HR = 0.754; 95% CI 0.366–1.552; p = 0.443) were not affected by ACEi compared to ARB therapy (not shown). In patients with LVEF < 35%, the risk of all-cause mortality (15% vs. 25%; log rank p = 0.408; HR = 0.711; 95% CI 0.315–1.602; p = 0.410) (Figure 5, right panel), composite arrhythmic endpoint (HR = 0.572; 95% CI 0.298–1.096; p = 0.092) and cardiac rehospitalization (HR = 0.562; 95% CI 0.274–1.149; p = 0.114) was equally distributed among patients with ACEi or ABB therapy (not shown).

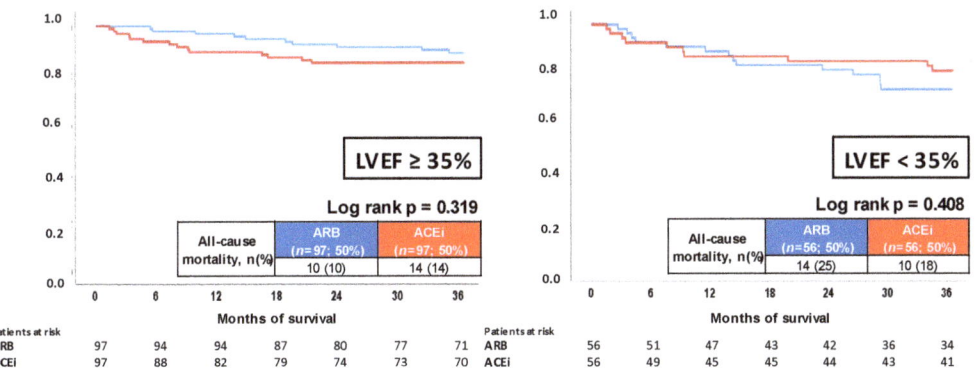

Figure 5. Prognostic impact of ACEi versus ARB treatment on all-cause mortality in patients with LVEF ≥ 35% (**left panel**); and LVEF < 35% (**right panel**) within propensity-score matched cohorts.

4. Discussion

The present study evaluates the prognostic impact of ACEi versus ARB treatment on the primary endpoint of all-cause mortality, as well as on secondary endpoints, such as a composite arrhythmic endpoint (i.e., recurrence of ventricular tachyarrhythmias, appropriate ICD therapies, SCD) and cardiac rehospitalization at three years in patients surviving index episodes of ventricular tachyarrhythmias.

This study suggests a comparable risk of all-cause mortality in patients treated with ACEi compared to ARB. ACEi and ARB had a comparable effect on the composite arrhythmic endpoint. Decreased risk of cardiac rehospitalization was no longer observed in patients treated with ACEi after propensity score matching.

The class I recommendation of ACEi/ARB for prevention of ventricular tachyarrhythmias relies on studies investigating the prognosis of ACEi/ARB in patients with HF and LVEF ≤ 40% for primary prevention of sudden cardiac death [6,8]. However, by preventing adverse cardiac remodeling, inhibitors of the renin angiotensin aldosterone system may also reduce the risk of arrhythmic events in patients with HF and AMI due to reduced cardiac fibrosis, lowering the risk of arrhythmic border zones [16]. In contrast to ACEi, ARB increases circulating angiotensin II levels by unopposed stimulation of the angiotensin II receptor, which increases plaque instability and the risk of thrombus formation [17].

However, real-life comparisons of ACEi and ARB are limited and mainly restricted to patients with AMI and systolic HF [6]. For instance, a recent meta-analysis including six randomized HF or AMI trials suggested a comparable risk of AMI, HF-related hospitalization, mortality, cardiovascular events and stroke in patients treated with ACEi as compared to ARB [18]. Furthermore, prognosis of patients treated with ACEi versus ARB was investigated within a study by Her et al., including over 13,000 patients with AMI undergoing percutaneous coronary intervention (PCI). At three years of follow-up, ACEi treatment was associated with a decreased risk of major adverse cardiac events (MACE), repeated revascularization and HF-related hospitalization when compared to ARB therapy [19]. In contrast, comparable risk of death, recurrent AMI, revascularization and risk of MACE was reported within a propensity-matched cohort including 3811 diabetics with ST-segment AMI at two years [20]. The present study, however, has a different point of view, including only patients with ventricular tachyarrhythmias, that have highest risk of death and recurrent arrhythmic events. No differences regarding all-cause mortality and the composite endpoint were observed, suggesting no additional benefit of ACEi regarding arrhythmic endpoints as compared to treatment with ARB. Due to the small number of patients with AMI in the present study (i.e., only 22 patients with ARB), further sub-analysis comparing ACEi and ARB were beyond the scope of the present study.

Focusing on patients without impaired LVEF, the prognostic role of ACEi and ARB was comprehensively investigated in 3006 patients with acute coronary syndrome and preserved ejection fraction (i.e., LVEF $\geq$ 40%). A comparable risk of all-cause mortality, as well as similar rates of the composite endpoint (i.e., death, AMI and HF) were demonstrated in patients treated with ACEi as compared to ARB [21]. These comparable effects may rely on the comparable effect of ACEi and ARB reducing the synthesis of angiotensin II, which represents a cornerstone in the pathogenesis of arrhythmic events on a structural, cellular and electrophysiological level [17].

In conclusion, the present study did not observe long-term differences in all-cause mortality in patients treated with ACEi or ARB.

Study Limitations

This observational and retrospective registry-based analysis reflects a realistic picture of consecutive health-care supply of high-risk patients presenting with ventricular tachyarrhythmias. Pharmacological therapies were based on discharge medication at the index event. Changes in pharmacological treatment (i.e., discontinuation, dose adjustment) as well as side effects occurring during follow-up were not available for the present study. Furthermore, episodes of recurrent ventricular tachyarrhythmias, appropriate ICD therapies and cardiac rehospitalization were assessed at our institution only. Some remaining selection bias due to inhomogeneous distribution of baseline characteristics and comorbidities, as well as unmeasured cofounding among patients treated with ACEi or ARB may not be excluded despite multivariable Cox regression analyses and propensity score matching. The present results need to be re-evaluated within an even larger and more representative multi-center registry data or even RCT.

Author Contributions: Conceptualization, T.S., M.B. and I.A.; methodology, T.S. and M.A.; software, T.S. and M.B.; validation, T.S., M.B., T.B., K.M. and K.W.; formal analysis, T.S. and K.W.; investigation, T.S., M.B. and I.A.; resources, M.B. and I.A.; data curation, T.B., K.M., M.A. and K.W.; writing—original draft preparation, T.S.; writing—review and editing, T.S., M.B., I.A., K.M., T.B. and K.W.; visualization, T.S.; supervision, M.B. and I.A.; project administration, M.B. and I.A. All authors have read and agreed to the published version of the manuscript.

Funding: This research received no external funding.

Institutional Review Board Statement: The study was conducted according to the guidelines of the Declaration of Helsinki, and approved by the Institutional Ethics Committee of Mannheim (2016-612N-MA).

Informed Consent Statement: Not applicable.

Data Availability Statement: The datasets used and/or analyzed during the current study are available from the corresponding author on reasonable request.

Conflicts of Interest: The authors declare no conflict of interest.

References

1. Pfeffer, M.A.; Braunwald, E.; Moyé, L.A.; Basta, L.; Brown, E.J.; Cuddy, T.E.; Davis, B.R.; Geltman, E.M.; Goldman, S.; Flaker, G.C.; et al. Effect of Captopril on Mortality and Morbidity in Patients with Left Ventricular Dysfunction after Myocardial Infarction—Results of the survival aNd ventricular enlargement trial. *N. Engl. J. Med.* **1992**, *327*, 669–677. [CrossRef] [PubMed]
2. Køber, L.; Torp-Pedersen, C.; Carlsen, J.E.; Bagger, H.; Eliasen, P.; Lyngborg, K.; Videbæk, J.; Cole, D.S.; Auclert, L.; Pauly, N.C.; et al. A Clinical Trial of the Angiotensin-Converting–Enzyme Inhibitor Trandolapril in Patients with Left Ventricular Dysfunction after Myocardial Infarction. *N. Engl. J. Med.* **1995**, *333*, 1670–1676. [CrossRef] [PubMed]
3. Ambrosioni, E.; Borghi, C.; Magnani, B. The Effect of the Angiotensin-Converting–Enzyme Inhibitor Zofenopril on Mortality and Morbidity after Anterior Myocardial Infarction. *N. Engl. J. Med.* **1995**, *332*, 80–85. [CrossRef] [PubMed]
4. Granger, C.B.; Mcmurray, J.; Yusuf, S.; Held, P.; Michelson, E.L.; Olofsson, B.; Östergren, J.; A Pfeffer, M.; Swedberg, K. Effects of candesartan in patients with chronic heart failure and reduced left-ventricular systolic function intolerant to angiotensin-converting-enzyme inhibitors: The CHARM-Alternative trial. *Lancet* **2003**, *362*, 772–776. [CrossRef]
5. Makkar, K.M.; A Sanoski, C.; A Spinler, S. Role of Angiotensin-Converting Enzyme Inhibitors, Angiotensin II Receptor Blockers, and Aldosterone Antagonists in the Prevention of Atrial and Ventricular Arrhythmias. *Pharmacotherapy* **2009**, *29*, 31–48. [CrossRef]

6. Priori, S.G.; Blomström-Lundqvist, C.; Mazzanti, A.; Blom, N.; Borggrefe, M.; Camm, J.; Elliott, P.M.; Fitzsimons, D.; Hatala, R.; Hindricks, G. 2015 ESC Guidelines for the management of patients with ventricular arrhythmias and the prevention of sudden cardiac death: The Task Force for the Management of Patients with Ventricular Arrhythmias and the Prevention of Sudden Cardiac Death of the European Society of Cardiology (ESC)Endorsed by: Association for European Paediatric and Congenital Cardiology (AEPC). *Eur. Heart J.* **2015**, *36*, 2793–2867. [CrossRef] [PubMed]
7. Domanski, M.J.; Exner, D.V.; Borkowf, C.B.; Geller, N.L.; Rosenberg, Y.; Pfeffer, M.A. Effect of angiotensin converting enzyme inhibition on sudden cardiac death in patients following acute myocardial infarction: A meta-analysis of randomized clinical trials. *J. Am. Coll. Cardiol.* **1999**, *33*, 598–604. [CrossRef]
8. Al-Khatib, S.M.; Stevenson, W.G.; Ackerman, M.J.; Bryant, W.J.; Callans, D.J.; Curtis, A.B.; Deal, B.J.; Dickfeld, T.; Field, M.E.; Fonarow, G.C.; et al. 2017 AHA/ACC/HRS Guideline for Management of Patients with Ventricular Arrhythmias and the Prevention of Sudden Cardiac Death: A Report of the American College of Cardiology/American Heart Association Task Force on Clinical Practice Guidelines and the Heart Rhythm Society. *J. Am. Coll. Cardiol.* **2018**, *72*, e91–e220. [CrossRef]
9. Schupp, T.; Behnes, M.; Weiß, C.; Nienaber, C.; Lang, S.; Reiser, L.; Bollow, A.; Taton, G.; Reichelt, T.; Ellguth, D.; et al. Beta-Blockers and ACE Inhibitors Are Associated with Improved Survival Secondary to Ventricular Tachyarrhythmia. *Cardiovasc. Drugs Ther.* **2018**, *32*, 353–363. [CrossRef]
10. Singh, S.N.; Karasik, P.; E Hafley, G.; Pieper, K.S.; Lee, K.L.; Wyse, D.; E Buxton, A. Electrophysiologic and clinical effects of angiotensin-converting enzyme inhibitors in patients with prior myocardial infarction, nonsustained ventricular tachycardia, and depressed left ventricular function. *Am. J. Cardiol.* **2001**, *87*, 716–720. [CrossRef]
11. de Diego, C.; González-Torres, L.; Núñez, J.M.; Inda, R.C.; Martin-Langerwerf, D.A.; Sangio, A.D.; Chochowski, P.; Casasnovas, P.; Blazquéz, J.C.; Almendral, J. Effects of angiotensin-neprilysin inhibition compared to angiotensin inhibition on ventricular arrhythmias in reduced ejection fraction patients under continuous remote monitoring of implantable defibrillator devices. *Heart Rhythm.* **2018**, *15*, 395–402. [CrossRef] [PubMed]
12. AlJaroudi, W.A.; Refaat, M.M.; Habib, R.H.; Al-Shaar, L.; Singh, M.; Gutmann, R.; Bloom, H.L.; Dudley, S.C.; Ellinor, P.T.; Saba, S.F.; et al. Effect of Angiotensin-Converting Enzyme Inhibitors and Receptor Blockers on Appropriate Implantable Cardiac Defibrillator Shock in Patients with Severe Systolic Heart Failure (from the GRADE Multicenter Study). *Am. J. Cardiol.* **2015**, *115*, 924–931. [CrossRef] [PubMed]
13. Zhang, Y.; Fonarow, G.C.; Sanders, P.W.; Farahmand, F.; Allman, R.M.; Aban, I.B.; Love, T.E.; Levesque, R.; Kilgore, M.L.; Ahmed, A. A Propensity-Matched Study of the Comparative Effectiveness of Angiotensin Receptor Blockers Versus Angiotensin-Converting Enzyme Inhibitors in Heart Failure Patients Age ≥65 Years. *Am. J. Cardiol.* **2011**, *108*, 1443–1448. [CrossRef]
14. Salvador, G.L.; Marmentini, V.M.; Cosmo, W.R.; Junior, E.L. Angiotensin-converting enzyme inhibitors reduce mortality compared to angiotensin receptor blockers: Systematic review and meta-analysis. *Eur. J. Prev. Cardiol.* **2017**, *24*, 1914–1924. [CrossRef] [PubMed]
15. Chen, R.; Suchard, M.A.; Krumholz, H.M.; Schuemie, M.J.; Shea, S.; Duke, J.; Pratt, N.; Reich, C.G.; Madigan, D.; You, S.C.; et al. Comparative First-Line Effectiveness and Safety of ACE (Angiotensin-Converting Enzyme) Inhibitors and Angiotensin Receptor Blockers: A Multinational Cohort Study. *Hypertension* **2021**, *78*, 591–603. [CrossRef]
16. Heart Outcomes Prevention Evaluation Study Investigators. Effects of ramipril on cardiovascular and microvascular outcomes in people with diabetes mellitus: Results of the HOPE study and MICRO-HOPE substudy. *Lancet* **2000**, *355*, 253–259, Erratum in *Lancet* **2000**, *356*, 860.
17. Strauss, M.H.; Hall, A.S. Angiotensin receptor blockers may increase risk of myocardial infarction: Unraveling the ARB-MI paradox. *Circulation* **2006**, *114*, 838–854. [CrossRef]
18. Ohtsubo, T.; Shibata, R.; Kai, H.; Okamoto, R.; Kumagai, E.; Kawano, H.; Fujiwara, A.; Kitazono, T.; Murohara, T.; Arima, H. Angiotensin-converting enzyme inhibitors versus angiotensin receptor blockers in hypertensive patients with myocardial infarction or heart failure: A systematic review and meta-analysis. *Hypertens. Res.* **2019**, *42*, 641–649. [CrossRef]
19. Her, A.-Y.; Choi, B.G.; Rha, S.-W.; Kim, Y.H.; Choi, C.U.; Jeong, M.H. The impact of angiotensin-converting-enzyme inhibitors versus angiotensin receptor blockers on 3-year clinical outcomes in patients with acute myocardial infarction without hypertension. *PLoS ONE* **2020**, *15*, e0242314. [CrossRef]
20. Choi, S.Y.; Choi, B.G.; Rha, S.-W.; Byun, J.K.; Shim, M.S.; Li, H.; Mashaly, A.; Choi, C.U.; Park, C.G.; Seo, H.S.; et al. Angiotensin-converting enzyme inhibitors versus angiotensin II receptor blockers in acute ST-segment elevation myocardial infarction patients with diabetes mellitus undergoing percutaneous coronary intervention. *Int. J. Cardiol.* **2017**, *249*, 48–54. [CrossRef]
21. Cespón-Fernández, M.; Raposeiras-Roubín, S.; Abu-Assi, E.; Pousa, I.M.; Queija, B.C.; Paz, R.J.C.; Erquicia, P.D.; Rodríguez, L.M.D.; Rodríguez, E.L.; Busto, M.C.; et al. Angiotensin-Converting Enzyme Inhibitors Versus Angiotensin II Receptor Blockers in Acute Coronary Syndrome and Preserved Ventricular Ejection Fraction. *Angiology* **2020**, *71*, 886–893. [CrossRef] [PubMed]

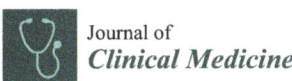

Article

Metabolic Syndrome, Gamma-Glutamyl Transferase, and Risk of Sudden Cardiac Death

Yun Gi Kim [1,†], Kyungdo Han [2,†], Joo Hee Jeong [1], Seung-Young Roh [1], Yun Young Choi [1], Kyongjin Min [1], Jaemin Shim [1], Jong-Il Choi [1,*] and Young-Hoon Kim [1]

[1] Division of Cardiology, Department of Internal Medicine, Korea University Anam Hospital, Korea University College of Medicine, Seoul 02841, Korea; tmod0176@gmail.com (Y.G.K.); jessica0115@naver.com (J.H.J.); rsy008@gmail.com (S.-Y.R.); yych60@naver.com (Y.Y.C.); mkj880628@naver.com (K.M.); jaemins@korea.ac.kr (J.S.); yhkmd@unitel.co.kr (Y.-H.K.)
[2] Department of Statistics and Actuarial Science, Soongsil University, Seoul 06978, Korea; hkd917@naver.com
* Correspondence: jongilchoi@korea.ac.kr; Tel.: +82-2-920-5445; Fax: +82-2-927-1478
† These authors contributed equally to this work.

Abstract: Background: Metabolic syndrome is associated with a significantly increased risk of sudden cardiac death (SCD). However, whether temporal changes in the metabolic syndrome status are associated with SCD is unknown. We aimed to determine whether metabolic syndrome and gamma-glutamyl transferase (ɤ-GTP), including their temporal changes, are associated with the risk of SCD. Methods: We performed a nationwide population-based analysis using the Korean National Health Insurance Service. People who underwent a national health check-up in 2009 and 2011 were enrolled. The influence of metabolic syndrome and ɤ-GTP on SCD risk was evaluated. Results: In 2009, 4,056,423 (848,498 with metabolic syndrome) people underwent health screenings, 2,706,788 of whom underwent follow-up health screenings in 2011. Metabolic syndrome was associated with a 50.7% increased SCD risk (adjusted hazard ratio (aHR) = 1.507; $p < 0.001$). The SCD risk increased linearly as the metabolic syndrome diagnostic criteria increased. The ɤ-GTP significantly impacted the SCD risk; the highest quartile had a 51.9% increased risk versus the lowest quartile (aHR = 1.519; $p < 0.001$). A temporal change in the metabolic syndrome status and ɤ-GTP between 2009 and 2011 was significantly correlated with the SCD risk. Having metabolic syndrome in 2009 or 2011 indicated a lower SCD risk than having metabolic syndrome in 2009 and 2011 but a higher risk than having no metabolic syndrome. People with a ≥20-unit increase in ɤ-GTP between 2009 and 2011 had an 81.0% increased SCD risk versus those with a change ≤5 units (aHR = 1.810; $p < 0.001$). Conclusions: Metabolic syndrome and ɤ-GTP significantly correlated with an increased SCD risk. SCD was also influenced by temporal changes in the metabolic syndrome status and ɤ-GTP, suggesting that appropriate medical treatment and lifestyle modifications may reduce future SCD risk.

Keywords: gamma-glutamyl transferase; metabolic syndrome; sudden cardiac death

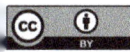

1. Introduction

Sudden cardiac death (SCD) is an emergent medical condition that requires timely intervention to bring the victim back to life [1,2]. However, since all SCD cases occur outside the hospital, immediate professional intervention is virtually impossible [2–5]. The SCD survival rates are still not satisfactory, even in the most developed regions of the world, whereas neurologically intact survival rates are even lower [6,7]. The immediate management of SCD is the cornerstone of SCD treatment. However, ensuring the adequate training of the general population for cardiopulmonary resuscitation and the dissemination of automated external defibrillators requires enormous medical resources. Therefore, understanding and meticulously managing the risk factors for SCD require greater attention.

The underlying causes of SCD include coronary artery disease, primary myocardial or electrical disorders such as hypertrophic cardiomyopathy and Brugada syndrome, and valvular heart disease [3,8]. Metabolic syndrome, which is characterized by abdominal obesity, dyslipidemia, an elevated fasting glucose, and high blood pressure, is an established risk factor for coronary artery disease and SCD [9,10]. Hess et al. revealed that the risk of SCD increased by 70% in people with metabolic syndrome [10]. However, the total sample number was not large at 13,168 people with 357 SCD events. Furthermore, the impact of metabolic syndrome management is not fully understood. Gamma-glutamyl transferase (γ-GTP) is linked with obesity, physical inactivity, hypertension, dyslipidemia, and glucose intolerance, suggesting it can be a good marker for metabolic syndrome [11–13]. Since the presence of metabolic syndrome is associated with an elevated risk of SCD, γ-GTP may have predictive value for the occurrence of SCD. However, the impact of γ-GTP and changes in γ-GTP on SCD remain to be elucidated.

Here, we aimed to evaluate the impact of: (i) metabolic syndrome, (ii) control of the metabolic syndrome, (iii) γ-GTP, and changes in γ-GTP on the risk of SCD through a nationwide population-based analysis.

2. Patients and Methods

2.1. Study Design

The Korean National Health Insurance Service (K-NHIS) database was used in this study. Since all citizens of South Korea are mandatory K-NHIS subscribers, its data represents the entire Korean population. The K-NHIS offers a nationwide regular health screening to its subscribers, including measurements of height, weight, waist circumference, and blood pressure; a self-reported questionnaire about alcohol consumption, smoking status, and physical activity level; and various laboratory tests, such as the blood cell count; renal function; liver function; fasting blood glucose; and lipid profile (total cholesterol, high-density lipoprotein, and triglycerides). Prior claims of various International Classification of Disease, tenth edition (ICD-10) diagnostic codes such as diabetes mellitus (DM), hypertension, dyslipidemia, or heart failure, and a prescription history of various drugs, are also recorded in the K-NHIS database. Therefore, the presence of metabolic syndrome can be identified for all K-NHIS subscribers who have undergone the nationwide health screening. The level of γ-GTP, a marker for metabolic syndrome, is included in the liver function test [14,15]. It is measured in international units per liter (IU/L), as with prior studies [11–13].

This study enrolled patients who underwent a nationwide health screening in 2009. People who were previously diagnosed with SCD and were aged less than 20 years at the 2009 health screening were excluded. Clinical follow-up data were available until December 2018. Since the K-NHIS is a nationwide mandatory and exclusive health care insurance system of the Republic of Korea, there were no follow-up losses, except for immigrants.

To identify baseline medical history variables such as hypertension and DM, the data obtained from January 2002 to December 2008 were used as the screening period, and the robustness of our coding strategy was validated via multiple prior studies [16–20]. Sequential nationwide health screenings are recommended for K-NHIS subscribers. We identified people who underwent a nationwide health screening in 2011 from among those who had undergone a nationwide health screening in 2009. Therefore, sequential alterations in the metabolic syndrome status and γ-GTP were available for the analysis.

The current study was approved by the Institutional Review Board of Korea University Medicine Anam Hospital (IRB number: 2021AN0185) and official review committee of the K-NHIS. Considering the retrospective nature of this study, the requirement for written informed consent was waived. The ethical guidelines of the 2013 Declaration of Helsinki and legal medical regulations of the Republic of Korea were strictly undertaken throughout the study.

2.2. Primary Outcome Endpoint

The occurrence of SCD was the main outcome of this study. The ICD-10 codes used to identify SCD were as follows: I46.0 (cardiac arrest with successful resuscitation), I46.1 (sudden cardiac arrest), I46.9 (cardiac arrest, cause unspecified), I49.0 (ventricular fibrillation and flutter), R96.0 (instantaneous death), and R96.1 (death occurring less than 24 h from symptom onset). Only claims accompanied by a declaration of death or cardiopulmonary resuscitation were included. In-hospital cardiac arrest was not the scope of this study; therefore, only claims that were coded during an emergency department visit were selected. Not all SCD events were of cardiac origin, and SCD events were not counted as a primary outcome endpoint if the participants had a prior diagnosis of asphyxia, gastrointestinal bleeding, cerebral hemorrhage, ischemic stroke, sepsis, anaphylaxis, trauma, suffocation, lightning strike, electric shock, drowning, or burn within 6 months of the diagnosis of SCD. The incidence of SCD was defined as the number of events per 1000 person/years of follow-up. The impacts of metabolic syndrome, γ-GTP, and their alterations over time on SCD incidence were evaluated. The incidence of SCD was defined as the number of events per 1000 person/years of follow-up.

2.3. Metabolic Syndrome

The National Cholesterol Education Program Adult Treatment Panel III criteria for metabolic syndrome was used in this study [21]. Metabolic syndrome was defined as the presence of three or more of the following criteria: (i) waist circumference $\geq$102 cm (men; $\geq$90 cm for East Asian men) or $\geq$88 cm (women; $\geq$80 cm for East Asian women), (ii) blood pressure $\geq$130/85 mmHg or on pharmacologic treatment, (iii) fasting blood glucose $\geq$100 mg/dL or on pharmacologic treatment, (iv) fasting triglyceride level $\geq$150 mg/dL or on pharmacologic treatment, and (v) fasting high-density lipoprotein cholesterol level $\leq$40 mg/dL (men) or $\leq$50 mg/dL (women) or on pharmacologic treatment.

2.4. Definitions

Diabetes mellitus and impaired fasting glucose were defined based on either the fasting blood glucose (FBG) level (FBG $\geq$ 126 mg/dL for DM and FBG 100–125 mg/dL for impaired fasting glucose) or a claim of relevant ICD-10 codes by a physician. Hypertension and prehypertension were also identified by measured blood pressure and ICD-10 codes for hypertension and prehypertension. Blood pressure criteria were systolic blood pressure (SBP) <120 mmHg and diastolic blood pressure (DBP) <80 mmHg for non-hypertension, either 120 $\leq$ SBP < 140 or 80 $\leq$ DBP < 90 for prehypertension, and either SBP $\geq$ 140 or DBP $\geq$ 90 for hypertension. Chronic kidney disease (CKD) was defined as estimated glomerular filtration rate < 60 mL/min/1.73 m^2, which was calculated by the Modification of Diet in Renal Disease (MDRD) equation. A self-questionnaire acquired during the 2009 health check-up was used to define regular physical activity. People who had one or more sessions in a week with high (such as running, climbing, or intense bicycle activities) or moderate physical activity (such as walking fast, tennis, or moderate bicycle activities) were classified as having regular physical activity. The robustness of the aforementioned definitions was validated in our prior studies [16,17,22].

2.5. Statistical Analysis

Continuous variables were expressed as the mean $\pm$ standard deviation, and the Student's *t*-test was used for statistical comparisons. Categorical variables were compared using the chi-square test or Fisher's exact test, as appropriate. The cumulative incidence of SCD was depicted by a Kaplan–Meier curve analysis, and intergroup differences were compared using the log-rank *t*-test. Raw and adjusted hazard ratios (aHRs) with 95% confidence intervals (CIs) were calculated using a Cox-regression analysis. Since γ-GTP was non-normally distributed, it was analyzed as a continuous variable in the Cox-regression analysis. We divided our cohort into quartile groups, and the HR for each group was calculated through a Cox-regression analysis, with the lowest quartile group as a reference group. Bonferroni correction was performed to adjust for the influence of multiple comparisons (if more than three groups are compared to each other). People with missing data were excluded from the study. Statistical significance was defined as p-values ≤ 0.05 in two-tailed tests. All statistical analyses were performed using SAS version 9.2 (SAS Institute, Cary, NC, USA).

3. Results

3.1. Study Population

Among people who underwent nationwide health screening in 2009, 50% of them were randomly selected and a total of 4,234,341 people were enrolled in this analysis. Due to a prior diagnosis of SCD and missing data, 491 and 177,427 people were excluded from the study, respectively. In terms of the baseline demographics (health screening in 2009), 4,056,423 people were analyzed, 2,706,788 among whom underwent a follow-up health screening in 2011. The flow of the study is summarized in Figure 1. The baseline demographics of the patients who did or did not experience SCD are summarized in Table 1. In brief, people who experienced SCD during the follow-up period were significantly older; had larger waist circumferences; were more likely to be male and smokers; had a higher prevalence of hypertension, DM, dyslipidemia, and chronic kidney disease; and had higher ɤ-GTP levels.

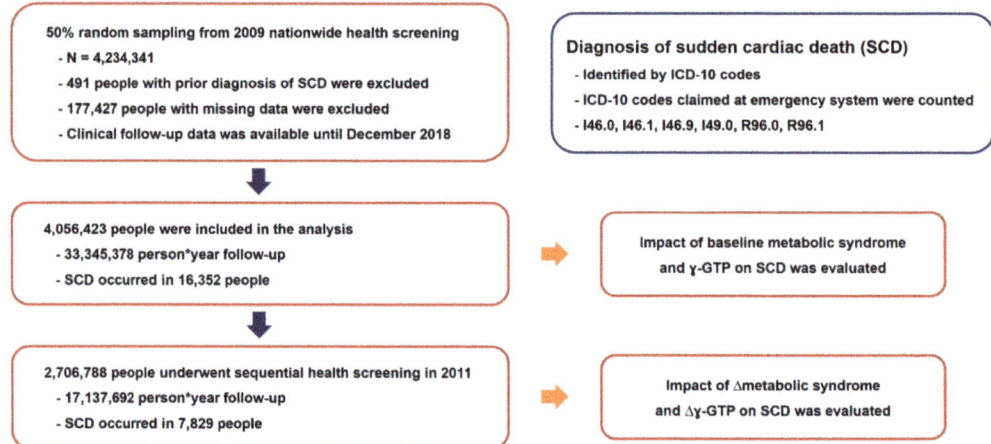

Figure 1. Study flow. ɤ-GTP: gamma-glutamyl transferase; ICD-10: International Classification of Disease, tenth edition; SCD: sudden cardiac death.

Table 1. Baseline characteristics of SCD victims.

	SCD		p-Value
	No 4,040,071	Yes 16,352	
Male sex	2,221,898 (55.0%)	11,633 (71.1%)	<0.001
Age (year)	47.0 ± 14.1	62.0 ± 13.2	<0.001
Body mass index (kg/m^2)	23.7 ± 3.2	23.8 ± 3.4	0.138
Waist circumference (cm)	80.2 ± 9.5	83.5 ± 8.9	<0.001
Smoking history			<0.001
Never-smoker	2,399,679 (59.4%)	7916 (48.4%)	
Ex-smoker	581,485 (14.4%)	3128 (19.1%)	
Current-smoker	1,058,907 (26.2%)	5308 (32.5%)	

Table 1. Cont.

	SCD		p-Value
	No 4,040,071	Yes 16,352	
Alcohol consumption			<0.001
Non-drinker	2,077,053 (51.4%)	9534 (58.3%)	
Mild-drinker	1,641,427 (40.6%)	5263 (32.2%)	
Heavy-drinker	321,591 (8.0%)	1555 (9.5%)	
Regular Exercise	733,609 (18.2%)	3148 (19.3%)	<0.001
Income (lowest 20% group)	704,587 (17.4%)	3075 (18.8%)	<0.001
Diabetes mellitus	349,134 (8.6%)	4264 (26.1%)	<0.001
Serum glucose (mg/dL)	97.2 ± 23.8	110.0 ± 41.5	<0.001
Hypertension	1,082,382 (27.0%)	9331 (57.1%)	<0.001
Systolic blood pressure (mmHg)	122.4 ± 15.0	129.3 ± 17.2	<0.001
Diastolic blood pressure (mmHg)	76.3 ± 10.0	78.9 ± 11.0	<0.001
Dyslipidemia	732,983 (18.1%)	4610 (28.2%)	<0.001
Cholesterol (mg/dL)	195.3 ± 41.1	195.1 ± 44.3	0.549
High density lipoprotein (mg/dL)	56.5 ± 32.9	53.6 ± 30.9	<0.001
Low density lipoprotein (mg/dL)	121.2 ± 214.2	115.0 ± 97.8	<0.001
Chronic kidney disease	275,854 (6.8%)	2740 (16.8%)	<0.001
eGFR (mL/min/1.73 m^2)	87.6 ± 44.9	80.4 ± 34.7	<0.001

eGFR: estimated glomerular filtration rate; SCD: sudden cardiac death.

3.2. Metabolic Syndrome

Baseline characteristics of the people with and without metabolic syndrome are summarized in Table 2. In brief, people with metabolic syndrome were older; had higher body mass index and waist circumference, had a higher prevalence of male sex, hypertension, DM, dyslipidemia, and chronic kidney disease. Among the 848,498 people with metabolic syndrome (with 6,897,608 person/years of follow-up), 6546 SCD events occurred with an incidence of 0.949 cases per 1000 person/years of follow-up. In people without metabolic syndrome, 9,806 SCD events occurred during 26,447,770 person/years of follow-up for an incidence of 0.371 (Table 3). After multivariate adjustment, the metabolic syndrome was associated with a 50.7% increased SCD risk (aHR = 1.507; 95% CI = 1.456–1.560; $p < 0.001$; Table 2). Metabolic syndrome was diagnosed based on the fulfillment of five criteria. The number of criteria fulfilled was linearly associated with the occurrence of SCD, with more criteria being associated with a greater risk (Table 3). People who met all five criteria for metabolic syndrome had a 2.956-fold increased risk of SCD compared with those who met no criteria (aHR = 2.956; 95% CI = 2.707–3.227; $p < 0.001$; Table 3). The SCD risk gradually increased as the number of fulfilled criteria for metabolic syndrome increased (Table 3).

Table 2. Baseline characteristics of patients with versus without metabolic syndrome.

	Metabolic Syndrome		p Value
	No 3,207,925	Yes 848,498	
Male sex	1,717,481 (53.6%)	516,050 (60.8%)	<0.001
Age	45.0 ± 13.6	55.0 ± 12.9	<0.001
Age group, years			<0.001
20–29	480,147 (15.0%)	21,469 (2.5%)	
30–39	687,795 (21.4%)	91,015 (10.7%)	
40–49	898,205 (28.0%)	167,654 (19.8%)	
50–59	627,768 (19.6%)	233,180 (27.5%)	
60–69	337,250 (10.5%)	211,238 (24.9%)	
70–79	152,342 (4.8%)	109,341 (12.9%)	
80+	24,418 (0.8%)	14,601 (1.7%)	

Table 2. Cont.

	Metabolic Syndrome		p Value
	No 3,207,925	Yes 848,498	
Body mass index	23.1 ± 2.9	26.0 ± 3.2	<0.001
Waist circumference	78.3 ± 8.5	87.9 ± 9.0	<0.001
Smoking status			<0.001
Non-smoker	1,940,944 (60.5%)	466,651 (55.0%)	
Ex-smoker	428,522 (13.4%)	156,091 (18.4%)	
Current smoker	838,459 (26.1%)	225,756 (26.6%)	
Alcohol consumption			<0.001
Non-drinker	1,639,224 (51.1%)	447,363 (52.7%)	
Mild drinker	1,341,119 (41.8%)	305,571 (36.0%)	
Heavy drinker	227,582 (7.1%)	95,564 (11.3%)	
Regular exercise	569,089 (17.7%)	167,668 (19.8%)	<0.001
Income (lower 20%)	564,051 (17.6%)	143,611 (16.9%)	<0.001
Diabetes mellitus	117,925 (3.7%)	235,473 (27.8%)	<0.001
Diabetes mellitus stage			<0.001
Non-diabetic	2,541,796 (79.2%)	242,335 (28.6%)	
Impaired fasting glucose	548,204 (17.1%)	370,690 (43.7%)	
New-onset	53,175 (1.7%)	67,408 (7.9%)	
<5 years	32,167 (1.0%)	87,320 (10.3%)	
≥5 years	32,583 (1.0%)	80,745 (9.5%)	
Fasting blood glucose (mg/dL)	92.9 ± 17.7	113.5 ± 34.6	<0.001
Hypertension	536,787 (16.7%)	554,926 (65.4%)	<0.001
Hypertension stage			<0.001
Non-hypertensive	1,340,278 (41.8%)	45,699 (5.4%)	
Pre-hypertension	1,330,860 (41.5%)	247,873 (29.2%)	
Hypertension without medication	210,930 (6.6%)	125,149 (14.8%)	
Hypertension with medication	325,857 (10.2%)	429,777 (50.7%)	
Systolic blood pressure	119.8 ± 14.0	132.4 ± 14.7	<0.001
Diastolic blood pressure	74.9 ± 9.5	81.7 ± 10.1	<0.001
Dyslipidemia	300,945 (9.4%)	436,648 (51.5%)	<0.001
Dyslipidemia stage (mg/dL)			<0.001
Total cholesterol < 240	2,906,980 (90.6%)	411,850 (48.5%)	
Total cholesterol ≥ 240	257,907 (8.0%)	90,765 (10.7%)	
Total cholesterol ≥ 240 with medication	43,038 (1.3%)	345,883 (40.8%)	
Cholesterol level (mg/dL)	192.3 ± 38.4	206.5 ± 48.5	<0.001
High-density lipoprotein (mg/dL)	57.5 ± 31.8	52.8 ± 36.7	<0.001
Low-density lipoprotein (mg/dL)	122.1 ± 232.1	117.8 ± 122.1	<0.001
Chronic kidney disease	182,472 (5.7%)	96,122 (11.3%)	<0.001
Estimated glomerular filtration rate	88.8 ± 46.6	83.0 ± 37.4	<0.001
Gamma-glutamyl transferase (IU/L)	23.81 (23.79-23.82)	38.86 (38.80-38.93)	<0.001

Data are shown as n (%), mean ± standard deviation, or median (95% confidence interval). IU/L: international units per liter.

Table 3. Impact of metabolic syndrome on SCD.

	n	SCD	Follow-Up Duration (Person/Years)	Incidence	Hazard Ratio with 95% Confidence Interval	
					Univariate	Multivariate
Metabolic syndrome						
No	3,207,925	9806	26,447,770	0.371	1 (reference)	1 (reference)
Yes	848,498	6546	6,897,608	0.949	2.558 (2.480–2.640)	1.507 (1.456–1.560)
Number of metabolic syndrome criteria met						
0	1,261,043	1806	10,465,831	0.173	1 (reference)	1 (reference)
1	1,127,888	3819	9,285,122	0.411	2.383 (2.254–2.521)	1.378 (1.302–1.459)
2	818,994	4181	6,696,816	0.624	3.619 (3.424–3.824)	1.677 (1.583–1.776)
3	509,764	3378	4,153,728	0.813	4.712 (4.451–4.990)	1.975 (1.858–2.100)
4	259,869	2287	2,107,073	1.085	6.288 (5.911–6.688)	2.367 (2.214–2.531)
5	78,865	881	636,807	1.383	8.008 (7.388–8.680)	2.956 (2.707–3.227)

Incidence is per 1000 person/years of follow-up. SCD: sudden cardiac death. The multivariate model was adjusted for age, sex, body mass index, smoking status, alcohol consumption, regular physical activity, and income level.

3.3. ɤ-GTP

In this nationwide cohort, ɤ-GTP levels were significantly higher in people with metabolic syndrome (median value 23.81, versus 38.86; $p < 0.001$; Table 2). People were classified into four groups according to serum ɤ-GTP concentration. The prevalence of metabolic syndrome in the highest ɤ-GTP level quartile was significantly higher than that in the lowest quartile (9.4% versus 44.1%; $p < 0.001$). Compared with people in the first (lowest ɤ-GTP level) quartile, those in the third (aHR = 1.158; 95% CI = 1.098–1.222; $p < 0.001$; Table 4) and fourth (highest ɤ-GTP level; aHR = 1.519; 95% CI = 1.437–1.605; $p < 0.001$; Table 4) quartiles showed significantly increased risks of SCD.

Table 4. Impact of ɤ-GTP level on SCD development.

	n	SCD	Follow-Up Duration (Person/Years)	Incidence	Hazard Ratio with 95% Confidence Interval	
					Univariate	Multivariate
ɤ-GTP						
Q1 (lowest)	987,003	2314	8,162,351	0.284	1 (reference)	1 (reference)
Q2	1,066,117	3727	8,789,346	0.424	1.496 (1.420–1.575)	1.055 (1.000–1.112)
Q3	996,270	4447	8,184,478	0.543	1.918 (1.824–2.017)	1.158 (1.098–1.222)
Q4 (highest)	1,007,033	5864	8,209,202	0.714	2.528 (2.409–2.652)	1.519 (1.437–1.605)

Incidence is per 1000 person/years of follow-up. ɤ-GTP, gamma-glutamyl transferase; SCD, sudden cardiac death, the multivariate model was adjusted for age, sex, body mass index, waist circumference, smoking status, alcohol consumption, regular physical activity, income level, hypertension, diabetes mellitus, dyslipidemia, and chronic kidney disease.

3.4. Temporal Changes

Compared with people without metabolic syndromes in both 2009 and 2011, those who developed metabolic syndrome in 2011 (without metabolic syndrome in 2009) had a 31.6% increased risk of SCD (aHR = 1.316; 95% CI = 1.215–1.426; $p < 0.001$; Table 5; Figure 2). People who had metabolic syndrome in both 2009 and 2011 had a 59.1% increased risk of SCD (aHR = 1.591; 95% CI = 1.503–1.684; $p < 0.001$; Table 5 and Figure 2). However, the

SCD risk was significantly lower if metabolic syndrome recovered in 2011 (aHR = 1.310; 95% CI = 1.207–1.423; $p < 0.001$; Table 5 and Figure 2).

Table 5. Impact of changes in metabolic syndrome status on SCD development.

	n	SCD	Follow-Up Duration (Person/Years)	Incidence	Hazard Ratio with 95% Confidence Interval	
					Univariate	Multivariate
Metabolic syndrome						
No (in 2009) → No (in 2011)	1,967,483	4,080	12,479,939	0.327	1 (reference)	1 (reference)
No → Yes	189,148	733	1,193,749	0.614	1.877 (1.735–2.030)	1.316 (1.215–1.426)
Yes → No	169,640	702	1,068,427	0.657	2.009 (1.854–2.176)	1.310 (1.207–1.423)
Yes → Yes	380,517	2,314	2,395,577	0.966	2.946 (2.800–3.101)	1.591 (1.503–1.684)

Incidence is per 1000 person/years of follow-up. SCD: sudden cardiac death. The multivariate model was adjusted for age, sex, body mass index, smoking status, alcohol consumption, regular physical activity, and income level.

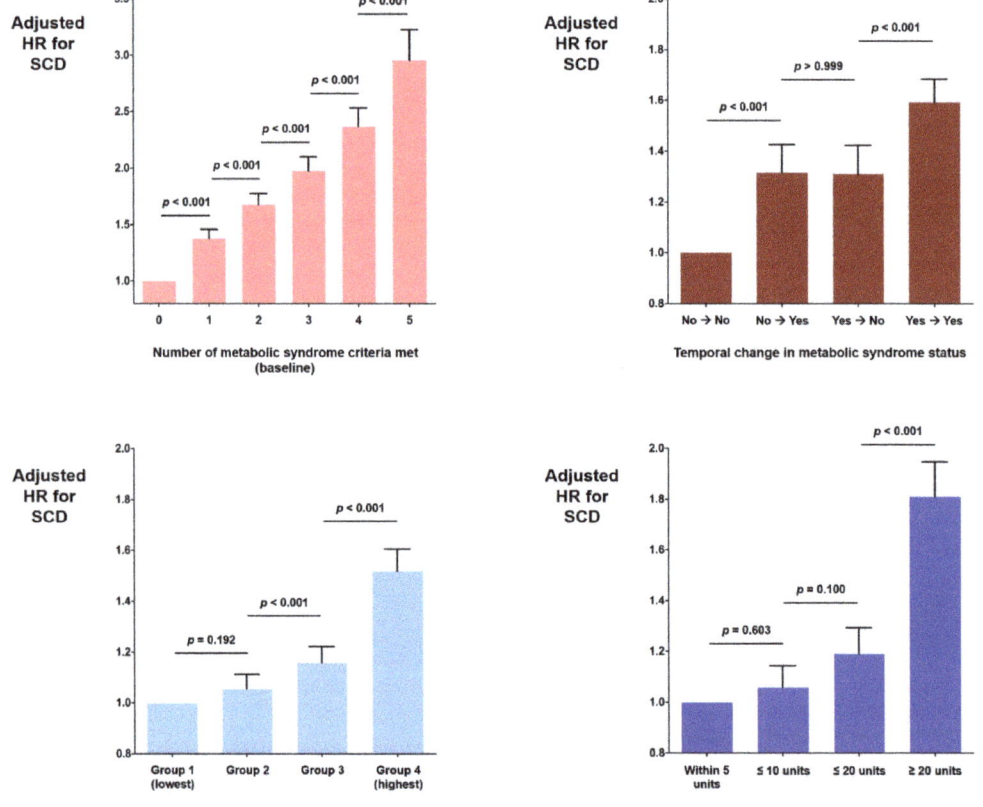

Figure 2. Impact of metabolic syndrome and ɤ-GTP on SCD. The risk of SCD increased linearly according to the number of metabolic syndrome criteria met and serum ɤ-GTP level (**left panels**). Temporal changes in the metabolic syndrome status and serum level of ɤ-GTP significantly influenced the SCD risk (**right panels**). The whiskers indicate 95% confidence intervals. p-values are presented with Bonferroni correction. ɤ-GTP, gamma-glutamyl transferase; HR, hazard ratio; SCD, sudden cardiac death.

Temporal changes in the ɤ-GTP level were also associated with SCD risk. Compared with people who maintained a change of the ɤ-GTP level within five units, people who had a more than 20-unit increase between 2009 and 2011 had an 81.0% increased SCD risk (aHR = 1.810; 95% CI = 1.683–1.947; $p < 0.001$; Figure 2). People with a change in the ɤ-GTP level of 10–20 units showed a 19.0% increased SCD risk (aHR = 1.190; 95% CI = 1.094–1.294; $p < 0.001$; Figure 2).

4. Discussion

This nationwide cohort-based study demonstrated that (i) metabolic syndrome was associated with a significantly increased SCD risk, (ii) the more number of criteria for metabolic syndrome fulfilled, the higher the SCD risk, (iii) the successful management of metabolic syndrome was associated with an alleviated SCD risk, (iv) people with uncontrolled metabolic syndrome were at higher SCD risk, (v) an increased ɤ-GTP level was significantly associated with an increased SCD risk, and (vi) a temporal increase in the ɤ-GTP level was significantly associated with an increased SCD risk.

Metabolic syndrome is an increasingly prevalent medical condition. This study revealed that metabolic syndrome, especially when uncontrolled, increases one's SCD risk. Furthermore, the successful management of metabolic syndrome may reduce the risk of SCD, indicating the importance of lifestyle modifications and medical treatment in people with metabolic syndrome. The prognosis of people with SCD is poor, and its primary prevention is especially important considering the intrinsic limitations in its management [6,7,23,24]. Our results can provide important clues for reducing SCD-related healthcare burdens.

4.1. Metabolic Syndrome

Metabolic syndrome is a cluster of central obesity, dyslipidemia, glucose intolerance, and elevated blood pressure [25]. Empana et al. reported a 68% increased risk of sudden death attributable to metabolic syndrome in middle-aged men [26]. Hess et al. also reported a 70% increased risk of sudden cardiac death among participants of the ARIC (Atherosclerosis Risk in Communities) study [10]. Our results are in accordance with those of the aforementioned studies, and our participants with metabolic syndrome showed a 50.7% increased risk of SCD. However, the current study is distinguished by the following points: (i) it included a significantly large number of participants, (ii) we simultaneously analyzed ɤ-GTP, and (iii) we analyzed the temporal changes in metabolic syndrome. The data of 4,056,423 people were analyzed, 848,498 of whom had metabolic syndrome. The total number of SCD events was 16,352, which was sufficient for various analyses. We divided our participants into six groups according to the number of metabolic syndrome criteria fulfilled and revealed that the SCD risk was the highest among those who met all five criteria. A linear increase in the SCD risk was noted as the number of fulfilled criteria increased, suggesting that there are no clear cut-off criteria, but rather, every aspect of metabolic syndrome matters. The clinical impact of temporal changes in the metabolic syndrome status is another strong aspect of this study. People with metabolic syndrome in the 2009 and 2011 nationwide health screenings were at the highest risk of SCD. People with newly developed metabolic syndrome in 2011 showed a 31.6% increased risk of SCD compared to those without metabolic syndrome in 2009 or 2011. Importantly, people who did not have metabolic syndrome in 2011 were at a significantly lower risk of developing SCD than those who had metabolic syndrome in both 2009 and 2011, suggesting that the adequate management of metabolic syndrome can have a significant therapeutic effect on reducing SCD risk.

4.2. Gamma-GTP

The serum ɤ-GTP level is routinely measured in nationwide health screening programs in South Korea; here, we were able to analyze large amounts of ɤ-GTP data. People with the highest ɤ-GTP level quartile were at a 51.9% increased risk of SCD compared with those in the lowest quartile. The association between ɤ-GTP and metabolic syndrome was described in prior studies of participants with higher ɤ-GTP levels showing a significantly higher risk of metabolic syndrome [14,27]. However, the association between ɤ-GTP level and SCD has not been described until now. The highest quartile group in our study, by definition, comprised 25% of the general population, and these people demonstrated a 51.9% increased SCD risk. This group vulnerable to SCD is not a small specific subgroup, suggesting that the ɤ-GTP level can be a very useful serum marker for identifying people at high risk for SCD. Furthermore, we demonstrated here that a temporal increase in the ɤ-GTP level of more than 20 units was associated with an 81.0% increased risk of developing SCD.

Insulin resistance is the suspected underlying mechanism linking ɤ-GTP and metabolic syndrome [14,27]. The prevalence of metabolic syndrome, number of its components, and insulin resistance increased as the ɤ-GTP level increased in a prior study of 3246 Korean people [28]. Kawamoto et al. reported that the association between ɤ-GTP and metabolic syndrome was significantly attenuated after the adjustment for markers of insulin resistance, suggesting that such an association is correlated with insulin resistance [14]. Insulin resistance is also the underlying pathophysiology of metabolic syndrome [29], and it may be the cause of the increased risk of SCD developing among the people with metabolic syndrome and high ɤ-GTP levels in this study. Whether improvements in insulin resistance can decrease the SCD risk will be an important area of future research.

An increased level of ɤ-GTP might also reflect the degree of inflammation, an important pathophysiology of atherosclerosis, explaining the potential association between high ɤ-GTP and increased risk of SCD observed in our study [14,30]. A prior study revealed that ɤ-GTP can increase low-density lipoprotein oxidation through hydrolyzing extracellular glutathione into more potent iron reductants, another possible mechanism linking ɤ-GTP, atherosclerosis, and SCD [31].

4.3. Limitations

This study has several limitations. Despite prior validation of our coding strategies, coding inaccuracies can arise from retrospective analyses of nationwide health insurance organization data [16,20,32,33]. The use of an exclusive cohort, which consisted solely of East Asian people, limited the generalizability of our findings. Additionally, liver function can affect the serum level of ɤ-GTP. However, we were not able to obtain liver function tests, such as the liver enzyme level, bilirubin level, alkaline phosphatase, or prothrombin time. Finally, we were able to assess the occurrence but not the result of SCD development.

5. Conclusions

The risk of SCD is significantly increased in people with metabolic syndrome, and the number of fulfilled metabolic syndrome diagnostic criteria and temporal changes in its status are significantly associated with the risk of SCD. The baseline level and temporal changes in ɤ-GTP, a serum marker for metabolic syndrome, are also significantly associated with the future risk of SCD. Our findings indicate that efforts to control metabolic syndrome and ɤ-GTP levels can reduce the risk of SCD.

Author Contributions: J.-I.C. had full access to all data in this study and takes responsibility for its integrity and analytical accuracy. The study concept and design were developed by Y.G.K., Y.Y.C., K.H., J.-I.C. and Y.-H.K. The data analysis and interpretation were performed by Y.G.K., Y.Y.C., K.H., J.H.J., S.-Y.R., K.M., Y.Y.C. and J.-I.C. The manuscript was drafted by Y.G.K., K.H. and J.-I.C. The statistical analysis was performed by Y.G.K., K.H. and J.-I.C. The data collection was performed by Y.G.K., K.H., J.S. and J.-I.C. All authors have read and agreed to the published version of the manuscript.

Funding: This work was supported by a National Research Foundation of Korea (NRF) grant funded by the Korean government (MSIT, Ministry of Science, and ICT) (No. 2021R1A2C2011325 to J.I.C.). The funder had no role in data collection, analysis, or interpretation, trial design, patient recruitment, or any other aspect pertinent to the study.

Institutional Review Board Statement: The current study was approved by the Institutional Review Board of Korea Univer-sity Medicine Anam Hospital (IRB number: 2021AN0185) and official review committee of the K-NHIS.

Informed Consent Statement: Considering the retrospective nature of this study, the requirement for written informed consent was waived.

Data Availability Statement: The raw data underlying this article cannot be shared publicly due to privacy reasons and legal regulations of the Republic of Korea. The raw data is stored and analyzed only in the designated server managed by the K-NHIS.

Conflicts of Interest: The authors have no conflict of interest and no relationships with the industry.

Abbreviations

aHR = adjusted hazard ratio; BMI = body mass index; CI = confidence interval; DM = diabetes mellitus; ɣ-GTP = gamma-glutamyl transferase; ICD = International Classification of Disease; K-NHIS = Korean National Health Insurance Service; SCD = sudden cardiac death.

References

1. Myat, A.; Song, K.J.; Rea, T. Out-of-hospital cardiac arrest: Current concepts. *Lancet* **2018**, *391*, 970–979. [CrossRef]
2. McCarthy, J.J.; Carr, B.; Sasson, C.; Bobrow, B.J.; Callaway, C.W.; Neumar, R.W.; Ferrer, J.M.E.; Garvey, J.L.; Ornato, J.P.; Gonzales, L.; et al. Out-of-Hospital Cardiac Arrest Resuscitation Systems of Care: A Scientific Statement From the American Heart Association. *Circulation* **2018**, *137*, e645–e660. [CrossRef] [PubMed]
3. Kelly, E.M.; Pinto, D.S. Invasive Management of Out of Hospital Cardiac Arrest. *Circ. Cardiovasc. Interv.* **2019**, *12*, e006071. [CrossRef] [PubMed]
4. Ong, M.E.H.; Perkins, G.D.; Cariou, A. Out-of-hospital cardiac arrest: Prehospital management. *Lancet* **2018**, *391*, 980–988. [CrossRef]
5. Hassager, C.; Nagao, K.; Hildick-Smith, D. Out-of-hospital cardiac arrest: In-hospital intervention strategies. *Lancet* **2018**, *391*, 989–998. [CrossRef]
6. Culley, L.L.; Rea, T.D.; Murray, J.A.; Welles, B.; Fahrenbruch, C.E.; Olsufka, M.; Eisenberg, M.S.; Copass, M.K. Public access defibrillation in out-of-hospital cardiac arrest: A community-based study. *Circulation* **2004**, *109*, 1859–1863. [CrossRef]
7. Kim, C.; Fahrenbruch, C.E.; Cobb, L.A.; Eisenberg, M.S. Out-of-hospital cardiac arrest in men and women. *Circulation* **2001**, *104*, 2699–2703. [CrossRef]
8. Kim, Y.G.; Oh, S.K.; Choi, H.Y.; Choi, J.I. Inherited arrhythmia syndrome predisposing to sudden cardiac death. *Korean J. Intern. Med.* **2021**, *36*, 527–538. [CrossRef]
9. Kurl, S.; Laaksonen, D.E.; Jae, S.Y.; Makikallio, T.H.; Zaccardi, F.; Kauhanen, J.; Ronkainen, K.; Laukkanen, J.A. Metabolic syndrome and the risk of sudden cardiac death in middle-aged men. *Int. J. Cardiol.* **2016**, *203*, 792–797. [CrossRef]
10. Hess, P.L.; Al-Khalidi, H.R.; Friedman, D.J.; Mulder, H.; Kucharska-Newton, A.; Rosamond, W.R.; Lopes, R.D.; Gersh, B.J.; Mark, D.B.; Curtis, L.H.; et al. The Metabolic Syndrome and Risk of Sudden Cardiac Death: The Atherosclerosis Risk in Communities Study. *J. Am. Heart Assoc.* **2017**, *6*, e006103. [CrossRef]
11. Nannipieri, M.; Gonzales, C.; Baldi, S.; Posadas, R.; Williams, K.; Haffner, S.M.; Stern, M.P.; Ferrannini, E. Liver enzymes, the metabolic syndrome, and incident diabetes: The Mexico City diabetes study. *Diabetes Care* **2005**, *28*, 1757–1762. [CrossRef] [PubMed]
12. Perry, I.J.; Wannamethee, S.G.; Shaper, A.G. Prospective study of serum gamma-glutamyltransferase and risk of NIDDM. *Diabetes Care* **1998**, *21*, 732–737. [CrossRef]
13. Lee, D.S.; Evans, J.C.; Robins, S.J.; Wilson, P.W.; Albano, I.; Fox, C.S.; Wang, T.J.; Benjamin, E.J.; D'Agostino, R.B.; Vasan, R.S. Gamma glutamyl transferase and metabolic syndrome, cardiovascular disease, and mortality risk: The Framingham Heart Study. *Arterioscler. Thromb. Vasc. Biol.* **2007**, *27*, 127–133. [CrossRef] [PubMed]
14. Kawamoto, R.; Kohara, K.; Tabara, Y.; Miki, T.; Otsuka, N. Serum gamma-glutamyl transferase levels are associated with metabolic syndrome in community-dwelling individuals. *J. Atheroscler. Thromb.* **2009**, *16*, 355–362. [CrossRef] [PubMed]
15. Rantala, A.O.; Lilja, M.; Kauma, H.; Savolainen, M.J.; Reunanen, A.; Kesaniemi, Y.A. Gamma-glutamyl transpeptidase and the metabolic syndrome. *J. Intern. Med.* **2000**, *248*, 230–238. [CrossRef]
16. Kim, Y.G.; Han, K.D.; Choi, J.I.; Choi, Y.Y.; Choi, H.Y.; Boo, K.Y.; Kim, D.Y.; Lee, K.N.; Shim, J.; Kim, J.S.; et al. Non-genetic risk factors for atrial fibrillation are equally important in both young and old age: A nationwide population-based study. *Eur. J. Prev. Cardiol.* **2021**, *28*, 666–676. [CrossRef]

17. Kim, Y.G.; Han, K.D.; Kim, D.Y.; Choi, Y.Y.; Choi, H.Y.; Roh, S.Y.; Shim, J.; Kim, J.S.; Choi, J.I.; Kim, Y.H. Different Influence of Blood Pressure on New-Onset Atrial Fibrillation in Pre- and Postmenopausal Women: A Nationwide Population-Based Study. *Hypertension* **2021**, *77*, 1500–1509. [CrossRef]
18. Kim, Y.G.; Han, K.D.; Choi, J.I.; Choi, Y.Y.; Choi, H.Y.; Shim, J.; Kim, Y.H. Premature ventricular contraction is associated with increased risk of atrial fibrillation: A nationwide population-based study. *Sci. Rep.* **2021**, *11*, 1601. [CrossRef]
19. Roh, S.Y.; Choi, J.I.; Kim, M.S.; Cho, E.Y.; Kim, Y.G.; Lee, K.N.; Shim, J.; Kim, J.S.; Kim, Y.H. Incidence and etiology of sudden cardiac arrest in Koreans: A cohort from the national health insurance service database. *PLoS ONE* **2020**, *15*, e0242799. [CrossRef]
20. Kim, Y.G.; Han, K.D.; Choi, J.I.; Yung Boo, K.; Kim, D.Y.; Oh, S.K.; Lee, K.N.; Shim, J.; Kim, J.S.; Kim, Y.H. Impact of the Duration and Degree of Hypertension and Body Weight on New-Onset Atrial Fibrillation: A Nationwide Population-Based Study. *Hypertension* **2019**, *74*, e45–e51. [CrossRef]
21. Grundy, S.M.; Cleeman, J.I.; Daniels, S.R.; Donato, K.A.; Eckel, R.H.; Franklin, B.A.; Gordon, D.J.; Krauss, R.M.; Savage, P.J.; Smith, S.C., Jr.; et al. Diagnosis and management of the metabolic syndrome: An American Heart Association/National Heart, Lung, and Blood Institute Scientific Statement. *Circulation* **2005**, *112*, 2735–2752. [CrossRef] [PubMed]
22. Roh, S.-Y.; Choi, J.-I.; Park, S.H.; Kim, Y.G.; Shim, J.; Kim, J.-S.; Do Han, K.; Kim, Y.-H. The 10-year trend of out-of-hospital cardiac arrests: A Korean nationwide population-based study. *Korean Circ. J.* **2021**, *51*, 866–874. [CrossRef] [PubMed]
23. Holzer, M.; Sterz, F.; Darby, J.M.; Padosch, S.A.; Kern, K.B.; Böttiger, B.W.; Polderman, K.H.; Girbes, A.R.J.; Holzer, M.; Bernard, S.A.; et al. Mild therapeutic hypothermia to improve the neurologic outcome after cardiac arrest. *N. Engl. J. Med.* **2002**, *346*, 549–556.
24. de Vreede-Swagemakers, J.J.; Gorgels, A.P.; Dubois-Arbouw, W.I.; van Ree, J.W.; Daemen, M.J.; Houben, L.G.; Wellens, H.J. Out-of-hospital cardiac arrest in the 1990's: A population-based study in the Maastricht area on incidence, characteristics and survival. *J. Am. Coll. Cardiol.* **1997**, *30*, 1500–1505. [CrossRef]
25. Haffner, S.; Taegtmeyer, H. Epidemic obesity and the metabolic syndrome. *Circulation* **2003**, *108*, 1541–1545. [CrossRef]
26. Empana, J.P.; Duciemetiere, P.; Balkau, B.; Jouven, X. Contribution of the metabolic syndrome to sudden death risk in asymptomatic men: The Paris Prospective Study I. *Eur. Heart J.* **2007**, *28*, 1149–1154. [CrossRef]
27. Kawamoto, R.; Tabara, Y.; Kohara, K.; Miki, T.; Kusunoki, T.; Takayama, S.; Abe, M.; Katoh, T.; Ohtsuka, N. High-sensitivity C-reactive protein and gamma-glutamyl transferase levels are synergistically associated with metabolic syndrome in community-dwelling persons. *Cardiovasc. Diabetol.* **2010**, *9*, 87. [CrossRef]
28. Kang, Y.H.; Min, H.K.; Son, S.M.; Kim, I.J.; Kim, Y.K. The association of serum gamma glutamyltransferase with components of the metabolic syndrome in the Korean adults. *Diabetes Res. Clin. Pract.* **2007**, *77*, 306–313. [CrossRef]
29. Ura, N.; Saitoh, S.; Shimamoto, K. Clinical diagnosis of metabolic syndrome 1. Metabolic syndrome and insulin resistance. *Intern. Med.* **2007**, *46*, 1283–1284. [CrossRef]
30. Hotamisligil, G.S. Inflammatory pathways and insulin action. *Int. J. Obes. Relat. Metab. Disord.* **2003**, *27* (Suppl 3), S53–S55. [CrossRef]
31. Paolicchi, A.; Minotti, G.; Tonarelli, P.; Tongiani, R.; De Cesare, D.; Mezzetti, A.; Dominici, S.; Comporti, M.; Pompella, A. Gamma-glutamyl transpeptidase-dependent iron reduction and LDL oxidation–a potential mechanism in atherosclerosis. *J. Investig. Med.* **1999**, *47*, 151–160. [PubMed]
32. Kim, Y.G.; Han, K.D.; Choi, J.I.; Boo, K.Y.; Kim, D.Y.; Oh, S.K.; Lee, K.N.; Shim, J.; Kim, J.S.; Kim, Y.H. The impact of body weight and diabetes on new-onset atrial fibrillation: A nationwide population based study. *Cardiovasc. Diabetol.* **2019**, *18*, 128. [CrossRef] [PubMed]
33. Kim, Y.G.; Han, K.D.; Choi, J.I.; Boo, K.Y.; Kim, D.Y.; Lee, K.N.; Shim, J.; Kim, J.S.; Kim, Y.H. Frequent drinking is a more important risk factor for new-onset atrial fibrillation than binge drinking: A nationwide population-based study. *Europace* **2020**, *22*, 216–224. [CrossRef] [PubMed]

Article

Can Blood Ammonia Level, Prehospital Time, and Return of Spontaneous Circulation Predict Neurological Outcomes of Out-of-Hospital Cardiac Arrest Patients? A Nationwide, Retrospective Cohort Study

Tsuyoshi Nojima [1,2], Hiromichi Naito [1,*], Takafumi Obara [1], Kohei Ageta [1], Hiromasa Yakushiji [1,3], Tetsuya Yumoto [1], Noritomo Fujisaki [1] and Atsunori Nakao [1]

1. Department of Emergency, Critical Care and Disaster Medicine, Okayama University Graduate School of Medicine, Dentistry and Pharmaceutical Sciences, Okayama 700-8558, Japan; t.nojima1002@gmail.com (T.N.); dainosinn@gmail.com (T.O.); ageage1982@gmail.com (K.A.); amorihamorih1111@yahoo.co.jp (H.Y.); tyumoto@cc.okayama-u.ac.jp (T.Y.); ntfujisaki@gmail.com (N.F.); qq-nakao@okayama-u.ac.jp (A.N.)
2. Department of Primary Care and Medical Education, Okayama University Graduate School of Medicine, Dentistry and Pharmaceutical Sciences, Okayama 700-8558, Japan
3. Yakushiji Jikei Hospital, Okayama 719-1126, Japan
* Correspondence: naito-hiromichi@s.okayama-u.ac.jp; Tel.: +81-86-235-7427

Abstract: Background: This study aimed to test if blood ammonia levels at hospital arrival, considering prehospital time and the patient's condition (whether return of spontaneous circulation [ROSC] was achieved at hospital arrival), can predict neurological outcomes after out-of-hospital cardiac arrest (OHCA). Methods: This was a retrospective cohort study on data from a nationwide OHCA registry in Japan. Patients over 17 years old and whose blood ammonia levels had been recorded were included. The primary outcome was favorable neurological outcome at 30 days after OHCA. Blood ammonia levels, prehospital time, and the combination of the two were evaluated using the receiver operating characteristic curve to predict favorable outcomes. Then, cut-off blood ammonia values were determined based on whether ROSC was achieved at hospital arrival. Results: Blood ammonia levels alone were sufficient to predict favorable outcomes. The overall cut-off ammonia value for favorable outcomes was 138 μg/dL; values were different for patients with ROSC (96.5 μg/dL) and those without ROSC (156 μg/dL) at hospital arrival. Conclusions: Our results using patient data from a large OHCA registry showed that blood ammonia levels at hospital arrival can predict neurological outcomes, with different cut-off values for patients with or without ROSC at hospital arrival.

Keywords: ammonia; cardiopulmonary resuscitation; neurological outcome; biomarkers

1. Introduction

Despite improvement in managing out-of-hospital cardiac arrest (OHCA), the proportion of patients with favorable neurological outcomes after suffering OHCA remains low [1]. Identifying neurologically intact survivors at an early stage is a high priority so clinicians can better inform families who need to make decisions about patient care and avoid early withdrawal of aggressive care because of "perceived" unfavorable neurological prognoses [2]. Current guidelines recommend that neurological prognostic tests are reviewed 72 h after the onset of cardiac arrest (CA), because no single test or clinical sign is satisfactorily to predict neurological outcomes early after CA [2,3].

To determine neurological outcomes, serum biomarkers appear more objective and feasible compared with physical examinations such as pupillary reflex to light, corneal reflexes, and motor response or physiological tests including electroencephalogram (EEG) and evoked potentials [4–8]. Several studies have demonstrated that serum ammonia levels could be a useful biomarker for predicting the neurological outcomes of OHCA patients [9,10]. To the extent that liver function is preserved, an elevation of blood ammonia levels in CA patients is supposed to be attributed to suppression of the glycolytic pathway in red blood cells resulting from prolonged acidosis and hypoxia [11,12]. Theoretically, blood ammonia levels thus may be affected by prehospital time and differ significantly between patients with and those without return of spontaneous circulation (ROSC) at hospital arrival. We therefore hypothesized that blood ammonia level combined with these factors may be a better predictive indicator of favorable patient outcomes after OHCA.

Accordingly, the objectives of this study, which included 7426 OHCA cases from a nationwide registry in Japan, were to (1) evaluate whether blood ammonia levels at hospital arrival in conjugation with total prehospital time outperform blood ammonia levels alone in predicting favorable neurological outcomes after OHCA, and (2) determine cut-off blood ammonia levels to predict these outcomes, stratified by patients who either did or did not achieve ROSC at hospital arrival.

2. Materials and Methods

2.1. Study Design

This was a retrospective, observational, cohort study using data from the Japanese Association for Acute Medicine (JAAM) OHCA Registry. The Okayama University Ethics Committee approved the study (K2106-008) and waived the requirement for informed consent.

2.2. Data Collection

The JAAM OHCA Registry is a prospective, multicenter, web-based registry started in 2005. In 2021, it was expanded to 101 tertiary hospitals in Japan that provide critical and emergency care with the goal of better understanding the characteristics and treatment of OHCA patients [13]. All OHCA patients transported directly to participating facilities are registered in the database. Data collection and design of the JAAM OHCA registry have been previously described in detail [14]. Prehospital data, including time measurements (transportation date, transportation time, on-scene time, response time, total prehospital time, prehospital treatment time) for OHCA patients were collected by emergency medical services (EMS) personnel using radio-controlled watches and subsequently entered into the national registry of the Fire and Disaster Management Agency. Total prehospital time was defined as the time from EMS call to hospital arrival. Physicians at each hospital are responsible for using a form to collect and record data including each patient's baseline characteristics (age, sex, cause of CA, etc.), information on prehospital setting (witnessed collapse, bystander cardiopulmonary resuscitation [CPR]), and treatments/outcomes at hospital (initial rhythm at hospital arrival, ROSC or sustained CA at hospital arrival, blood test results on hospital arrival, outcomes in hospital, etc.). The registry does not include any information about comorbidities such as hypertension, diabetes, cardiovascular disease, chronic kidney disease, and chronic liver disease. Blood ammonia levels were obtained at hospital arrival if applicable. Cerebral performance category (CPC) scale score at 30 days was used to determine neurological outcomes. Finally, data from the JAAM OHCA registry was integrated with data from the prehospital registry of the Fire and Disaster Management Agency and in-hospital data.

2.3. The Emergency Medical Services System in Japan

The EMS system in Japan has been described in detail elsewhere [15]. Briefly, all emergency calls (via 119 in Japan) are handled by local operations centers that dispatch the nearest ambulance to the scene. Each vehicle is staffed by three or four EMS personnel, at least one of whom is highly trained and known as an emergency life-saving technician (ELST). ELSTs can perform advanced airway management including supraglottic airway placement. In addition, specially trained ELSTs are allowed to perform endotracheal intubation and adrenaline administration under real-time medical direction by physicians.

EMS personnel are obligated to resuscitate and transport OHCA patients to the hospital unless obvious signs of death are present.

2.4. Participants, Groups, and Endpoints

All patients with OHCA of cardiac and noncardiac causes treated from 1 July 2014 to 31 December 2017 in the JAAM OHCA registry were eligible for inclusion in the study. Patients over 17 years of age whose blood ammonia levels had been recorded at hospital arrival were included in the study. Patients with unknown ages were excluded.

Patients were divided into two groups based on CPC scores 30 days after OHCA; the favorable outcomes group and the poor outcomes group was comprised of patients with CPC scores of 1 or 2 and 3 through 5, respectively.

The primary outcome was favorable neurological outcome. The impact of blood ammonia levels on the primary outcome was determined using multiple logistic regression analysis. Then, prognostic performance for a favorable neurological outcome was determined using the receiver operating characteristic (ROC) curve.

The relationship between blood ammonia levels and total prehospital time was examined for favorable or poor neurological outcomes. Then, the relationship between blood ammonia levels and total prehospital time was examined separately for the ROSC group and the non-ROSC group at the time of hospital arrival. For further analysis, patients were stratified into groups for OHCA with cardiac causes and OHCA with noncardiac causes.

2.5. Statistical Analysis

Continuous variables are described using medians with interquartile ranges. Categorical variables are described using numbers and percentages. We used multiple logistic regression analysis to identify independent predictors of favorable neurological outcomes. In addition to age, sex, total prehospital time, and blood ammonia levels on arrival, clinically relevant factors and covariates based on the results of univariate analysis were used to adjust for outcomes in multivariate logistic regression. The results of logistic regression are described using odds ratios (OR) with 95% confidence intervals (CI). Prognostic performance (area under the curve; sensitivity; specificity) was examined using total prehospital time and blood ammonia level at hospital arrival, respectively. The cut-off values for favorable outcomes were examined for blood ammonia levels and transportation time using Youden's index. The association between time and blood ammonia level was determined with linear logistic regression and 95% CI. Stata version 16 (StataCorp LP, College Station, TX, USA) was used for the analysis.

3. Results
3.1. Patient Characteristics

A total of 34,754 OHCA patients were registered during the study period. After eligibility screening, 7426 patients were included. Favorable neurological outcomes were seen in 364 patients; poor neurological outcomes were seen in 7062 patients at 30 days after CA (Figure 1).

Participants' characteristics are shown in Table 1. The median age was 76 (64–84), and 4538 (61%) patients were male. Of the 7426 patients, 3181 (47%) had collapse witnessed by bystanders; bystander CPR was performed on 3202 (47%), and public automated external defibrillator (AED) was used at the scene on 149 (2.2%). Shockable rhythms, including pulseless ventricular tachycardia or ventricular fibrillation, were observed in 392 (5.3%) patients. The overall median total prehospital time was 34 (28–41) minutes, and median total prehospital times were 31 (25–39) minutes in the favorable outcomes group and 34 (28–42) minutes in the poor outcomes group. The overall median blood ammonia level at hospital arrival was 253 (125–438) μg/dL, and median blood ammonia levels were 70 (42–122) μg/dL in the favorable outcomes group and 265 (138–452) μg/dL in the poor outcomes group. ROSC on arrival was observed in 910 patients (12%).

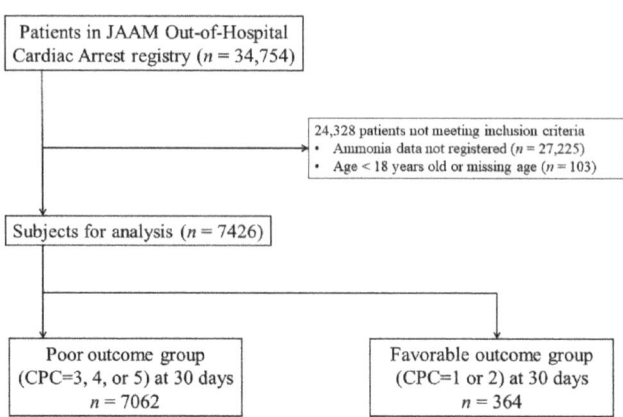

Figure 1. Flow diagram of patients analyzed. The favorable outcome group comprised patients with CPC scale scores of 1 or 2. The poor outcome group comprised patients with CPC scale sores of 3, 4, and 5. CPC: cerebral performance category, JAAM: Japanese Association for Acute Medicine.

Table 1. Patient characteristics and outcomes at 30 days.

	All Participants (n = 7426)	Favorable Outcomes (CPC 1–2) at 30 Days (n = 364)	Poor Outcomes (CPC 3–5) at 30 Days (n = 7062)	p-Value
Age (year), median (IQR)	76 (64–84)	63 (48–73)	76 (65–85)	<0.01
Male, n (%)	4538 (61%)	281 (77%)	4257 (60%)	<0.01
Total prehospital time * (min), median (IQR)	34 (28–41)	31 (25–39)	34 (28–42)	<0.01
Witnessed collapse, n (%)	3181 (43%)	259 (71%)	2922 (41%)	<0.01
Bystander CPR, n (%)	3202 (43%)	183 (50%)	3019 (43%)	<0.01
AED used by bystander, n (%)	149 (2.0%)	78 (21%)	71 (1.0%)	<0.01
Adrenaline used by EMS	2278 (31%)	35 (9.6%)	2243 (32%)	<0.01
Cardiac cause, n (%)	3719 (50%)	302 (83%)	3417 (48%)	<0.01
Initial rhythm at hospital arrival				
VF/pulseless VT, n (%)	392 (5.3%)	69 (19%)	323 (4.6%)	<0.01
PEA/asystole, n (%)	6124 (82%)	46 (13%)	6078 (86%)	<0.01
ROSC during transport, n (%)	910 (12%)	249 (68%)	661 (9.4%)	<0.01
Blood ammonia level (μg/dL), median (IQR)	253 (125–438)	70 (42–122)	265 (138–452)	<0.01
Potassium (mEq/L), median (IQR)	6.0 (4.6–7.9)	3.8 (3.4–4.2)	6.1 (4.8–8.1)	<0.01
Lactate (mg/dL), median (IQR)	118 (74–156)	64 (17–117)	119 (75–156)	<0.01
TTM, n (%)	634 (8.5%)	203 (56%)	431 (6.1%)	<0.01
Patients admitted to the hospital, n (%)	2457 (33%)	N/A	N/A	
Survival at 30 days, n (%)	738 (10%)	N/A	N/A	

Abbreviations: cardiopulmonary resuscitation (CPR); interquartile range (IQR); automated external defibrillator (AED); emergency medical services (EMS); ventricular fibrillation (VF); ventricular tachycardia (VT); pulseless electrical activity (PEA); return of spontaneous circulation (ROSC); targeted temperature management (TTM).
* Total prehospital time was defined as the time span from awareness to hospital arrival.

3.2. Impact of Blood Ammonia Level and Time on Favorable Neurological Outcomes

Multivariable logistic regression analysis for favorable neurological outcomes was performed and used blood ammonia levels and total prehospital time with other variables (age, sex, witnessed collapse, bystander CPR, AED use on scene, adrenaline use on scene, electrocardiogram on arrival, potassium and lactate levels at hospital arrival, and cardiogenic arrest) as adjustments. Lower blood ammonia levels indicated more favorable neurological outcomes (adjusted OR: 0.991, 95% CI: 0.989–0.993) and shorter total prehospital time indicated more favorable neurological outcomes (adjusted OR: 0.996, 95% CI: 0.997–0.997) (Table 2).

Table 2. Univariable and multivariable logistic regression analysis of blood ammonia level and total prehospital time for favorable neurological outcomes.

	Crude OR (95% CI)	Adjusted OR (95% CI)
Blood ammonia level at hospital arrival	0.988 (0.987–0.990)	0.995 (0.994–0.998)
Total prehospital time	0.996 (0.996–0.997)	0.993 (0.981–1.006)

Abbreviations: odds ratio (OR); confidence interval (CI). Adjustments for multivariable logistic regression: age, sex, witnessed collapse, bystander cardiopulmonary resuscitation, automated external defibrillator use on scene, adrenaline use on scene, electrocardiogram on arrival, potassium and lactate levels at hospital arrival, and cardiogenic cause.

3.3. Prognostic Performance of Blood Ammonia Levels

Figure 2 demonstrates the prognostic performance of blood ammonia levels. The areas under the ROC curve for total prehospital time and blood ammonia levels for the prediction of poor outcomes were 0.587 (95% CI: 0.551–0.622) and 0.849 (95% CI: 0.829–0.869), respectively. The cut-off values for each variable using Youden's index were as follows: total prehospital time, 31.5 min (sensitivity 0.61, specificity 0.53, positive predictive value 0.96, negative predictive value 0.07), and blood ammonia levels, 138 µg/dL (sensitivity 0.75, specificity 0.80, positive predictive value 0.99, negative predictive value 0.16, positive likelihood ratio 3.74). The area under the ROC curve for blood ammonia levels at hospital arrival in combination with total prehospital time was 0.849 (95% CI: 0.829–0.870), which was similar to the ROC curve for blood ammonia levels alone.

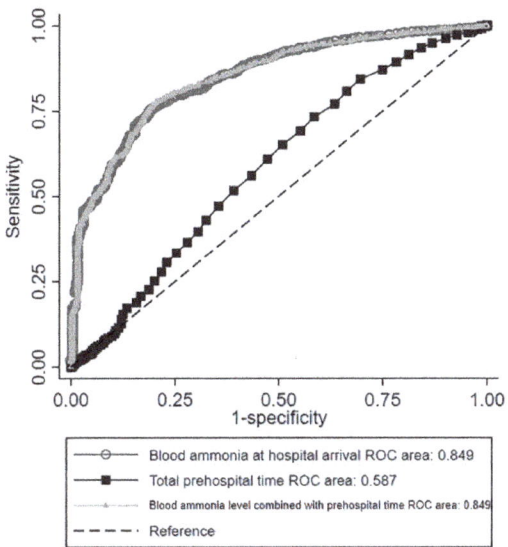

Figure 2. ROC curve for predicting poor outcomes with blood ammonia level (circle), total prehospital time (square), and blood ammonia level combined with total prehospital time (triangle). The areas under the ROC curve are shown in the box. The ROC curve of blood ammonia level at hospital arrival and of blood ammonia level combined with total prehospital time are almost identical. Abbreviations: receiver operating characteristic (ROC).

3.4. Correlation between Blood Ammonia Level and Total Prehospital Time

Figure 3 depicts the correlation between the blood ammonia levels and the duration of total prehospital time in the favorable outcomes group and the poor outcomes group. The favorable outcomes group showed a slight trend towards increase in blood ammonia levels as prehospital time increased, while a stronger correlation was noted in the poor outcomes group; blood ammonia levels were markedly increased as a result of prolonged prehospital time. The blood ammonia levels of patients in the poor outcomes group were significantly higher compared to those in the favorable outcomes group, regardless of the duration of total prehospital time.

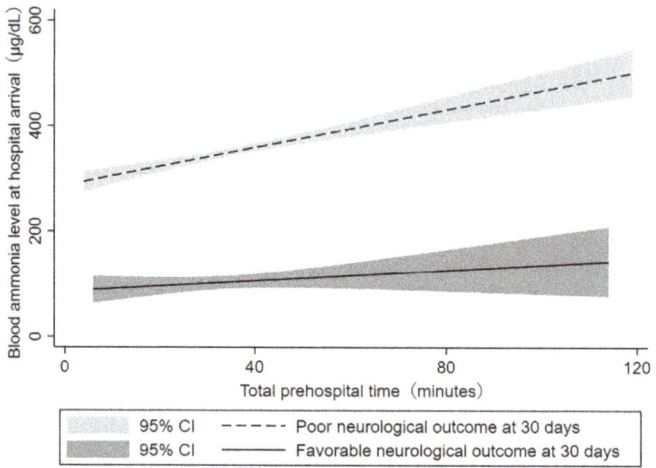

Figure 3. Relationship between blood ammonia level and total prehospital time. The blood ammonia level at hospital arrival increased with total prehospital time. The blood ammonia level in the favorable neurological outcomes group was lower than that in the poor neurological outcomes group. Abbreviations: confidence interval (CI).

To further examine the impact of blood ammonia levels on patient outcomes based on the assumption that sustained CA could lead to hyperammonemia, the patients were divided into groups for those who had achieved ROSC and those who did not achieve ROSC at hospital arrival. Table 3 shows the basic demographics of the two groups. Blood ammonia levels were significantly lower in patients with ROSC compared to those without ROSC at the time of hospital arrival (103 vs. 278 µg/dL, $p < 0.01$). The patients who had achieved ROSC had better functional outcomes compared to those who had sustained CA (27 vs. 1.8%, $p < 0.01$). In patients who had obtained ROSC at hospital arrival, the blood ammonia levels of each outcome were almost constant regardless of total prehospital time (Figure 4A). Blood ammonia levels were significantly lower in patients with favorable outcomes compared to those with poor outcomes (70 vs. 265 µg/dL, $p < 0.01$). In patients who had sustained CA at the time of hospital arrival, blood ammonia levels were positively correlated with total prehospital time for both favorable and poor outcomes (Figure 4B). Similarly, for the group that had sustained CA, blood ammonia levels were significantly lower in patients with favorable outcomes than in those with poor outcomes (149 vs. 365 µg/dL, $p < 0.01$). The blood ammonia level cut-off points for favorable outcomes in the ROSC group and the sustained CA group were 96.5 µg/dL (sensitivity 0.65, specificity 0.76), and 156 µg/dL (sensitivity 0.56, specificity 0.64), respectively.

Table 3. Patient characteristics in the ROSC group and the sustained CA group at the time of hospital arrival.

	All Participants (n = 7426)	ROSC at Time of Hospital Arrival (n = 910)	Sustained CA at Hospital Arrival (n = 6516)	p-Value
Age (year), median (IQR)	76 (64–84)	74 (62–83)	76 (64–84)	0.012
Male, n (%)	4538 (61%)	576 (63%)	3962 (61%)	0.15
Total prehospital time * (min), median (IQR)	34 (28–41)	34 (29–41)	34 (28–41)	0.08
Witnessed collapse, n (%)	3181 (43%)	526 (58%)	2655 (41%)	<0.01
Bystander CPR, n (%)	3202 (43%)	411 (45%)	2791 (43%)	<0.01
AED used by bystander, n (%)	149 (2.0%)	76 (8.4%)	73 (1.1%)	<0.01
Adrenalin used by EMS	2278 (31%)	380 (42%)	1898 (29%)	<0.01
Cardiac cause, n (%)	3719 (50%)	426 (47%)	3293 (51%)	0.035
Initial rhythm at hospital arrival				
VF/pulseless VT, n (%)	392 (5.3%)	N/A	392 (6 %)	N/A
PEA/Asystole, n (%)	6124 (82%)	N/A	6124 (94%)	N/A
ROSC during transport, n (%)	910 (12%)	910 (100%)	N/A	N/A
Blood ammonia level (µg/dL), median (IQR)	253 (125–438)	103 (54–206)	278 (148–472)	<0.01
Potassium (mEq/L), median (IQR)	6.0 (4.6–7.9)	3.9 (3.5–4.8)	6.3 (4.9–8.2)	<0.01
Lactate (mg/dL), median (IQR)	118 (74–156)	81 (38–110)	119 (75–156)	<0.01
TTM, n (%)	634 (8.5%)	246 (27%)	388 (6.0%)	<0.01
Patients admitted to the hospital, n (%)	2457 (33%)	788 (87%)	1669 (26%)	<0.01
Survival at 30 days, n (%)	738 (10%)	419 (46%)	319 (4.9%)	<0.01
Favorable neurological outcome at 30 days, n (%)	364 (4.9%)	249 (27%)	115 (1.8%)	<0.01

Abbreviations: return of spontaneous circulation (ROSC); cardiac arrest (CA); interquartile range (IQR); cardiopulmonary resuscitation (CPR); automated external defibrillator (AED); emergency medical services (EMS); ventricular fibrillation (VF); ventricular tachycardia (VT); pulseless electrical activity (PEA); targeted temperature management (TTM). * Total prehospital time was defined as the time span from awareness to hospital arrival.

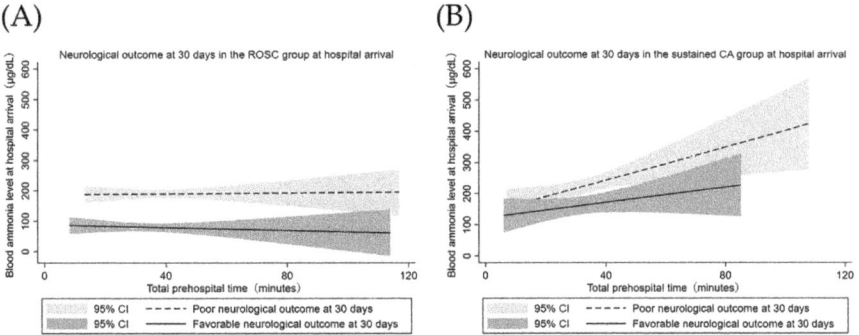

Figure 4. Relationship between blood ammonia level at hospital arrival and total prehospital time in the ROSC group (A) and the sustained CA group (B). In the ROSC patients, the blood ammonia levels of each outcome were almost constant regardless of total prehospital time. The blood ammonia level was lower in patients with favorable outcomes compared to those with poor outcomes. In the sustained CA patients, blood ammonia levels continued to increase in correlation with transportation time for both outcomes. Abbreviations: return of spontaneous circulation (ROSC); cardiopulmonary arrest (CA); confidence interval (CI).

3.5. Cardiac Causes vs. Noncardiac Causes

Further analysis was performed to determine whether there were differences between patients with OHCA from cardiac vs. those with OHCA from noncardiac causes. Patients were divided into two groups: the cardiac causes group and the noncardiac causes group. Patients' characteristics are presented in Table S1. Multivariable logistic regression analysis revealed that lower blood ammonia levels were associated with favorable neurological outcomes in both the cardiac causes group and the noncardiac causes group (Table S2). The areas under the ROC curve for the cardiac causes group and the noncardiac causes group for prediction of poor outcome were 0.856 (95% CI: 0.836–0.875) and 0.805 (95% CI: 0.757–0.853), respectively. The cut-off values for each variable using Youden's index were as follows: cardiac causes group, 138 µg/dL (sensitivity 0.76, specificity 0.82), and noncardiac causes group, 133 µg/dL (sensitivity 0.75, specificity 0.71) (Figure S1). Finally, the relationship between blood ammonia levels at hospital arrival and total prehospital time is shown for the cardiac causes and noncardiac causes groups (Figure S2). These results indicate that blood ammonia levels at hospital arrival may be a reliable predictor of neurological outcomes regardless of the cause of OHCA, whether cardiac or noncardiac. Furthermore, blood ammonia may have more precisely predicted neurological outcomes in the cardiac causes group compared with the noncardiac causes group.

4. Discussion

In this registry-based study of OHCA patients in Japan, we examined the hypothesis that blood ammonia levels at hospital arrival in conjugation with total prehospital time were superior to blood ammonia levels alone for prediction of favorable neurological outcomes at 30 days after OHCA. There may have been fewer patients with favorable neurological outcomes due to selection bias; however, blood ammonia levels alone were sufficient to identify those with favorable outcomes. The cut-off ammonia level for favorable outcomes in the overall study cohort was 138 µg/dL. This cut-off value varied depending on whether ROSC was achieved at the time of hospital arrival: it was 96.5 µg/dL for patients with ROSC at hospital arrival and 156 µg/dL for patients with sustained CA, respectively.

Given the assumption that blood ammonia levels would increase in proportion with ischemic duration, our results showed that the patients who had achieved ROSC had a lower cut-off ammonia level for favorable outcomes compared to patients with sustained CA. In a previous study, Shinozaki et al. found that blood ammonia levels at hospital admission was an independent predictor of favorable outcomes at six months after OHCA with a cut-off value of 170 µg/dL, which is a bit higher than the findings for our patients with sustained CA [16]. Similarly, other studies have revealed that blood ammonia levels below 100 µg/dL were associated with favorable outcomes at 30 days following OHCA [9,17], although these studies did not consider whether or not the patients had achieved ROSC at hospital arrival. Thus, our data suggest that blood ammonia levels should be interpreted based on additional findings, including the presence or absence of ROSC at hospital arrival.

A prior study showed that longer prehospital resuscitation time was associated with a lower chance of favorable neurological survival [18]. In contrast to this study, we observed that total prehospital time was unable to precisely predict patients with favorable outcomes. Although there is no plausible explanation for this discrepancy, the diagnostic performance of blood ammonia levels plus total prehospital time did not add any advantages in predicting favorable outcomes compared with blood ammonia levels alone. Prehospital time as a surrogate for ischemic duration was examined in only one study. Nagamine reported that blood ammonia levels were elevated in parallel with increased prehospital time; all patients in that study fully recovered without neurological sequelae unless ammonia levels exceeded 180 µg/dL [17].

Physical examinations, EEG, evoked potentials, imaging tests, and biomarkers are tools commonly used for neurological prognostication after CA. No single test among these is adequate for precise evaluation; multimodal prognostication is recommended to assess comatose patients [3]. Blood ammonia levels combined with lactate levels have previously been shown to improve prognostic performance. Additionally, it should be noted that blood ammonia levels did well at prognosticating neurological outcomes in children after CA, performing better than early EEG or computed tomography [19]. Measuring blood ammonia levels after OHCA can be useful as a multimodal method for determining neurological outcomes.

Ammonia, a component of the physiological buffer system that maintains pH homeostasis, is metabolized with the ornithine cycle, muscle, and astrocytes [19]. Serum ammonia can increase due to numerous causes. Patients with liver dysfunction cannot metabolize ammonia, leading to its accumulation. In patients with normal liver function, hyperammonemia can be due to drug toxicities and infections can be due to urease-producing bacteria, urea cycle disorders, acidosis, hyperalimentation, renal tubular acidosis, and increased muscle activity [20]. Likewise, blood ammonia levels increase in patients with CA due to both excessive ammonia production and metabolism dysfunction. CA and consequent interruption of blood flow for ammonia metabolization in tissue cause metabolic acidosis due to aerobic respiration due to oxygen deprivation and accumulation of end products such as hydrogen ions, lactate, and carbon dioxide. Respiratory and metabolic acidosis induce the release of ammonia from red blood cells, and ammonia damages the brain [21]. Furthermore, mitochondrial dysfunction associated with acidosis results in deterioration of glycolysis metabolism (the Krebs cycle) and the ornithine cycle [12]. Decreased metabolism results in persistent hyperammonemia, leading to a vicious cycle; hyperammonemia further damages the brain.

Hypoxia with CA increases blood ammonia concentration and brain cell damage associated with metabolic degradation. Based on evidence that hypoxic brain injury increases blood neuron specific enolase (NSE) concentrations [5,6,8], international guidelines recommend NSE use as part of a multimodal prognosis [8,22]. S100B is another biomarker often used for neuroprognostication in CA patients. However, the blood tests for NSE and S-100B have the disadvantage of lack of feasibility, because these tests are not always available in ordinary emergency laboratories. Ammonia is more easily measured than NSE and S-100B for prognostication in emergency centers.

The strength of this study was that it was a nationwide registry-based investigation on a larger population. Previous studies have already shown that blood ammonia levels were a strong predictor of favorable neurological outcomes [9,10,16,17]. Our study provides a confirmation on a rather large population though with a limited number of patients with favorable neurological outcomes. Further analysis was performed focusing on total prehospital time and ROSC at hospital arrival, which provided some novel insights into clinical interpretation. The cut-off ammonia levels values differed for patients with or without ROSC. Interestingly, total prehospital time did not have any impact on blood ammonia levels in patients with ROSC at hospital arrival. These findings should be considered when interpreting the ammonia levels of OHCA patients.

This study has some limitations. First, the influence of pre-existing diseases such as cardiovascular disease or chronic liver disease that potentially affect outcomes was not considered [23]. In particular, patients with underlying chronic liver disease may have had higher blood ammonia levels compared with those without underlying chronic liver disease. However, this can be almost ignored, presumably given the minority of these patients with chronic liver disease [24]. Second, there may have been a selection bias because the only patients with recorded blood ammonia levels were included in this investigation. Third, the quality of CPR during prehospital management was not considered. Fourth, the time at which blood samples were collected may have differed among the facilities, although overall they were obtained soon after hospital arrival. Fifth, there was little detailed information regarding hospital treatment. Sixth, the prehospital time was used to study this question, instead of low-flow time (from collapse to ROSC), because it was impossible to determine exact low-flow time of unwitnessed CA patients. Low-flow time may be longer than prehospital time. Finally, our findings may not be generalized outside of this population due to relatively lower numbers of patients with favorable neurological outcomes, presumably due to the specific EMS system in Japan and the age distribution of the Japanese population.

5. Conclusions

The results from our study on data from a large OHCA registry showed that blood ammonia level measured at hospital arrival can predict neurological prognosis at 30 days after OHCA, and these cut-off values were different for patients with ROSC and those without ROSC at hospital arrival. Blood ammonia levels gradually increased with increasing total prehospital time. However, the blood ammonia levels of the patients who had achieved ROSC at arrival were almost constant regardless of total prehospital time. The overall cut-off ammonia level for favorable outcomes was 138 µg/dL, and the cutoff values for patients with ROSC at hospital arrival was 96.5 µg/dL and 156 µg/dL for patients with sustained CA.

Supplementary Materials: The following supporting information can be downloaded at: https://www.mdpi.com/article/10.3390/jcm11092566/s1, Table S1: Characteristics of patients in the cardiac causes group and the noncardiac causes group at hospital arrival. Abbreviations: interquartile range (IQR); cardiopulmonary resuscitation (CPR); automated external defibrillator (AED); emergency medical services (EMS); ventricular fibrillation (VF); ventricular tachycardia (VT); pulseless electrical activity (PEA); return of spontaneous circulation (ROSC); targeted temperature management (TTM). * Total prehospital time was defined as the time span from awareness to hospital arrival. Table S2: Univariable and multivariable logistic regression analysis of blood ammonia levels for favorable neurological outcomes based upon whether the causes of cardiac arrest were cardiac or noncardiac. Abbreviations: odds ratio (OR); confidence interval (CI); cerebral performance category. Adjustments for multivariable logistic regression: age, sex, witnessed collapse, bystander cardiopulmonary resuscitation, automated external defibrillator used on the scene, adrenaline used on scene, electrocardiogram on arrival, and potassium, lactate, and ammonia levels at hospital arrival. Figure S1: ROC curve for predicting poor outcomes with blood ammonia levels in the cardiac causes group (A) and the noncardiac causes group (B). The areas under the ROC curve for the cardiac causes group and the noncardiac causes group for the prediction of poor outcomes were 0.856 (95% CI: 0.836–0.875) and 0.805 (95% CI: 0.757–0.853), respectively. Abbreviations: receiver operating characteristic (ROC). Figure S2: Relationship between blood ammonia levels and total prehospital time in the cardiac causes group (A) and the noncardiac causes group (B). Blood ammonia levels at hospital arrival increased with total prehospital time. Blood ammonia levels at hospital arrival were a reliable predictor in both the cardiac causes group and the noncardiac causes group. Blood ammonia level measured at hospital arrival more precisely predicted neurological outcomes in the cardiac causes group compared to the noncardiac causes group. Abbreviation: confidence interval (CI).

Author Contributions: Conceptualization: T.N., H.N., H.Y., K.A., T.Y., N.F. and A.N.; formal analysis: T.N., H.N. and T.O.; investigation: T.N., H.N. and T.O.; methodology: T.N., T.Y. and H.N.; writing-original draft: T.N., H.N., T.Y. and A.N; writing-review and editing: T.N., H.N., T.O., H.Y., N.F. and A.N. All authors have read and agreed to the published version of the manuscript.

Funding: This research received no external funding.

Institutional Review Board Statement: The ethics committee of Okayama University approved this study (K2106-008).

Informed Consent Statement: The ethics committee of Okayama University waived the requirement for informed consent.

Data Availability Statement: The data in this study was from the Japanese Association for Acute Medicine (JAAM) OHCA Registry database. JAAM approves the sharing of data with interested researchers.

Acknowledgments: We thank Kaoru Masuda for assistance with collecting data. We thank Christine Burr for editing the manuscript.

Conflicts of Interest: The authors declare no conflict of interest.

References

1. Geocadin, R.G.; Callaway, C.W.; Fink, E.L.; Golan, E.; Greer, D.M.; Ko, N.U.; Lang, E.; Licht, D.J.; Marino, B.S.; McNair, N.D.; et al. Standards for Studies of Neurological Prognostication in Comatose Survivors of Cardiac Arrest: A Scientific Statement From the American Heart Association. *Circulation* **2019**, *140*, e517–e542. [CrossRef] [PubMed]
2. Elmer, J.; Torres, C.; Aufderheide, T.P.; Austin, M.A.; Callaway, C.W.; Golan, E.; Herren, H.; Jasti, J.; Kudenchuk, P.J.; Scales, D.C.; et al. Association of early withdrawal of life-sustaining therapy for perceived neurological prognosis with mortality after cardiac arrest. *Resuscitation* **2016**, *102*, 127–135. [CrossRef] [PubMed]

3. Nolan, J.P.; Sandroni, C.; Bottiger, B.W.; Cariou, A.; Cronberg, T.; Friberg, H.; Genbrugge, C.; Haywood, K.; Lilja, G.; Moulaert, V.R.M.; et al. European Resuscitation Council and European Society of Intensive Care Medicine guidelines 2021: Post-resuscitation care. *Intensive Care Med.* **2021**, *47*, 369–421. [CrossRef] [PubMed]
4. Sandroni, C.; D'Arrigo, S.; Cacciola, S.; Hoedemaekers, C.W.E.; Kamps, M.J.A.; Oddo, M.; Taccone, F.S.; Di Rocco, A.; Meijer, F.J.A.; Westhall, E.; et al. Prediction of poor neurological outcome in comatose survivors of cardiac arrest: A systematic review. *Intensive Care Med.* **2020**, *46*, 1803–1851. [CrossRef] [PubMed]
5. Jakkula, P.; Skrifvars, M.B.; Pettila, V.; Hastbacka, J.; Reinikainen, M. NSE concentrations and haemolysis after cardiac arrest. *Intensive Care Med.* **2019**, *45*, 741–742. [CrossRef] [PubMed]
6. Chung-Esaki, H.M.; Mui, G.; Mlynash, M.; Eyngorn, I.; Catabay, K.; Hirsch, K.G. The neuron specific enolase (NSE) ratio offers benefits over absolute value thresholds in post-cardiac arrest coma prognosis. *J. Clin. Neurosci.* **2018**, *57*, 99–104. [CrossRef] [PubMed]
7. Sondag, L.; Ruijter, B.J.; Tjepkema-Cloostermans, M.C.; Beishuizen, A.; Bosch, F.H.; van Til, J.A.; van Putten, M.; Hofmeijer, J. Early EEG for outcome prediction of postanoxic coma: Prospective cohort study with cost-minimization analysis. *Crit. Care* **2017**, *21*, 111. [CrossRef]
8. Calderon, L.M.; Guyette, F.X.; Doshi, A.A.; Callaway, C.W.; Rittenberger, J.C. The Post Cardiac Arrest Service. Combining NSE and S100B with clinical examination findings to predict survival after resuscitation from cardiac arrest. *Resuscitation* **2014**, *85*, 1025–1029. [CrossRef]
9. SOS-KANTO 2012 Study Group. Initial Blood Ammonia Level Is a Useful Prognostication Tool in Out-of-Hospital Cardiac Arrest-Multicenter Prospective Study (SOS-KANTO 2012 Study). *Circ. J.* **2017**, *81*, 1839–1845. [CrossRef]
10. Lin, C.H.; Chi, C.H.; Wu, S.Y.; Hsu, H.C.; Chang, Y.H.; Huang, Y.Y.; Chang, C.J.; Hong, M.Y.; Chan, T.Y.; Shih, H.I. Prognostic values of blood ammonia and partial pressure of ammonia on hospital arrival in out-of-hospital cardiac arrests. *Am. J. Emerg. Med.* **2013**, *31*, 8–15. [CrossRef]
11. Yang, D.; Ryoo, E.; Kim, H.J. Combination of Early EEG, Brain CT, and Ammonia Level Is Useful to Predict Neurologic Outcome in Children Resuscitated From Cardiac Arrest. *Front. Pediatrics* **2019**, *7*, 223. [CrossRef] [PubMed]
12. Khacho, M.; Tarabay, M.; Patten, D.; Khacho, P.; MacLaurin, J.G.; Guadagno, J.; Bergeron, R.; Cregan, S.P.; Harper, M.E.; Park, D.S.; et al. Acidosis overrides oxygen deprivation to maintain mitochondrial function and cell survival. *Nat. Commun.* **2014**, *5*, 3550. [CrossRef] [PubMed]
13. JAAM OHCA Registry. Available online: http://www.jaamohca-web.com (accessed on 14 September 2011).
14. Irisawa, T.; Matsuyama, T.; Iwami, T.; Yamada, T.; Hayakawa, K.; Yoshiya, K.; Noguchi, K.; Nishimura, T.; Uejima, T.; Yagi, Y.; et al. The effect of different target temperatures in targeted temperature management on neurologically favorable outcome after out-of-hospital cardiac arrest: A nationwide multicenter observational study in Japan (the JAAM-OHCA registry). *Resuscitation* **2018**, *133*, 82–87. [CrossRef]
15. Naito, H.; Yumoto, T.; Yorifuji, T.; Tahara, Y.; Yonemoto, N.; Nonogi, H.; Nagao, K.; Ikeda, T.; Sato, N.; Tsutsui, H. Improved outcomes for out-of-hospital cardiac arrest patients treated by emergency life-saving technicians compared with basic emergency medical technicians: A JCS-ReSS study report. *Resuscitation* **2020**, *153*, 251–257. [CrossRef] [PubMed]
16. Shinozaki, K.; Oda, S.; Sadahiro, T.; Nakamura, M.; Hirayama, Y.; Watanabe, E.; Tateishi, Y.; Nakanishi, K.; Kitamura, N.; Sato, Y.; et al. Blood ammonia and lactate levels on hospital arrival as a predictive biomarker in patients with out-of-hospital cardiac arrest. *Resuscitation* **2011**, *82*, 404–409. [CrossRef]
17. Nagamine, K. Does Blood Ammonia Level at Time of Initial Treatment Predict the Outcome of Patients in Cardiopulmonary Arrest on Arrival? *Nihon Kyukyu Igakukai Zasshi* **2005**, *16*, 283–288. [CrossRef]
18. Nagao, K.; Nonogi, H.; Yonemoto, N.; Gaieski, D.F.; Ito, N.; Takayama, M.; Shirai, S.; Furuya, S.; Tani, S.; Kimura, T.; et al. Duration of Prehospital Resuscitation Efforts After Out-of-Hospital Cardiac Arrest. *Circulation* **2016**, *133*, 1386–1396. [CrossRef]
19. Cooper, A.J.; Plum, F. Biochemistry and physiology of brain ammonia. *Physiol. Rev.* **1987**, *67*, 440–519. [CrossRef]
20. Dasarathy, S.; Mookerjee, R.P.; Rackayova, V.; Rangroo Thrane, V.; Vairappan, B.; Ott, P.; Rose, C.F. Ammonia toxicity: From head to toe? *Metab. Brain Dis.* **2017**, *32*, 529–538. [CrossRef]
21. Braissant, O.; McLin, V.A.; Cudalbu, C. Ammonia toxicity to the brain. *J. Inherit. Metab. Dis.* **2013**, *36*, 595–612. [CrossRef]
22. Wihersaari, L.; Tiainen, M.; Skrifvars, M.B.; Bendel, S.; Kaukonen, K.M.; Vaahersalo, J.; Romppanen, J.; Pettila, V.; Reinikainen, M. Usefulness of neuron specific enolase in prognostication after cardiac arrest: Impact of age and time to ROSC. *Resuscitation* **2019**, *139*, 214–221. [CrossRef] [PubMed]
23. Hirlekar, G.; Jonsson, M.; Karlsson, T.; Hollenberg, J.; Albertsson, P.; Herlitz, J. Comorbidity and survival in out-of-hospital cardiac arrest. *Resuscitation* **2018**, *133*, 118–123. [CrossRef] [PubMed]
24. Roedl, K.; Wallmüller, C.; Drolz, A.; Horvatits, T.; Rutter, K.; Spiel, A.; Ortbauer, J.; Stratil, P.; Hubner, P.; Weiser, C.; et al. Outcome of in- and out-of-hospital cardiac arrest survivors with liver cirrhosis. *Ann. Intensive Care* **2017**, *7*, 103. [CrossRef] [PubMed]

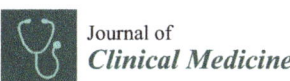

Article

The Use of Levosimendan after Out-of-Hospital Cardiac Arrest and Its Association with Outcome—An Observational Study

Susanne Rysz [1,2], Malin Jonsson Fagerlund [1,3], Johan Lundberg [4,5], Mattias Ringh [6], Jacob Hollenberg [6], Marcus Lindgren [7], Martin Jonsson [6], Therese Djärv [2,8] and Per Nordberg [1,6,*]

1. Function Perioperative Medicine and Intensive Care, Karolinska University Hospital, 171 76 Stockholm, Sweden; susanne.rysz@regionstockholm.se (S.R.); malin.jonsson-fagerlund@regionstockholm.se (M.J.F.)
2. Department of Medicine Solna, Karolinska Institutet, 171 77 Stockholm, Sweden; therese.djarv@ki.se
3. Department of Physiology and Pharmacology, Karolinska Institutet, 171 77 Stockholm, Sweden
4. Department of Clinical Neuroscience, Karolinska Institutet, 171 77 Stockholm, Sweden; johan.lundberg@regionstockholm.se
5. Department of Neuroradiology, Karolinska University Hospital, 171 76 Stockholm, Sweden
6. Center for Resuscitation Science, Department of Clinical Science and Education, Karolinska Institutet Södersjukhuset, 118 83 Stockholm, Sweden; mattias.ringh@ki.se (M.R.); jacob.hollenberg@ki.se (J.H.); martin.k.jonsson@regionstockholm.se (M.J.)
7. Department of Medicine, Piteå Hospital, 941 50 Piteå, Sweden; marcus@tegenaria.com
8. Function Emergency Medicine, Karolinska University Hospital, 171 76 Stockholm, Sweden
* Correspondence: per.nordberg@ki.se

Citation: Rysz, S.; Fagerlund, M.J.; Lundberg, J.; Ringh, M.; Hollenberg, J.; Lindgren, M.; Jonsson, M.; Djärv, T.; Nordberg, P. The Use of Levosimendan after Out-of-Hospital Cardiac Arrest and Its Association with Outcome—An Observational Study. J. Clin. Med. 2022, 11, 2621. https://doi.org/10.3390/jcm11092621

Academic Editors: Michael Behnes and Tobias Schupp

Received: 30 March 2022
Accepted: 4 May 2022
Published: 6 May 2022

Publisher's Note: MDPI stays neutral with regard to jurisdictional claims in published maps and institutional affiliations.

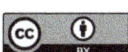

Copyright: © 2022 by the authors. Licensee MDPI, Basel, Switzerland. This article is an open access article distributed under the terms and conditions of the Creative Commons Attribution (CC BY) license (https://creativecommons.org/licenses/by/4.0/).

Abstract: Background: Levosimendan improves resuscitation rates and cardiac performance in animal cardiac arrest models. The aim of this study was to describe the use of levosimendan in out-of-hospital cardiac arrest (OHCA) patients and its association with outcome. Methods: A retrospective observational study of OHCA patients admitted to six intensive care units in Stockholm, Sweden, between 2010 and 2016. Patients treated with levosimendan within 24 h from admission were compared with those not treated with levosimendan. Propensity score matching and multivariable logistic regression analysis were used to assess the association between levosimendan treatment and 30-day mortality Results: Levosimendan treatment was initiated in 94/940 (10%) patients within 24 h. The proportion of men (81%, vs. 67%, $p = 0.007$), initial shockable rhythm (66% vs. 37%, $p < 0.001$), acute myocardial infarction, AMI (47% vs. 24%, $p < 0.001$) and need for vasoactive support (98% vs. 61%, $p < 0.001$) were higher among patients treated with levosimendan. After adjustment for age, sex, bystander cardiopulmonary resuscitation, witnessed status, initial rhythm and AMI, the odds ratio (OR) for 30-day mortality in the levosimendan group compared to the no-levosimendan group was 0.94 (95% Confidence interval [CI], 0.56–1.57, $p = 0.82$). Similar results were seen when using a propensity score analysis comparing patients with circulatory shock. Conclusions: In this observational study of OHCA patients, levosimendan was used in a limited patient group, most often in those with initial shockable rhythms, acute myocardial infarction and with a high need for vasopressors. In this limited patient cohort, levosimendan treatment was not associated with 30-day mortality. However, a better matching of patient factors and indications for use is required to derive conclusions on associations with outcome.

Keywords: cardiac arrest; intensive care; levosimendan; inotropy

1. Introduction

Out-of-hospital cardiac arrest (OHCA) affects more than 300,000 people annually in Europe, with a mortality rate of approximately 90% [1]. However, the systematic and broad introduction of basic and advanced cardiopulmonary life support in combination with a more standardised form of post-resuscitation care over the last decades has improved its prognosis [2–4]. To further increase survival and improved cardiac and neurologic function following OHCA, an exploration of pharmacological interventions beyond adrenaline and amiodarone is warranted [5,6].

Levosimendan is an inotropic substance used in acute severe heart failure (HF). Besides the inotropic effect due to calcium sensitization, levosimendan's pharmacological mechanisms also include vessel wall smooth muscle relaxation, and cell protection by activating ATP-sensitive potassium channels (K_{ATP}-channels) [7]. The lusitropic effect of levosimendan with reduced ventricular filling pressure and improved cardiac performance could add further potential advantages following OHCA, especially when considering that stunning and cardiogenic shock are common findings together with both systolic and diastolic dysfunction in cardiac-arrest patients [8–11]. Thus, levosimendan is one of several nonadrenergic vasoactive and inotropic agents that may be used to limit the reduced response to adrenergic agonists after prolonged stimulation, such as in cases of refractory circulatory shock [12].

Using an animal model, we have shown that these pharmacological effects might be beneficial when levosimendan is administered during resuscitation and in the post-resuscitation period following cardiac arrest [13]. Experimental studies with levosimendan in both ischemic and non-ischemic cardiac arrest models have shown promising results in terms of resuscitation rates, hemodynamic performance and survival [14–17]. However, in clinical practice, the use of levosimendan has not been studied properly in the context of circulatory shock following a cardiac arrest. There may be several reasons for this, including its vasodilating properties in patients in severe shock and its long half-life time. This may explain the limited data available on levosimendan use in OHCA patients [18]. The aim of this observational study was to describe the use of levosimendan in out-of-hospital cardiac arrest (OHCA) patients and its association with outcome.

2. Methods

2.1. Study Design and Ethics

We performed a retrospective observational study by extracting data from three different national registers (Swedish Registry for Cardiopulmonary Resuscitation (SRCR), Centricity critical care (CCC), and SWEDEHEART). The study was approved by Stockholm regional ethics committee (id: 2016/873-31/2) and was conducted according to the Helsinki declaration.

2.2. Study Population and Sub-Groups

Adult OHCA patients admitted to any of the six intensive care units (ICUs) in three tertiary hospitals in Stockholm, Sweden, and recorded in the Swedish register for cardiopulmonary resuscitation (SRCR) and the Swedeheart register between 2010–2016 were eligible for study inclusion. Patients receiving levosimendan >24 h from ICU admission were excluded.

A sub-group classification was further performed regarding initial rhythm (shockable versus non-shockable) and time to starting treatment with levosimendan from ICU admission (0–6 h, 6–12 h and 12–24 h).

2.3. Data Sources

2.3.1. The Swedish Register for Cardiopulmonary Resuscitation (SRCR)

The SRCR includes all Emergency Medical Service (EMS) organisations in Sweden and includes the vast majority of OHCA cases in Sweden in whom cardiopulmonary resuscitation (CPR) was attempted [19]. It is a national quality register administered by the National Board of Health and Welfare and has been previously described in detail [20]. The EMSs report data in accordance with Utstein guidelines [21]. The register predominantly contains pre-hospital variables and data on 30-day survival [22].

2.3.2. Centricity Critical Care (CCC)

Centricity Critical Care CCC (GE Healthcare) is a patient data system used in ICUs in Stockholm to collate vital parameters, blood gas analysis, administered medicines and fluids, and data from ventilators and other apparatus. The system is linked with a patient note system which contains administrative data and laboratory results. The collected information includes diagnosis and intervention codes and ICU-outcome.

2.3.3. The SWEDEHEART Register

The SWEDEHEART register components include SCAAR (Swedish Coronary Angiography and Angioplasty Register) and RIKS-HIA (Register of Information and Knowledge about Swedish Heart Intensive Care Admission). SCAAR contains information on patients from hospitals performing Coronary angiography and percutaneous coronary intervention in Sweden. Coronary angiographic data are collected in a predefined manner according to data registration standards for clinical practice.

2.4. Exposure and Outcome

The independent exposure variable was levosimendan treatment initiated within 24 h from ICU admission in OHCA patients. The outcome measure was 30-day mortality.

2.5. Statistical Analysis

Data are presented as the total number of patients and proportion (%) in each group. Differences between groups, including outcome, were assessed by using the Chi-square test for categorical data and Wilcoxon rank sum test for continuous data. The results were regarded as significant if these tests yielded a p-value of equal to or less than 0.05. Logistic regression was used to determine the association between levosimendan treatment and 30-day mortality. The following variables were included in the multivariable analysis: age (years), gender, bystander-CPR (yes/no), witnessed event (yes/no), acute myocardial infarction (yes/no) and initial rhythm (shockable versus non-shockable rhythm). The associations are presented as an odds ratio (OR) with 95% confident interval (CI). In addition, to assess outcome propensity, score matching was conducted using 1:1 matching (age, sex, witnessed arrest, shockable rhythm, myocardial infarction, EMS response time and bystander CPR rate) and nearest neighbor with a caliper width of 0,1 to assess outcome. All analyses were performed using Stata SE Stata SE (14.2 StataCorp LLC, College Station, TX, USA).

3. Results

Among 1015 OHCA admitted to the ICU between 10 January 2010 and 31 December 2016, a total of 940 patients were included in the study. Overall, 94 (10%) patients received levosimendan <24 h from admission, and 846 (90%) did not receive any levosimendan (Figure 1).

3.1. Patient Characteristics and Treatment in All Patients

Baseline demographic and resuscitation characteristics are shown in Table 1. In the levosimendan group there were more men compared to the group not treated with levosimendan (81% vs. 67%, $p = 0.007$) (Table 1). There were no differences between the groups regarding age. The proportions of patients with shockable rhythm (66% vs. 37%, $p < 0.001$), acute myocardial infarction (AMI) (47% vs. 24%, $p < 0.001$) and circulatory shock with the need for vasoactive support, e.g., Noradrenaline (98% vs. 61%, $p < 0.001$) were higher in the levosimendan group (Tables 1 and 2). The proportion of ST-elevation myocardial infarction (STEMI) among those with MI was higher in the levosimendan group (75% vs. 52%, $p = 0.005$) and percutaneous coronary intervention was higher in the levosimendan group (39% vs. 13%, $p < 0.001$) (Table 1). The median time to the initiation of levosimendan treatment was 6.1 h (IQR 2.4–10.1 h) with a median dose of 11.66 mg (IQR

10.66–13.40). The median length of stay in ICU was longer for the levosimendan group, with four vs. two days (IQR 2–7 vs. 1–4, $p < 0.001$) (Table 2).

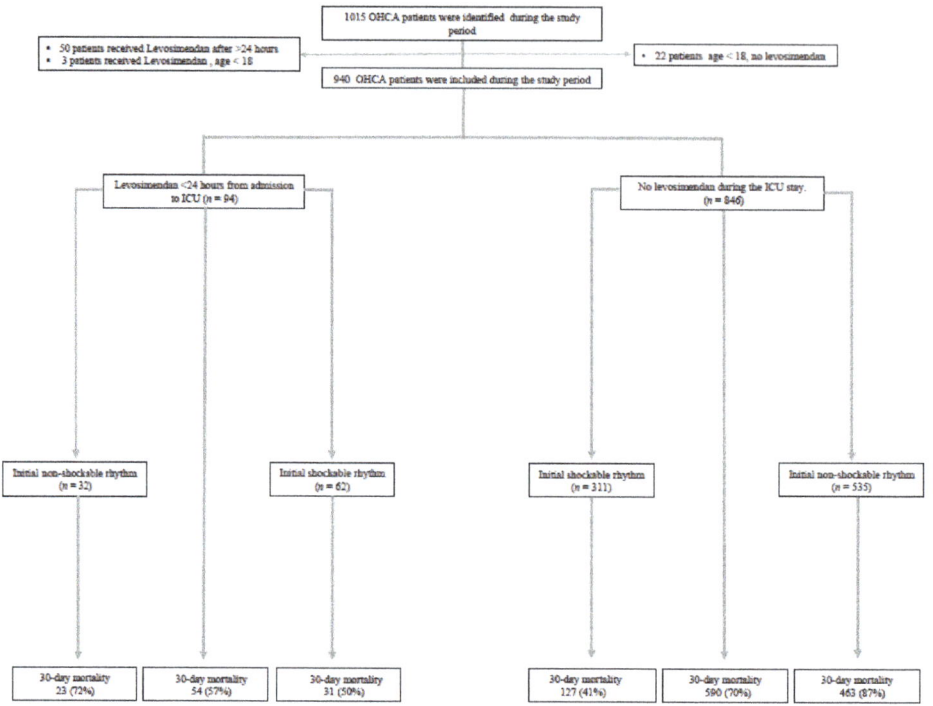

Figure 1. The CONSORT Flow Diagram of out-of hospital cardiac arrest patients admitted to the ICU in Stockholm, Sweden, 2010–2016. Abbreviations: OHCA = out-of-hospital-cardiac arrest; ICU = intensive care unit.

Table 1. Baseline characteristics in out-of-hospital-cardiac arrest patients admitted to the intensive care unit in Stockholm, Sweden, 2010–2016.

Characteristics	Levosimendan < 24 h (n = 94)	No Levosimendan (n = 846)	p-Value
Sex, n = (%)			
Male	76 (81)	568 (67)	0.007
Age, year			
Median, (IQR)	66 (60–74)	67 (56–77)	1.00
Acute myocardial ischemia, n = (%)			
Myocardial infarction, any	44 (47)	199 (24)	<0.001
STEMI	33 (75)	103 (52)	0.005
CPR-characteristics, n = (%)			
Shockable rhythm	62 (66)	311 (37)	<0.001
Witnessed event *	71/90 (79)	574/795 (72)	0.18
Bystander CPR *	53/90 (59)	364/792 (46)	0.02
Respons-time, minutes median (IQR) *	9 (7–14.5)	9 (7–13)	0.89
Coronary angiography with PCI	37 (39)	112 (13)	<0.001

Table 1. *Cont.*

Characteristics	Levosimendan < 24 h (n = 94)	No Levosimendan (n = 846)	p-Value
Patients with initial shockable rhythm			
Characteristics	Levosimendan < 24 h (n = 62)	No Levosimendan (n = 311)	
Sex, n = (%)			
Male	50 (81)	247 (79)	0.83
Age, year	12 (19)	64 (21)	
Median, (IQR)	66 (61–73)	66 (56–76)	0.68
Acute myocardial ischemia, n = (%)			
Acute myocardial infarction	38 (61)	132 (42)	0.007
STEMI	27 (71)	81 (61)	0.27
CPR-characteristics			
Witnessed event *	48/59 (81)	244/294 (83)	0.76
Bystander-CPR *	42/59 (71)	181/292 (62)	0.18
Respons-time, minutes median (IQR) *	10 (7–16)	9 (6–12)	0.24
Coronary angiography with PCI	32 (52)	90 (29)	0.001

Data are presented as median (IQR) for continuous measures, and n (%) for categorical measures. Abbreviations: STEMI = ST-elevation myocardial infarction; CPR = cardiopulmonary resuscitation; PCI = percutaneous coronary intervention. * missing values. In the variables with missing values we present nominator-denominator.

Table 2. Interventions and outcomes in out-of-hospital-cardiac arrest patients admitted to the intensive care unit in Stockholm, Sweden, 2010–2016.

Characteristics	Levosimendan < 24 h (n = 94)	No Levosimendan (n = 846)	p-Value
ICU-interventions and outcome			
Vasoactive/inotropic support, n= (%)			
Noradrenaline	92 (98)	515 (61)	<0.001
Adrenaline	14 (15)	55 (6)	0.003
Amiodarone	15 (16)	40 (5)	<0.001
Milrinone	14 (15)	6 (1)	<0.001
Dobutamine	18 (19)	65 (8)	<0.001
Arginine vasopressin	1 (1)	8 (1)	0.91
Cardiogenic shock *	13/58 (22)	52/326 (16)	0.23
TTM *	45/71 (63)	237/629 (38)	<0.001
ICU stay, days, median (IQR) *	4 (2–6)	2 (1–4)	<0.001
Mortality, 30-days, n = (%)	54 (57)	590 (70)	0.02
Patients with initial shockable rhythm			
Characteristics	Levosimendan < 24 h (n = 62)	No Levosimendan (n = 311)	
ICU-interventions and outcome			
Vasoactive/inptropic support, n = (%)			
Noradrenaline	62 (100)	222 (71)	<0.001
Adrenaline	8 (13)	10 (3)	0.001
Cordarone	9 (14)	25 (8)	0.11

Table 2. Cont.

Characteristics	Levosimendan < 24 h (n = 94)	No Levosimendan (n = 846)	p-Value
Milrinone	9 (14)	4 (1)	<0.001
Dobutamine	15 (24)	24 (8)	<0.001
Arginine vasopressin	1 (1,7)	0	0.03
Cardiogenic shock *	11/48 (23)	29/208 (14)	0.12
TTM *	35/49 (71)	163/258 (63)	0.27
ICU-stay days, median (IQR)	5 (3–6)	3 (1–6)	0.02
Mortality, 30-days, n = (%)	31 (50)	184 (59)	0.18

Data are presented as median (IQR) for continuous measures, and n (%) for categorical measures. Abbreviations: ICU = intensive care unit; TTM = targeted temperature management. * missing values. In the variables with missing values we present nominator-denominator.

3.2. Outcome in All Patients

The 30-day mortality rate was 57% (n = 54) in the group treated with levosimendan versus 70% (n = 590) in the group not treated with levosimendan (Table 2). The unadjusted OR for 30-day mortality was 0.59 (95% CI, 0.38–0.90, $p = 0.02$). When adjusted for age (year), sex, bystander-CPR (yes/no), witnessed event (yes/no), myocardial infarction (yes/no) and initial rhythm (shockable/non-shockable), the OR for 30-day mortality in the levosimendan group was 0.94 (95% CI, 0.56–1.57, $p = 0.82$) (Table 3 and Supplementary Table S1a).

Table 3. Multivariable regression analyses showing the association with Levosimendan treatment and 30-day mortality in out-of-hospital-cardiac arrest patients admitted to ICU in Stockholm, Sweden 2010–2016. All analyses were adjusted for age, sex bystander-CPR, witnessed event, myocardial infarction and initial rhythm.

Variable	Odds Ratio (95% CI)	p-Value
Levosimendan < 24 h	0.94 (0.56–1.57)	0.82
Levosimendan < 24 h in patients with shockable rhythm	1.35 (0.75–2.43)	0.32
Levosimendan start 0–6 h	0.43 (0.21–0.90)	0.03
Levosimendan start 6–12 h	2.89 (1.14–7.32)	0.03
Levosimendan start 12–24 h	1.06 (0.34–3.32)	0.916

Abbreviations: OHCA; out-of-hospital-cardiac arrest, ICU = intensive care unit; CPR = cardiopulmonary resuscitation; CI = confidence interval.

In the propensity score analysis, we studied patients with circulatory shock defined as patients needing noradrenaline. In this cohort, there was no association between treatment with Levosimendan and 30-day mortality, with 60% of patients in the control group requiring noradrenaline versus 59% of the patients treated with Levosimendan, $p = 1.0$ (Supplementary Table S2a,b).

3.3. Patient Characteristics and Treatment in Patients with Initial Shockable Rhythm

In the subgroup of patients with initial shockable rhythm (n = 373), 17% (n = 62) received levosimendan < 24 h and 83% (n = 311) did not (Table 1). There were no differences in baseline characteristics between the groups (Table 1). The proportion with MI (61% vs. 42%, $p < 0.007$) and the need for vasoactive support (100% vs. 71%, $p < 0.001$) were higher in the levosimendan group (Table 2). The proportion of STEMI among those with MI did not differ between the groups (71% vs. 61%, $p = 0.27$) (Table 1). The median time to the initiation of levosimendan treatment was 3.9 h (IQR 1.9–7.9). The ICU length of stay was longer for the levosimendan group, with a median time of five vs. three days (IQR 3–6 vs. 1–6, $p < 0.015$) (Table 2).

3.4. Outcome in Patients with Initial Shockable Rhythm

The 30-day mortality rate in this subgroup population of patients with initial shockable rhythm, was 50% (n = 31) in the levosimendan group vs. 41% (n = 127) in the group not treated with levosimendan (Table 2). The unadjusted OR 30-day mortality in the levosimendan group was 1.45 (95% CI, 0.84–2.50, p = 0.18) and the adjusted OR for 30-day mortality in the levosimendan group was 1.35 (95% CI, 0.75–2.43, p = 0.32), (Table 3, Supplementary Table S1b).

3.5. Exploratory Analyses

In an exploratory analysis of time to starting treatment with levosimendan, (0–6 h, 6–12 h and 12–24 h), the adjusted OR for 30-day mortality was 0.43 (95% CI, 0.21–0.89, p = 0.025) when levosimendan treatment was started 0–6 h from ICU admission compared to if treatment was started at a later stage (Table 3). Baseline demographic and resuscitation characteristics as well as ICU-interventions and outcome for these subgroups are shown in Supplementary Table S3a,b.

4. Discussion

We conducted a registry-based observational study with the aim of describing the usage and effects of levosimendan within 24 h from ICU-admission in OHCA patients. One of our main findings was that only 10% of the OHCA population received inotropic support with levosimendan in the first 24 h after ICU admission. In the population treated with levosimendan, we see primarily men, patients with an initial shockable rhythm and acute myocardial infarction. Further, we observed an association with a higher need for vasopressor agents and additional inotropic support in the group of patients treated with levosimendan. The outcome analyses must be regarded as exploratory due to the low number of patients treated with levosimendan and the limitations in adjusting for disease severity (e.g., severity of cardiogenic shock) and multiorgan failure. In the adjusted outcome analysis, no differences in 30-day mortality between the groups were observed. Similar findings were seen in the propensity score matching analysis where we selected patients with circulatory shock requiring noradrenaline. Within the group who received levosimendan, we could identify that initiating treatment with levosimendan within the first 6 h after ICU-admission was associated with improved 30-day survival compared to when initiating treatment at a later stage. However, when interpreting these findings, it is important to acknowledge that a better matching on disease severity, indication for use and other confounders that cannot be identified in this register data needs to be performed to derive any conclusions for outcome from this dataset.

In this study, the patients receiving Levosimendan most often had an underlying cardiac etiology with initial shockable rhythm and a high proportion of acute myocardial ischemia. Several of the mechanisms of action of levosimendan may mitigate the ischemic-reperfusion injuries that may ensue after these cardiac arrests. There are multiple interacting processes that contribute to the reversible deterioration of cardiac function after a cardiac arrest, leading to acute cardiac dysfunction superimposed on underlying structural heart disease. Ischemic reperfusion, catecholamines and cytokines, all constitute a threat to normal cardiovascular function. In addition to levosimendan as the main indication as an inodilator in acute severe HF, the activation of mitochondrial K_{ATP}-channels may be clinically advantageous after successful CPR. The activation of these channels potentially conveys a vital role in cardioprotection [23]. In addition, in cardiac surgery patients with acute kidney injury, levosimendan has been shown to improve renal blood flow via renal vasodilation, but with no or little effect on glomerular filtration rates [24]. The pre- and postconditioning properties of levosimendan have been investigated in experimental ischemia-reperfusion models indicating cardioprotective effects of the drug with a reduced infarction size and the recovery of myocardium at risk [25,26]. The effects seem to be linked to the combination of an improved hemodynamic performance and the activation of mitochondrial K$_{ATP}$-channels in myocytes. In addition, these effects have been observed in other cell types as well (i.e., brain, liver and kidneys) [27,28]. Thus, the different mechanisms of action compared to other inotropic agents may have important clinical implications. In particular, in patients with acute HF or in patients with pre-existing severe ventricular impairment undergoing planned myocardial stress, the administration of levosimendan may potentially be used to bridge the patient through the critical phase [29].

In the present cohort, we observed that patients, after the successful resuscitation of mostly ischemic-ventricular fibrillation cardiac arrest, were more frequently treated with levosimendan. Since shockable rhythms are associated with an improved outcome compared to other CA rhythms, these patients may be a specific group for whom full measures are taken more frequently. Interestingly, for the patients treated with levosimendan, first-hand inotropic treatment options were more often conventionally used inotropic drugs (i.e., dobutamine, adrenaline), usually used in combination with one or more vasopressors with levosimendan being a later inotropic alternative. The vasodilating property of levosimendan, with the potential to aggravate an already existing hypotension in situations with compromised hemodynamic functions, may be one reason for the delayed or lack of levosimendan use observed in this study. However, the use of vasodilation in cardiac arrest has been investigated previously. Yannopoulos et al. investigated sodium nitroprusside intra-arrest in a porcine model of ischemic cardiac arrest. In their study, sodium nitroprusside was associated with improved ROSC as well as short term survival [30]. Recently, in a blinded randomized placebo-controlled study in swine investigating the effects of the early administration (intra-arrest) of levosimendan vs. placebo on survival in an ischemic cardiac arrest model, we demonstrated that there was an increased survival of the animals treated with levosimendan [13]. Interestingly, there was a less pressing need for both inotropic and vasopressor support in the animals treated with levosimendan despite a tendency towards more pronounced vasodilatation in the same group.

The literature is sparse regarding circulatory targets and the timing of vasoactive support after cardiac arrest. However, persistent vasoactive support requirements lasting more than 24 h after ROSC due to non-receding myocardial dysfunction and vasoplegia are associated with poor outcome [31]. Our exploratory finding of an association between early levosimendan initiation (<6 h from ICU admission) and improved survival warrants further investigation. One possible explanation might be a reduced need for catecholaminergic inotropic support since catecholamine in high doses has been described to worsen myocardial function [31]. In this context, with acute and severe HF subsequent to an OHCA, levosimendan, administrated at an early stage during decompensation, may improve hemodynamic and cardiac recovery, thus preparing a patient for the administration of beta blockers, mineralocorticoid receptor antagonists, SGLT2 inhibitors and angiotensin-converting enzyme inhibitor/angiotensin receptor-neprilysin inhibitors [32].

This is in line with several animal studies demonstrating an overall beneficial effect of the early administration of levosimendan in experimental cardiac arrest. In these studies, levosimendan treatment was initiated either intra-arrest or near the arrest time [14–17]. These studies indicate promising hemodynamic and organ-protective effects intra-arrest as well as in the following post-resuscitation period. However, in the clinical setting, there are only a few case reports where the intra-arrest administration of levosimendan in refractory cardiac arrest has been described [33–36]. It is also worth mentioning that only in the last year, several experimental studies examining the effects of levosimendan after cardiac arrest or in I/R-arrest have been conducted, which may encourage future clinical trials on the topic.

There has been a debate regarding the potential pro-arrhythmic properties of levosimendan but without a clear resolution. In this study, the initiation of anti-arrhythmic treatment (i.e., amiodarone) did not differ in frequency before or after the initiation of levosimendan (data not shown).

Finally, we could not observe any differences in 30-day mortality between patients treated with levosimendan within 24 h after an OHCA compared to those who did not. Even though the present study may be limited by, as discussed previously, a high risk of "confounding by indication" for both groups, it may indicate that levosimendan treatment after OHCA could be an early alternative for hemodynamic support not associated with an increased risk of death, not even in situations of severe compromised hemodynamics. Further prospective studies are needed to determine the timing and effects of levosimendan on cardiac performance and the outcome in OHCA-patients.

5. Limitations

There are several limitations to this study. Missing data present a hazard for retrospective studies which implies that data may be scarce in variables that are important when matching groups, such as cardiogenic shock, multi organ failure and the severity of these two conditions. Comorbidities and demographic information were not included in this study, nor were data of neurological outcome or echocardiography assessment. The observational design precludes any causal association and might introduce the risk of selection bias and confounding by indication. Further, the different ICUs within this study may use different post-arrest management algorithms, which we have not included in the analysis since post-arrest algorithms are overlapping and hard to describe succinctly as a variable in regression analysis.

6. Conclusions

In this observational study of OHCA patients, levosimendan was used in a limited patient group, mostly in those with initial shockable rhythms, acute myocardial infarction and with a high need for vasopressors. In this limited patient cohort, levosimendan treatment was not associated with 30-day mortality. However, a better matching of patient factors and indications for use needs to be performed to derive conclusions on associations with outcome. Further prospective studies are needed to determine the effects of levosimendan on cardiac performance and outcome in OHCA patients.

Supplementary Materials: The following supporting information can be downloaded at: https://www.mdpi.com/article/10.3390/jcm11092621/s1, Table S1: Univariable and multivariable logistic regression analysis showing the association of different variables including levosimendan treatment (<24 h) and 30-day mortality in out-of-hospital-cardiac arrest patients admitted to the intensive care unit in Stockholm, Sweden, 2010–2016. Table S2: Baseline characteristics and outcome before and after propensity score matching. Table S3: Baseline characteristics in subgroups of time-to-treatment-start with levosimendan in out-of-hospital-cardiac arrest patients admitted to the intensive care unit in Stockholm, Sweden, 2010–2016.

Author Contributions: Conceptualization, S.R., M.J.F., J.L., M.R., J.H., T.D. and P.N.; Data curation, S.R. and M.L.; Formal analysis, S.R., J.L., M.J. and P.N.; Investigation, T.D.; Methodology, S.R., M.J.F., M.R., J.H., M.L., M.J., T.D. and P.N.; Resources, M.J.F. and P.N.; Supervision, M.J.F., J.L., T.D. and P.N.; Writing—original draft, S.R.; Writing—review & editing, M.J.F., J.L., M.R., J.H., M.L., M.J., T.D. and P.N. All authors have read and agreed to the published version of the manuscript.

Funding: This research was partly funded by the Swedish Heart and Lung Foundation with the grant number 20180412.

Institutional Review Board Statement: The study was conducted in accordance with the Declaration of Helsinki, and approved by the Regional Ethics Committee in Stockholm with the protocol code 2016/873-31/2 for studies involving humans.

Informed Consent Statement: Not applicable.

Data Availability Statement: The study present data from The Swedish Register for Cardiopulmonary Resuscitation, The Centricity Critical Care patient data and monitoring system in the Stockholm region, and The SWEDEHEART register. The data are not publicly available in accordance with ethical approval and institutional regulations of patient data management.

Conflicts of Interest: The authors declare no conflict of interest.

References

1. Wong, C.X.; Brown, A.; Lau, D.H.; Chugh, S.S.; Albert, C.M.; Kalman, J.M.; Sanders, P. Epidemiology of Sudden Cardiac Death: Global and Regional Perspectives. *Heart Lung Circ.* **2019**, *28*, 6–14. [CrossRef]
2. Hollenberg, J.; Herlitz, J.; Lindqvist, J.; Riva, G.; Bohm, K.; Rosenqvist, M.; Svensson, L. Improved survival after out-of-hospital cardiac arrest is associated with an increase in proportion of emergency crew—Witnessed cases and bystander cardiopulmonary resuscitation. *Circulation* **2008**, *118*, 389–396. [CrossRef] [PubMed]
3. Ong, M.E.H.; Perkins, G.D.; Cariou, A. Out-of-hospital cardiac arrest: Prehospital management. *Lancet* **2018**, *391*, 980–988. [CrossRef]
4. Nolan, J.P.; Soar, J.; Cariou, A.; Cronberg, T.; Moulaert, V.R.; Deakin, C.D.; Bottiger, B.W.; Friberg, H.; Sunde, K.; Sandroni, C. European Resuscitation Council and European Society of Intensive Care Medicine Guidelines for Post-resuscitation Care 2015: Section 5 of the European Resuscitation Council Guidelines for Resuscitation 2015. *Resuscitation* **2015**, *95*, 202–222. [CrossRef] [PubMed]
5. Perkins, G.D.; Kenna, C.; Ji, C.; Deakin, C.D.; Nolan, J.P.; Quinn, T.; Fothergill, R.; Gunson, I.; Pocock, H.; Rees, N.; et al. The effects of adrenaline in out of hospital cardiac arrest with shockable and non-shockable rhythms: Findings from the PACA and PARAMEDIC-2 randomised controlled trials. *Resuscitation* **2019**, *140*, 55–63. [CrossRef]
6. Kudenchuk, P.J.; Cobb, L.A.; Copass, M.K.; Cummins, R.O.; Doherty, A.M.; Fahrenbruch, C.E.; Hallstrom, A.P.; Murray, W.A.; Olsufka, M.; Walsh, T. Amiodarone for resuscitation after out-of-hospital cardiac arrest due to ventricular fibrillation. *N. Engl. J. Med.* **1999**, *341*, 871–878. [CrossRef]
7. Papp, Z.; Edes, I.; Fruhwald, S.; De Hert, S.G.; Salmenpera, M.; Leppikangas, H.; Mebazaa, A.; Landoni, G.; Grossini, E.; Caimmi, P.; et al. Levosimendan: Molecular mechanisms and clinical implications: Consensus of experts on the mechanisms of action of levosimendan. *Int. J. Cardiol.* **2012**, *159*, 82–87. [CrossRef]
8. Fredholm, M.; Jorgensen, K.; Houltz, E.; Ricksten, S.E. Inotropic and lusitropic effects of levosimendan and milrinone assessed by strain echocardiography-A randomised trial. *Acta Anaesthesiol. Scand.* **2018**, *62*, 1246–1254. [CrossRef] [PubMed]
9. Trambaiolo, P.; Bertini, P.; Borrelli, N.; Poli, M.; Romano, S.; Ferraiuolo, G.; Penco, M.; Guarracino, F. Evaluation of ventriculo-arterial coupling in ST elevation myocardial infarction with left ventricular dysfunction treated with levosimendan. *Int. J. Cardiol.* **2019**, *288*, 1–4. [CrossRef]
10. De Luca, L.; Sardella, G.; Proietti, P.; Battagliese, A.; Benedetti, G.; Di Roma, A.; Fedele, F. Effects of levosimendan on left ventricular diastolic function after primary angioplasty for acute anterior myocardial infarction: A Doppler echocardiographic study. *J. Am. Soc. Echocardiogr. Off. Publ. Am. Soc. Echocardiogr.* **2006**, *19*, 172–177. [CrossRef]
11. Dominguez-Rodriguez, A.; Samimi-Fard, S.; Garcia-Gonzalez, M.J.; Abreu-Gonzalez, P. Effects of levosimendan versus dobutamine on left ventricular diastolic function in patients with cardiogenic shock after primary angioplasty. *Int. J. Cardiol.* **2008**, *128*, 214–217. [CrossRef] [PubMed]
12. Belletti, A.; Landoni, G.; Lomivorotov, V.V.; Oriani, A.; Ajello, S. Adrenergic Downregulation in Critical Care: Molecular Mechanisms and Therapeutic Evidence. *J. Cardiothorac. Vasc. Anesth.* **2020**, *34*, 1023–1041. [CrossRef] [PubMed]
13. Rysz, S.; Lundberg, J.; Nordberg, P.; Eriksson, H.; Wieslander, B.; Lundin, M.; Fyrdahl, A.; Pernow, J.; Ugander, M.; Djärv, T.; et al. The effect of levosimendan on survival and cardiac performance in an ischemic cardiac arrest model—A blinded randomized placebo-controlled study in swine. *Resuscitation* **2020**, *150*, 113–120. [CrossRef] [PubMed]
14. Xanthos, T.; Bassiakou, E.; Koudouna, E.; Rokas, G.; Goulas, S.; Dontas, I.; Kouskouni, E.; Perrea, D.; Papadimitriou, L. Combination pharmacotherapy in the treatment of experimental cardiac arrest. *Am. J. Emerg. Med.* **2009**, *27*, 651–659. [CrossRef] [PubMed]
15. Koudouna, E.; Xanthos, T.; Bassiakou, E.; Goulas, S.; Lelovas, P.; Papadimitriou, D.; Tsirikos, N.; Papadimitriou, L. Levosimendan improves the initial outcome of cardiopulmonary resuscitation in a swine model of cardiac arrest. *Acta Anaesthesiol. Scand.* **2007**, *51*, 1123–1129. [CrossRef]
16. Malmberg, M.; Vahasilta, T.; Saraste, A.; Koskenvuo, J.W.; Parkka, J.P.; Leino, K.; Laitio, T.; Stark, C.; Heikkila, A.; Saukko, P.; et al. Intracoronary Levosimendan during Ischemia Prevents Myocardial Apoptosis. *Front. Physiol.* **2012**, *3*, 17. [CrossRef]
17. Cammarata, G.A.; Weil, M.H.; Sun, S.; Huang, L.; Fang, X.; Tang, W. Levosimendan improves cardiopulmonary resuscitation and survival by K(ATP) channel activation. *J. Am. Coll. Cardiol.* **2006**, *47*, 1083–1085. [CrossRef]
18. Varvarousi, G.; Stefaniotou, A.; Varvaroussis, D.; Aroni, F.; Xanthos, T. The role of Levosimendan in cardiopulmonary resuscitation. *Eur. J. Pharmacol.* **2014**, *740*, 596–602. [CrossRef]
19. Hasselqvist-Ax, I.; Riva, G.; Herlitz, J.; Rosenqvist, M.; Hollenberg, J.; Nordberg, P.; Ringh, M.; Jonsson, M.; Axelsson, C.; Lindqvist, J.; et al. Early cardiopulmonary resuscitation in out-of-hospital cardiac arrest. *N. Engl. J. Med.* **2015**, *372*, 2307–2315. [CrossRef]

20. Stromsoe, A.; Svensson, L.; Axelsson, A.B.; Claesson, A.; Goransson, K.E.; Nordberg, P.; Herlitz, J. Improved outcome in Sweden after out-of-hospital cardiac arrest and possible association with improvements in every link in the chain of survival. *Eur. Heart J.* **2015**, *36*, 863–871. [CrossRef]
21. Jacobs, I.; Nadkarni, V.; Bahr, J.; Berg, R.A.; Billi, J.E.; Bossaert, L.; Cassan, P.; Coovadia, A.; D'Este, K.; Finn, J.; et al. Cardiac arrest and cardiopulmonary resuscitation outcome reports: Update and simplification of the Utstein templates for resuscitation registries. A statement for healthcare professionals from a task force of the international liaison committee on resuscitation (American Heart Association, European Resuscitation Council, Australian Resuscitation Council, New Zealand Resuscitation Council, Heart and Stroke Foundation of Canada, InterAmerican Heart Foundation, Resuscitation Council of Southern Africa). *Resuscitation* **2004**, *63*, 233–249. [CrossRef] [PubMed]
22. Herlitz, J. Svenska Hjärt-och Lungräddningsregistret. Available online: https://hlrr.se (accessed on 15 January 2022).
23. Facundo, H.T.; Fornazari, M.; Kowaltowski, A.J. Tissue protection mediated by mitochondrial K+ channels. *Biochim. Biophys. Acta* **2006**, *1762*, 202–212. [CrossRef] [PubMed]
24. Tholen, M.; Ricksten, S.E.; Lannemyr, L. Effects of levosimendan on renal blood flow and glomerular filtration in patients with acute kidney injury after cardiac surgery: A double blind, randomized placebo-controlled study. *Crit. Care* **2021**, *25*, 207. [CrossRef] [PubMed]
25. du Toit, E.F.; Genis, A.; Opie, L.H.; Pollesello, P.; Lochner, A. A role for the RISK pathway and K(ATP) channels in pre- and post-conditioning induced by levosimendan in the isolated guinea pig heart. *Br. J. Pharm.* **2008**, *154*, 41–50. [CrossRef]
26. Scheiermann, P.; Beiras-Fernandez, A.; Mutlak, H.; Weis, F. The protective effects of levosimendan on ischemia/reperfusion injury and apoptosis. *Recent Pat Cardiovasc. Drug Discov.* **2011**, *6*, 20–26. [CrossRef]
27. Pollesello, P.; Papp, Z. The cardioprotective effects of levosimendan: Preclinical and clinical evidence. *J. Cardiovasc. Pharm.* **2007**, *50*, 257–263. [CrossRef]
28. Farmakis, D.; Alvarez, J.; Gal, T.B.; Brito, D.; Fedele, F.; Fonseca, C.; Gordon, A.C.; Gotsman, I.; Grossini, E.; Guarracino, F.; et al. Levosimendan beyond inotropy and acute heart failure: Evidence of pleiotropic effects on the heart and other organs: An expert panel position paper. *Int. J. Cardiol.* **2016**, *222*, 303–312. [CrossRef]
29. Cosentino, N.; Niccoli, G.; Fracassi, F.; Rebuzzi, A.; Agostoni, P.; Marenzi, G. Rationale, experimental data, and emerging clinical evidence on early and preventive use of levosimendan in patients with ventricular dysfunction. *Eur. Heart J. Cardiovasc. Pharm.* **2020**, *6*, 310–316. [CrossRef]
30. Yannopoulos, D.; Bartos, J.A.; George, S.A.; Sideris, G.; Voicu, S.; Oestreich, B.; Matsuura, T.; Shekar, K.; Rees, J.; Aufderheide, T.P. Sodium nitroprusside enhanced cardiopulmonary resuscitation improves short term survival in a porcine model of ischemic refractory ventricular fibrillation. *Resuscitation* **2017**, *110*, 6–11. [CrossRef]
31. Laurent, I.; Monchi, M.; Chiche, J.-D.; Joly, L.-M.; Spaulding, C.; Bourgeois, B.é.; Cariou, A.; Rozenberg, A.; Carli, P.; Weber, S.; et al. Reversible myocardial dysfunction in survivors of out-of-hospital cardiac arrest. *J. Am. Coll. Cardiol.* **2002**, *40*, 2110–2116. [CrossRef]
32. Severino, P.; D'Amato, A.; Prosperi, S.; Dei Cas, A.; Mattioli, A.V.; Cevese, A.; Novo, G.; Prat, M.; Pedrinelli, R.; Raddino, R.; et al. Do the Current Guidelines for Heart Failure Diagnosis and Treatment Fit with Clinical Complexity? *J. Clin. Med.* **2022**, *11*, 857. [CrossRef] [PubMed]
33. Carev, M.; Karanovic, N.; Kocen, D.; Bulat, C. Useful supplement to the best practice of using levosimendan in cardiac surgery patients: 2.5-mg intravenous bolus for cardiopulmonary resuscitation during perioperative cardiac arrest. *J. Cardiothorac. Vasc. Anesth.* **2013**, *27*, e75–e77. [CrossRef] [PubMed]
34. Toller, W.; Guarracino, F.; Landoni, G. Reply to Carev et al.: "Useful supplement to the best practice of using levosimendan in cardiac surgery patients: 2.5 mg intravenous bolus for cardiopulmonary resuscitation during perioperative cardiac arrest". *J. Cardiothorac. Vasc. Anesth.* **2013**, *27*, e77–e78. [CrossRef] [PubMed]
35. Krumnikl, J.J.; Toller, W.G.; Prenner, G.; Metzler, H. Beneficial outcome after prostaglandin-induced post-partum cardiac arrest using levosimendan and extracorporeal membrane oxygenation. *Acta Anaesthesiol. Scand.* **2006**, *50*, 768–770. [CrossRef]
36. Tsagalou, E.P.; Nanas, J.N. Resuscitation from adrenaline resistant electro-mechanical dissociation facilitated by levosimendan in a young man with idiopathic dilated cardiomyopathy. *Resuscitation* **2006**, *68*, 147–149. [CrossRef] [PubMed]

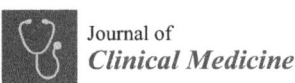

Article

Prognostic Value of Cardiac Troponin I in Patients with Ventricular Tachyarrhythmias

Ibrahim Akin [1], Michael Behnes [1,*], Julian Müller [2,3], Jan Forner [1], Mohammad Abumayyaleh [1], Kambis Mashayekhi [4], Muharrem Akin [5], Thomas Bertsch [6], Kathrin Weidner [1], Jonas Rusnak [1], Dirk Große Meininghaus [7], Maximilian Kittel [8] and Tobias Schupp [1]

[1] First Department of Medicine, University Medical Centre Mannheim (UMM), Faculty of Medicine Mannheim, University of Heidelberg, 68167 Mannheim, Germany; ibrahim.akin@umm.de (I.A.); jan.forner@umm.de (J.F.); mohammad.abumayyaleh@umm.de (M.A.); kathrin.weidner@umm.de (K.W.); jonas.rusnak@umm.de (J.R.); tobias.schupp@umm.de (T.S.)

[2] Clinic for Interventional Electrophysiology, Heart Centre Bad Neustadt, 97616 Bad Neustadt a. d. Saale, Germany; julianmueller240491@gmail.com

[3] Department of Cardiology and Angiology, Philipps-University Marburg, 35037 Marburg, Germany

[4] Department of Internal Medicine and Cardiology, Mediclin Heart Centre Lahr, 77933 Lahr, Germany; kambis.mashayekhi@universitaets-herzzentrum.de

[5] Department of Cardiology and Angiology, Hannover Medical School, 30625 Hannover, Germany; akin-muharrem@mh-hannover.de

[6] Institute of Clinical Chemistry, Laboratory Medicine and Transfusion Medicine, Nuremberg General Hospital, Paracelsus Medical University, 90419 Nuremberg, Germany; thomas.bertsch@nuernberg.de

[7] Department of Cardiology, Carl-Thiem-Klinikum Cottbus, 03048 Cottbus, Germany; med1@ck.de

[8] Institute for Clinical Chemistry, Faculty of Medicine Mannheim, Heidelberg University, 68167 Mannheim, Germany; maximilian.kittel@umm.de

* Correspondence: michael.behnes@umm.de; Tel.: +49-621-383-6239

Abstract: Besides the diagnostic role in acute myocardial infarction, cardiac troponin I levels (cTNI) may be increased in various other clinical conditions, including heart failure, valvular heart disease and sepsis. However, limited data are available regarding the prognostic role of cTNI in the setting of ventricular tachyarrhythmias. Therefore, the present study sought to assess the prognostic impact of cTNI in patients with ventricular tachyarrhythmias (i.e., ventricular tachycardia (VT) and fibrillation (VF)) on admission. A large retrospective registry was used, including all consecutive patients presenting with ventricular tachyarrhythmias from 2002 to 2015. The prognostic impact of elevated cTNI levels was investigated for 30-day all-cause mortality (i.e., primary endpoint) using Kaplan–Meier, receiver operating characteristic (ROC), multivariable Cox regression analyses and propensity score matching. From a total of 1104 patients with ventricular tachyarrhythmias and available cTNI levels on admission, 46% were admitted with VT and 54% with VF. At 30 days, high cTNI was associated with the primary endpoint (40% vs. 22%; log rank $p = 0.001$; HR = 2.004; 95% CI 1.603–2.505; $p = 0.001$), which was still evident after multivariable adjustment and propensity score matching (30% vs. 18%; log rank $p = 0.003$; HR = 1.729; 95% CI 1.184–2.525; $p = 0.005$). Significant discrimination of the primary endpoint was especially evident in VT patients (area under the curve (AUC) 0.734; 95% CI 0.645–0.823; $p = 0.001$). In contrast, secondary endpoints, including all-cause mortality at 30 months and a composite arrhythmic endpoint, were not affected by cTNI levels. The risk of cardiac rehospitalization was lower in patients with high cTNI, which was no longer observed after propensity score matching. In conclusion, high cTNI levels were associated with increased risk of all-cause mortality at 30 days in patients presenting with ventricular tachyarrhythmias.

Keywords: ventricular tachyarrhythmias; cardiac troponin I; biomarkers; sudden cardiac death; coronary artery disease

Citation: Akin, I.; Behnes, M.; Müller, J.; Forner, J.; Abumayyaleh, M.; Mashayekhi, K.; Akin, M.; Bertsch, T.; Weidner, K.; Rusnak, J.; et al. Prognostic Value of Cardiac Troponin I in Patients with Ventricular Tachyarrhythmias. *J. Clin. Med.* **2022**, *11*, 2987. https://doi.org/10.3390/jcm11112987

Academic Editor: Massimo Iacoviello

Received: 7 April 2022
Accepted: 23 May 2022
Published: 25 May 2022

Publisher's Note: MDPI stays neutral with regard to jurisdictional claims in published maps and institutional affiliations.

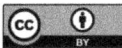

Copyright: © 2022 by the authors. Licensee MDPI, Basel, Switzerland. This article is an open access article distributed under the terms and conditions of the Creative Commons Attribution (CC BY) license (https://creativecommons.org/licenses/by/4.0/).

1. Introduction

Despite improvements in the treatment strategies of cardiovascular diseases, including better guideline adherence to pharmacological therapies, coronary revascularization strategies and increasing supply with an implantable cardioverter defibrillator (ICD), sudden cardiac death (SCD) still accounts for almost 50% of all cardiovascular deaths [1–3]. While congenital heart defects account for most SCD cases in younger patients, coronary artery disease (CAD) is the main cause for SCD-related deaths in patients over 35 years of age [4]. In more than 75% of cases, SCD occurs due to ventricular tachyarrhythmias (i.e., ventricular tachycardia (VT) or fibrillation (VF)). Commonly, VF is detected in patients with acute myocardial injury, leading to metabolic derangement and oxidative stress, whereas VT may occur more often in patients with structural heart disease (such as ischemic cardiomyopathy (ICMP)) and channelopathies [5]. However, in more than half of the patients, SCD occurs in patients without evidence of severe heart failure (HF). The mechanisms causing SCD are not fully understood, as outlined within recent European guidelines for the prevention of ventricular tachyarrhythmias and SCD [6,7]. Therefore, the identification of patients at high risk for SCD remains challenging [7]. Over the years, the identification of biomarkers for the identification of individuals at high risk for SCD (such as cardiac troponins, N-terminal pro-B-type natriuretic peptide (NT pro-BNP), Galectin-3 and soluble ST2) has gained greater significance [8–12].

Cardiac muscle contraction occurs as a result of increased intracellular Ca^{2+} levels, which affects the troponin complex—consisting of troponin C (cTNC), troponin T (cTNT) and troponin I (cTNI). The regulatory role of TNI consists in the inhibition of the Adenosine 5′-TriPhosphatase (ATPase) activity of the actomyosin complex and the modulation of cross-bridge formation and cardiac muscle contraction [13,14]. In particular, cTNT and cTNI are biomarkers of myocardial injury and are commonly released during myocardial necrosis in the presence of acute myocardial infarction (AMI) [15]. Myocardial necrosis causes the replacement of cardiac myocytes by fibrotic tissue, which further promotes adverse cardiac remodeling [16]. Elevated cTNI has already been shown to increase the risk of the composite endpoint of death, percutaneous coronary intervention (PCI) and AMI—especially in patients with a history of CAD—as observed in a study of 131 patients with supraventricular tachyarrhythmias [17]. In line with this finding, it was demonstrated that cTNT can function as a predictor of cardiac death, as was found among 70 patients with heart failure and left ventricular ejection fraction (LVEF) $\leq$ 35% at 2.2 years [18].

However, to the best of the authors' knowledge, no available study has investigated the prognostic role of cardiac troponins in patients admitted with ventricular tachyarrhythmias. Therefore, this study investigates the prognostic role of cTNI levels on 30-day all-cause mortality (primary endpoint) in patients presenting with index ventricular tachyarrhythmias. Secondary endpoints include a composite arrhythmic endpoint (i.e., recurrent ventricular tachyarrhythmias, appropriate ICD therapies and SCD) and cardiac rehospitalization at 30 months.

2. Materials and Methods

2.1. Data Collection and Documentation

The present study retrospectively included data from all consecutive patients presenting with ventricular tachyarrhythmias on hospital admission, from 2002 to 2015, at the First Department of Medicine, University Medical Centre Mannheim, Germany, as recently published [19]. Using the hospital information system, all relevant clinical data related to the index event were documented.

Ventricular tachyarrhythmias comprised VT and VF, as defined by current international guidelines [7]. Sustained VT was defined by a duration of >30 s or as causing hemodynamic collapse within 30 seconds. Nonsustained VT was defined by a duration of <30 s. Both were characterized by wide QRS complexes ($\geq$120 ms) at a rate greater than 100 beats per minute [7]. Ventricular tachyarrhythmias were documented by 12-lead electrocardiogram (ECG), ECG telemonitoring, ICD or—in the case of an unstable course or during cardiopulmonary resuscitation (CPR)—by external defibrillator monitoring. Documented VF was treated by external defibrillation and—in case of prolonged instability—with additional intravenous antiarrhythmic drugs during CPR.

The present study is derived from an analysis of the "Registry of Malignant Arrhythmias and Sudden Cardiac Death-Influence of Diagnostics and Interventions (RACE-IT)" and represents a single-center registry, including consecutive patients presenting with ventricular tachyarrhythmias and aborted cardiac arrest being acutely admitted to the University Medical Center Mannheim (UMM), Germany (clinicaltrials.gov; identifier: NCT02982473), from 2002 to 2015. The registry was carried out according to the principles of the declaration of Helsinki and was approved by the medical ethics committee II of the Medical Faculty Mannheim (Ethical Approval Number: 2016-612N-MA), University of Heidelberg, Germany.

2.2. Measurement of cTNI

During the study period from 2002 to 2015, cTNI testing was performed using three different cTNI assays. From 2002 to June 2006, the SIEMENS Dimension RxL CTNI assay was used for cTNI testing. The lowest detection limit of the assay was 0.004 ng/mL. The 99th percentile, measured from a healthy reference population, was 0.007 ng/mL, with a coefficient of variation (CV) of 15–22%. Thereafter, from June 2006 to December 2010, the Beckman Coulter Access AccuTNI assay was used, with the lowest detection limit being 0.01 ng/mL. The 99th percentile, measured from a healthy reference population, was 0.04 ng/mL, with a CV of 10%. From December 2010 to the end of the study period, cTNI was measured with the SIEMENS Dimension® Vista 1500™. The lowest detection limit of the assay was 0.015 ng/mL. The 99th percentile, measured from a healthy reference population, was 0.045 ng/mL, with a CV of 10% [20].

2.3. Definition of Study Groups, Inclusion and Exclusion Criteria

For the present analysis, risk stratification was performed according to a single cTNI measurement related to the index event. For each patient, only the cTNI measurement closest to the index event was used, with a maximum time frame of 24 h before and after the index event. First, risk stratification was performed, dichotomized according to the median cTNI level. Despite the use of three different cTNI assays during the study period, the median cTNI level for each cTNI assay was assessed. Patients were classified as "high cTNI" (in the presence of cTNI above the median cTNI level) and "low cTNI" (in the presence of cTNI below or equal the median cTNI level) for each of the cTNI assays. To better assess the prognostic value of incremental cTNI increase, quartile analyses were performed thereafter. Quartiles were calculated, separated by each cTNI assay. Accordingly, patients were classified as "low" (Q1), "low-intermediate" (Q2), "intermediate-high" (Q3) and "high" (Q4). Based on those quartiles, the prognostic impact of incremental cTNI increase was investigated within the entire study cohort, and thereafter within prespecified subgroups. Patients without cTNI measurement during the allowed time frame, as well as patients without complete follow-up data regarding mortality, were excluded. Each patient was included only once when presenting with the first episode of ventricular tachyarrhythmias.

2.4. Risk Stratification

Further risk stratification was performed according to the underlying cardiac pathology. Patients with non-AMI, ST-segment elevation myocardial infarction (STEMI), non-ST segment elevation myocardial infarction (NSTEMI), ischemic (ICMP) and nonischemic cardiomyopathy (NICMP), as well as patients with idiopathic ventricular tachyarrhythmias, were analyzed.

STEMI was defined as a novel rise in the ST segment in at least two contiguous leads, with ST-segment elevation $\geq$ 2.5 mm in men < 40 years, $\geq$ 2 mm in men $\geq$ 40 years, or $\geq$ 1.5 mm in women in leads V2–V3 and/or 1 mm in the other leads. Additional ECG criteria were new ST depression or inversion, T wave alterations, Q waves or new left bundle branch block [21]. NSTEMI was defined as the presence of an acute coronary syndrome with a troponin I increase of above the 99th percentile of a healthy reference population, in the absence of ST segment elevation, but with persistent or transient ST segment depression, inversion or alteration of T wave, or a normal ECG in the presence of a coronary culprit lesion. The culprit lesion was defined as an acute complete thrombotic occlusion for STEMI and as any relevant critical coronary stenosis for NSTEMI, with the potential need for coronary revascularization either by PCI or coronary artery bypass grafting (CABG). The presence of a coronary culprit lesion was mandatory for both diagnoses of NSTEMI and STEMI. Evidence of regional wall motion abnormalities was also included in AMI diagnosis, as far as was available. Values of left ventricular ejection fraction (LVEF) were retrieved from standardized transthoracic echocardiographic examinations, usually performed before hospital discharge in survivors, to assess realistic LVEF values beyond the acute phase of acute coronary ischemia during AMI. In minor part, and only if available, earlier LVEF values, assessed on admission or during intensive care, were retrieved from patients who died while already within the acute phase of AMI [22].

ICMP comprised all patients with LVEF < 55% and had either prior documented CAD or newly diagnosed CAD, as well as patients with AMI assessed by coronary angiography at index stay sufficient to cause myocardial dysfunction. Identification of CAD (defined as at least one relevant stenosis of one epicardial coronary artery of more than 50%) was based on the judgment of the investigating interventional cardiologist during routine care. All coronary angiograms and reports were reassessed post hoc by two independent interventional cardiologists to determine whether the CAD was sufficient for causality of myocardial dysfunction [23]. NICMP comprised all patients with LVEF < 55%, in the absence of CAD, valvular heart disease and congenital heart disease sufficient to cause the observed myocardial abnormality. The following types were allocated to the NICMP group: dilated cardiomyopathy (DCM), hypertrophic obstructive cardiomyopathy, arrhythmogenic right ventricular dysplasia (ARVD) and noncompaction cardiomyopathy (NCCMP) [23–26].

Patients presenting without AMI, ICMP and NICMP, and who had no evidence of impaired LVEF or structural heart disease, were classified as patients with "idiopathic ventricular tachyarrhythmias".

Finally, the prognostic impact of cTNI was investigated within different subgroups of patients with CAD, whereas only patients undergoing coronary angiography were included. Thus, multivessel disease (MVD) was characterized by significant stenosis of at least 2 major coronary vessels (defined as at least one relevant stenosis of one epicardial coronary artery of more than 50% and/or prior PCI of one coronary artery). The coronary chronic total occlusion (CTO) group comprised all patients with a native unrevascularized CTO in coronary vessels with a diameter >1.5 mm [27,28]. Identification of CTO and CAD was based on the judgment of the investigating interventional cardiologist during routine care. The CTO group also included patients with acute revascularization of non-CTO-vessels by PCI or CABG. Moreover, patients with an occluded bypass graft on the native CTO vessel were allocated to CTO group.

2.5. Study Endpoints

The primary endpoint was all-cause mortality at 30 days after index ventricular tachyarrhythmias. Secondary endpoints were all-cause deaths at 24 h, 30 months, cardiac death at 30 days, cardiac rehospitalization at 30 months and a composite arrhythmic endpoint (including recurrent ventricular tachyarrhythmias, appropriate ICD therapies and SCD) at 30 days and 30 months after index ventricular tachyarrhythmias. Overall follow-up period lasted until 2016. All-cause mortality was documented using our electronic hospital information system and by directly contacting state resident registration offices ("bureau of mortality statistics") across Germany. Identification of patients was verified by place of name, surname, day of birth and registered living address. Lost-to-follow-up rate was 1.7% (n = 48) regarding survival until the end of the follow-up period.

2.6. Statistical Methods

Quantitative data are presented as mean ± standard error of mean (SEM), median and interquartile ranges (IQR), as well as ranges depending on the distribution of the data and were compared using the Student's t test for normally distributed data, or the Mann–Whitney U test for nonparametric data. Deviations from a Gaussian distribution were tested by the Kolmogorov–Smirnov test. Spearman's rank correlation for nonparametric data was used to test univariate correlations. Qualitative data are presented as absolute and relative frequencies and were compared using the Chi^2 test or the Fisher's exact test, as appropriate.

Firstly, overall data of consecutive patients on admission are given for the entire unmatched cohort in order to present the real-life character of health-care supply at our institution between 2002 and 2015. Here, Kaplan–Meier method, as well as uni- and multivariable Cox regression models, were applied for the evaluation of all-cause mortality at 30 days after index ventricular tachyarrhythmias.

Secondly, propensity score matching was applied. Propensity scores (1:1) were created for the comparisons of "high cTNI" vs. "low TNI", including the entire study cohort and applying a nonparsimonious multivariable logistic regression model. Propensity scores were created according to the presence of the following independent variables: age, sex, diabetes, chronic kidney disease, CAD, LVEF, CPR, index ventricular tachyarrhythmia (i.e., VT/VF) and presence of an ICD. Based on the propensity score values counted by logistic regression, for each patient, one patient in the control group with a similar propensity score value was found (accepted difference of propensity score value: <5%). Univariable stratification was performed using the Kaplan–Meier method, with comparisons between groups using univariable hazard ratios (HR) given together with 95% confidence intervals.

Finally, the prognostic value of cTNI, assessed with the SIEMENS Dimension® Vista intelligent lab system, was investigated using receiver operating characteristic (ROC) analyses. ROC analyses were performed separately for both patients with index episodes of VT and VF. An optimum cutoff value was determined in accordance with the maximum Youden index. The Youden index, defined as the maximum of sensitivity + specificity −1, was used to determine the largest total diagnostic accuracy a biomarker can achieve [29,30].

The result of a statistical test was considered significant for $p < 0.05$. SPSS (Version 25, IBM Armonk, New York, NY, USA) was used for statistics.

3. Results

3.1. Entire Study Cohort

From 2422 patients with ventricular tachyarrhythmias on admission, 1318 patients without cTNI measurement related to the index event were excluded. Accordingly, the present study included 1104 patients with ventricular tachyarrhythmias and available cTNI measurement (Figure 1).

Within the entire study cohort, median cTNI levels were 0.700 ng/mL (IQR 0.370–3.125 ng/mL) for the SIEMENS Dimension® RxL CTNI assay, 0.800 ng/mL (IQR 0.300–3.515 ng/mL) for the Beckman Coulter Access AccuTNI assay and 0.610 ng/mL (IQR 0.380–2.2965 ng/mL for the SIEMENS Dimension® Vista 1500™ assay. Accordingly, cTNI did not significantly differ among the different cTNI assays ($p \geq 0.248$ for all comparisons). As illustrated in Figure 2, cTNI levels were significantly higher among nonsurvivors as compared to survivors at 30 days, irrespective of the applied cTNI assay ($p = 0.001$ for all comparisons).

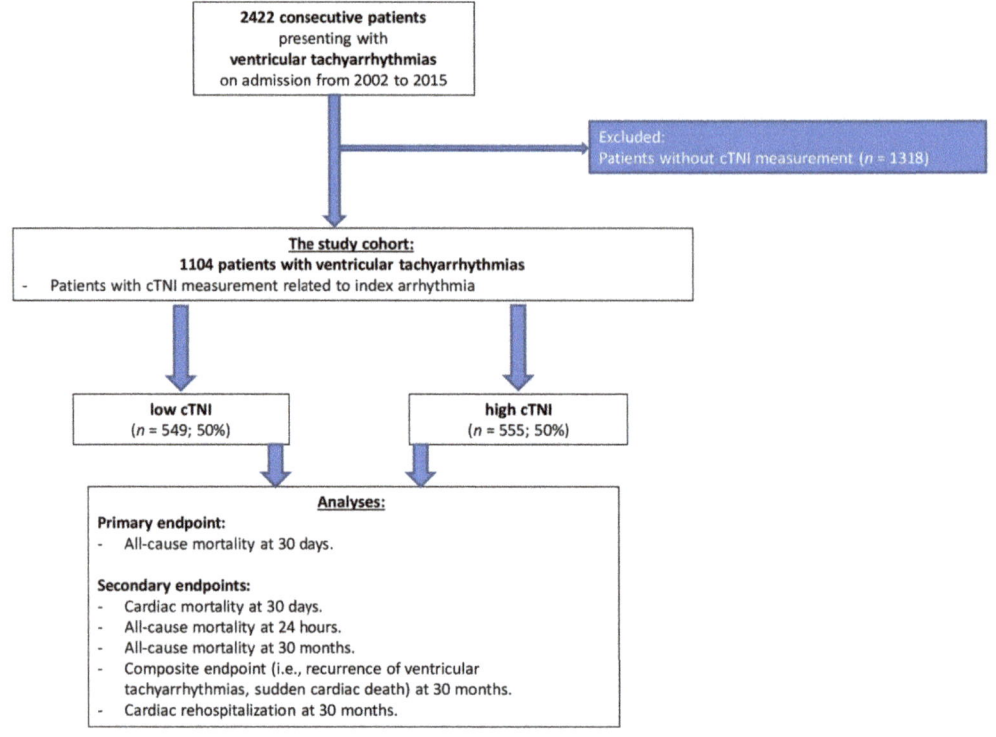

Figure 1. Study population. cTNI, cardiac troponin I.

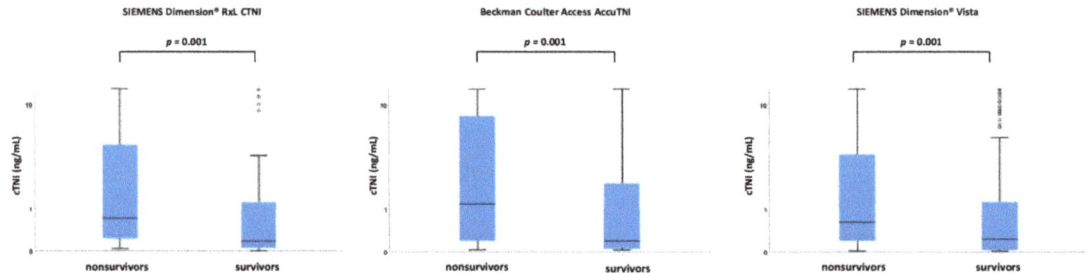

Figure 2. Box plots demonstrating distribution of cTNI levels depending on the applied assay, in patients with ventricular tachyarrhythmias, comparing survivors and nonsurvivors at 30 days.

Patients' characteristics within the entire, unmatched study cohort for the comparison of patients with high vs. low cTNI are outlined within Table 1 (left panel). Patients with high cTNI more frequently presented with VF as compared to patients with low cTNI (62% vs. 47%; $p = 0.001$). In contrast, cardiovascular risk factors and LVEF were equally distributed in both groups. Rates of CPR were higher in patents with elevated cTNI (70% vs. 49%; $p = 0.001$). Furthermore, patients with high cTNI were more frequently treated with beta blockers, ACE inhibitors, statins, amiodarone and aldosterone antagonists.

CAD-related findings are presented in Table 2 (left panel). Coronary angiography was more frequently performed in patients with high cTNI (75% vs. 63%; $p = 0.001$), who had higher rates of CAD (87% vs. 67%; $p = 0.001$). In line with this finding, the rate of PCI was significantly higher among patients with elevated cTNI (72% vs. 37%; $p = 0.001$).

Table 1. Baseline characteristics before and after propensity score matching.

Characteristic	Without Propensity Score Matching			With Propensity Score Matching		
	Low cTNI (n = 549; 50%)	High cTNI (n = 555; 50%)	p Value	Low cTNI (n = 238; 50%)	High cTNI (n = 238; 50%)	p Value
Age, median (range)	67 (16–94)	67 (15–97)	0.474	67 (19–94)	67 (15–91)	0.415
Male gender, n (%)	397 (72)	402 (72)	0.965	178 (75)	174 (73)	0.676
Ventricular tachyarrhythmias at index, n (%)						
Ventricular tachycardia	293 (53)	211 (38)	0.001	116 (49)	110 (46)	0.582
Ventricular fibrillation	256 (47)	344 (62)		122 (51)	128 (54)	
Underlying cardiac disease, n (%)						
Coronary artery disease	235 (43)	108 (19)	0.001	91 (39)	84 (35)	0.436
STEMI	31 (6)	141 (25)	0.001	24 (10)	43 (18)	0.012
NSTEMI	87 (16)	204 (37)	0.001	61 (26)	47 (20)	0.125
Nonischemic cardiomyopathy	24 (4)	16 (3)	0.186	15 (6)	16 (7)	0.853
Channelopathy	23 (4)	10 (2)	0.020	9 (4)	8 (3)	0.805
Idiopathic ventricular tachyarrhythmias	149 (27)	76 (24)	0.001	38 (16)	40 (17)	0.804
Cardiovascular risk factors, n (%)						
Arterial hypertension	311 (57)	320 (58)	0.735	137 (58)	139 (58)	0.853
Diabetes mellitus	124 (23)	151 (27)	0.076	60 (25)	63 (27)	0.753
Hyperlipidemia	143 (26)	138 (25)	0.652	63 (27)	71 (30)	0.415
Smoking	161 (29)	188 (34)	0.104	77 (32)	84 (35)	0.498
Cardiac family history	48 (9)	52 (9)	0.717	22 (9)	19 (12)	0.300
Comorbidities at index stay, n (%)						
Prior myocardial infarction	129 (24)	109 (20)	0.119	53 (22)	57 (24)	0.664
Prior coronary artery disease	224 (41)	197 (36)	0.070	101 (42)	103 (43)	0.853
Prior heart failure	126 (23)	91 (16)	0.001	65 (27)	57 (24)	0.401
Prior PCI	121 (22)	98 (18)	0.068	60 (25)	52 (22)	0.387
Atrial fibrillation	170 (31)	170 (31)	0.904	76 (32)	88 (37)	0.247
Cardiopulmonary resuscitation	271 (49)	390 (70)	0.001	130 (55)	144 (61)	
In hospital	97 (18)	142 (36)		49 (21)	48 (20)	0.377
Out of hospital	174 (32)	248 (47)		81 (35)	96 (40)	
Chronic kidney disease	296 (54)	384 (69)	0.001	148 (62)	157 (66)	0.390
COPD	53 (10)	50 (9)	0.713	19 (8)	23 (10)	0.518
LVEF, n (%)			0.073			0.531
>55%	142 (34)	114 (28)		71 (30)	69 (29)	
54–45%	49 (12)	68 (17)		29 (12)	37 (16)	
44–35%	78 (19)	86 (21)		47 (20)	53 (22)	

Table 1. Cont.

Characteristic	Without Propensity Score Matching			With Propensity Score Matching		
	Low cTNI (n = 549; 50%)	High cTNI (n = 555; 50%)	p Value	Low cTNI (n = 238; 50%)	High cTNI (n = 238; 50%)	p Value
<35%	147 (35)	133 (33)	-	91 (38)	79 (33)	-
No evidence of LVEF	-	-	-	-	-	-
Cardiac therapies at index, n (%)						
Electrophysiological examination	100 (18)	47 (5)	**0.001**	34 (14)	16 (7)	**0.007**
VT ablation therapy	21 (4)	11 (2)	0.068	11 (5)	7 (3)	0.336
Presence of an ICD at discharge, n (%)	210 (50)	121 (37)	**0.001**	86 (46)	78 (48)	0.659
Medication at discharge, n (%)						
Beta blocker	332 (79)	291 (90)	**0.001**	164 (87)	144 (88)	0.657
ACE inhibitor	257 (61)	237 (73)	**0.001**	122 (65)	113 (69)	0.343
ARB	58 (14)	23 (7)	**0.003**	25 (13)	13 (8)	0.110
Statin	259 (62)	257 (79)	**0.001**	129 (68)	117 (72)	0.472
Amiodarone	51 (12)	56 (17)	**0.046**	24 (13)	34 (21)	**0.040**
Digitalis	41 (10)	20 (6)	0.078	18 (10)	15 (9)	0.918
Aldosterone antagonist	54 (13)	38 (12)	0.652	25 (13)	26 (16)	0.469

ACE, angiotensin converting enzyme; ARB, angiotensin receptor blocker; CAD, coronary artery disease; COPD, chronic obstructive pulmonary disease; cTNI, cardiac troponin I; left ventricular ejection fraction; NSTEMI, non-ST-segment elevation myocardial infarction; PCI, percutaneous coronary intervention; SEM, standard error of mean; VT, ventricular tachycardia. Bold type indicates $p < 0.05$.

Table 2. CAD-related findings.

Characteristic	Without Propensity Score Matching						With Propensity Score Matching					
	Low cTNI (n = 549; 50%)		High cTNI (n = 555; 50%)			p Value	Low cTNI (n = 238; 50%)		High cTNI (n = 238; 50%)			p Value
Coronary angiography, n (%)	344	(63)	417	(75)		**0.001**	161	(68)	180	(76)		0.053
No evidence of CAD	112	(33)	53	(13)			36	(22)	40	(22)		
1-vessel disease	78	(23)	115	(28)		**0.001**	48	(30)	43	(24)		0.456
2-vessel disease	84	(24)	139	(33)			43	(27)	61	(34)		
3-vessel disease	70	(20)	110	(26)			34	(21)	36	(20)		
Significant stenosis of coronary vessels, n (%)												
Right coronary artery	151	(44)	221	(53)		**0.012**	76	(47)	86	(48)		0.916
Left main trunk	17	(5)	32	(8)		0.126	9	(6)	12	(7)		0.680
Left anterior descending	156	(45)	246	(59)		**0.001**	89	(55)	91	(51)		0.383
Left circumflex	104	(30)	180	(43)		**0.001**	54	(34)	69	(39)		0.358
Chronic total occlusion	74	(22)	81	(19)		0.477	42	(26)	43	(24)		0.639
Presence of CABG	44	(13)	35	(8)		**0.048**	16	(10)	23	(13)		0.411
PCI, n (%)	127	(37)	300	(72)		**0.001**	76	(47)	89	(49)		0.680
Right coronary artery	57	(17)	106	(25)		**0.003**	31	(19)	36	(20)		0.863
Left main trunk	6	(2)	20	(5)		**0.021**	3	(2)	3	(2)		1.000
Left anterior descending	64	(19)	153	(37)		**0.001**	41	(26)	47	(26)		0.892
Left circumflex	28	(8)	72	(17)		**0.001**	19	(12)	17	(9)		0.480
CABG	3	(0.9)	4	(1)		1.000	1	(0.6)	2	(1)		1.000
Sent to CABG, n (%)	10	(3)	7	(2)		0.254	5	(3)	5	(3)		1.000
Thrombus aspiration, n (%)	23	(7)	69	(17)		**0.001**	18	(11)	21	(12)		0.888
CPR during coronary angiography, n (%)	23	(7)	44	(11)		0.061	8	(5)	9	(5)		0.990

CABG, coronary artery bypass grafting; CAD, coronary artery disease; CPR, cardiopulmonary resuscitation; PCI, percutaneous coronary intervention. Bold type indicates p < 0.05.

3.2. Survival Analyses within the Entire Study Cohort

Median follow-up time in the entire study cohort was 1.7 years (IQR 8 days–5.0 years). At 30 days, the all-cause mortality (primary endpoint) occurred in 40% of patients with high cTNI and in 20% of patients presenting with low cTNI (Figure 3).

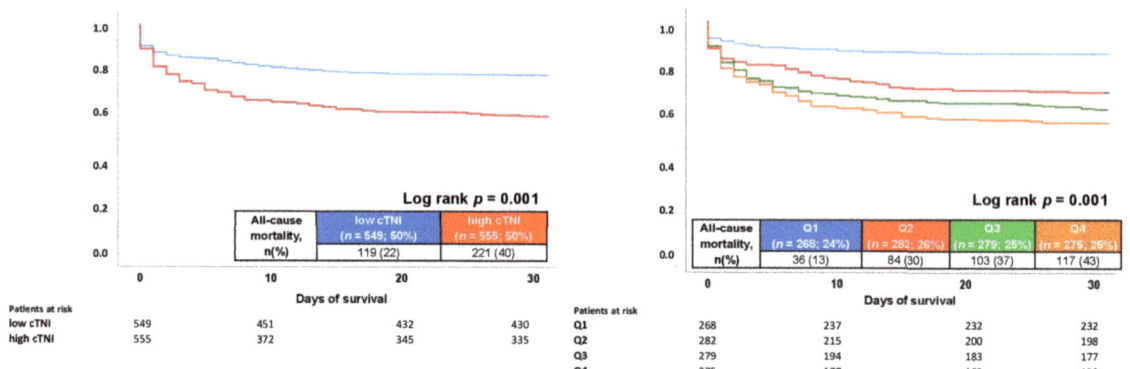

Figure 3. Kaplan–Meier analysis comparing patients with high cTNI to patients with low cTNI (**left** panel), as well as within a quartile analysis (**right** panel), with regard to 30-day all-cause mortality (primary endpoint) within the entire unmatched study cohort.

Accordingly, elevated cTNI levels were associated with increased 30-day all-cause mortality (primary endpoint) in patients with ventricular tachyarrhythmias (HR = 2.004; 95% CI 1.603–2.505; $p = 0.001$) (Table 3, left). Furthermore, cardiac death was more common in patients with high cTNI (31% vs. 17%; $p = 0.001$). In line with this finding, higher rates of all-cause mortality at 24 hours (22% vs. 13%; $p = 0.001$) and 30 months (52% vs. 38%; $p = 0.001$) were seen in patients with high cTNI. The risk of the composite arrhythmic endpoint (i.e., recurrent ventricular tachyarrhythmias, appropriate ICD therapies and SCD) and cardiac rehospitalization at 30 months were not affected by cTNI within the unmatched study cohort. Notably, median intensive care unit (ICU) time was longer in patients with high cTNI (4 days (interquartile range (IQR) 2–10 days) vs. 4 days (IQR 1–8 days); $p = 0.001$), along with a shorter median follow-up time (624 vs. 1079 days) (Table 3, left panel).

Table 3. Endpoints and follow-up data before and after propensity score matching.

Characteristics	Without Propensity Score Matching				With Propensity Score Matching			
	Low cTNI (n = 549; 50%)		High cTNI (n = 555; 50%)		Low cTNI (n = 238; 50%)		High cTNI (n = 238; 50%)	
				p Value				p Value
Primary endpoint, n (%)								
All-cause mortality, at 30 days	119	(22)	221	(40)	**0.001**	43	(18)	71	(30)	**0.003**
Secondary endpoints, n (%)								
All-cause mortality, at 24 h	73	(13)	121	(22)	**0.001**	27	(11)	37	(16)	0.179
Cardiac death, at 30 days *	91/108	(17)	172/198	(31)	**0.001**	35/40	(15)	51/61	(21)	0.057
All-cause mortality, at 30 months	206	(38)	287	(52)	**0.001**	85	(36)	101	(42)	0.133
Cardiac rehospitalization, at 30 months	67	(12)	40	(7)	**0.005**	31	(13)	19	(8)	0.073
Composite arrhythmic endpoint (recurrence of ventricular tachyarrhythmias, sudden cardiac death), at 30 days	100	(21)	107	(23)	0.524	36	(15)	45	(19)	0.272
Composite arrhythmic endpoint (recurrence of ventricular tachyarrhythmias, sudden cardiac death), at 30 months	148	(27)	168	(30)	0.223	57	(24)	65	(27)	0.401
Follow-up times, n (%)								
Hospitalization total; days (median (IQR))	12 (7–20)		11 (5–22)		0.693	13 (8–23)		13 (7–24)		0.422
ICU time; days (median (IQR))	4 (1–8)		4 (2–10)		**0.001**	4 (1–9)		5 (2–10)		0.174
Follow-up; days (mean; median (range))	1183; 795 (0–4655)		891; 263 (0–4624)		**0.001**	1258; 1079 (0–4357)		1006; 624 (0–4626)		**0.008**

ICU, invasive care unit; IQR, interquartile range. * Mode of death was unknown in 14% of the patients at 30 days. Level of significance is $p \leq 0.05$. Bold type indicates $p \leq 0.05$.

Despite significant differences regarding the distribution of index tachyarrhythmias and comorbidities among patients with and without elevated cTNI levels, additional propensity score-matched analyses were performed (n = 238 patients with high and low cTNI). After propensity score matching (Tables 1 and 2, right panels), no further differences were observed regarding age, distribution of VT/VF and cardiovascular risk factors. Especially for LVEF, distribution of CAD and ICD rates were comparable in both groups. After propensity score matching, cTNI was still associated with increased risk of 30-day all-cause mortality (30% vs. 18%; log rank p = 0.003; HR = 1.729; 95% CI 1.184–2.525; p = 0.005) (Table 3; right panel; Figure 4). However, rates of all-cause mortality at 24 hours (16% vs. 11%; p = 0.179) and 30 months (42% vs. 36%; p = 0.133), as well as risk of the composite arrhythmic endpoint (19% vs. 15%; p = 0.272) and cardiac rehospitalization (8% vs. 13%; p = 0.073), did not differ in patients with and without elevated cTNI levels following propensity score matching (Table 3; right panel). Furthermore, follow-up times were significantly shorter (median 1006 vs. 1258 days; p = 0.001) in patients with high cTNI, whereas hospitalization and ICU times did not differ among patients with high or low cTNI (Table 3; right panel).

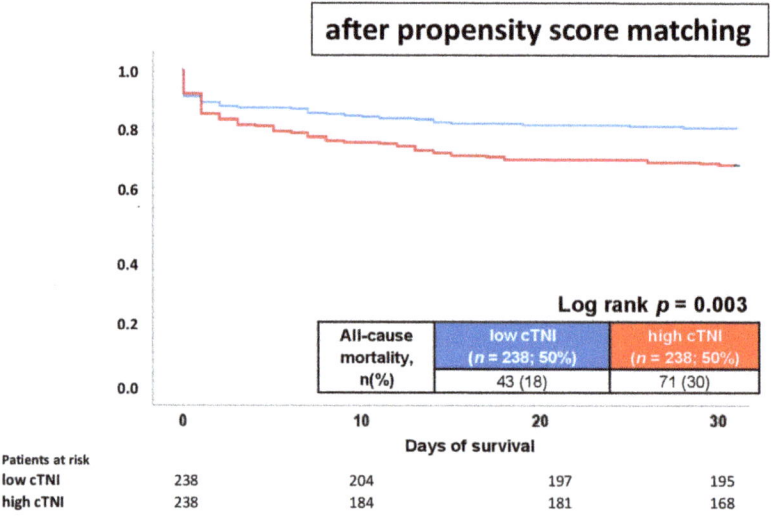

Figure 4. Kaplan–Meier analysis comparing patients with high cTNI to patients with low cTNI with regard to 30-day all-cause mortality (primary endpoint) within the propensity-matched cohort.

Subsequently, quartile analyses were performed within the entire, unmatched study cohort, whereas the following groups were analyzed: Q1: SIEMENS Dimension® RxL CTNI assay < 0.370 ng/mL; Beckman Coulter Access AccuTNI < 0.300 ng/mL; SIEMENS Dimension® Vista 1500™ < 0.380 ng/mL; Q2: SIEMENS Dimension® RxL CTNI assay 0.370–0.700 ng/mL; Beckman Coulter Access AccuTNI 0.300–0.800 ng/mL; SIEMENS Dimension® Vista 1500™ 0.380–610 ng/mL; Q3: SIEMENS Dimen-sion® RxL CTNI assay > 0.700–3.125 ng/mL; Beckman Coulter Access AccuTNI > 0.800–3.515 ng/mL; SIEMENS Dimension® Vista 1500™ > 0.610–2.2965 ng/mL; Q4: SIEMENS Dimension® RxL CTNI assay >3.125 ng/mL; Beckman Coulter Access AccuTNI > 3.515 ng/mL; SIEMENS Dimension® Vista 1500™ > 2.2965 ng/mL.

When analyzed as quartile analyses within the entire, unmatched study cohort, patients with high cTNI were associated with highest all-cause mortality at 30 days (HR = 3.639; 95% CI 2.504–5.288; p = 0.001), followed by patients with intermediate-high cTNI (HR = 3.071; 95% CI 2.101–4.489; p = 0.001) and low-intermediate cTNI (HR = 2.387; 95% CI 1.615–3.527; p = 0.001), as compared to patients with low cTNI (Figure 3; right panel).

3.3. Survival Analyses within Prespecified Subgroups

When focusing on prespecified subgroups within the unmatched study cohort, increased risk of mortality at 30 days in patients with high cTNI was observed in both patients admitted with index episodes of VT (HR = 2.694; 95% CI 1.762–4.121; p = 0.001) and VF (HR = 1.496; 95% CI 1.151–1.944; p = 0.004) (Figure 5).

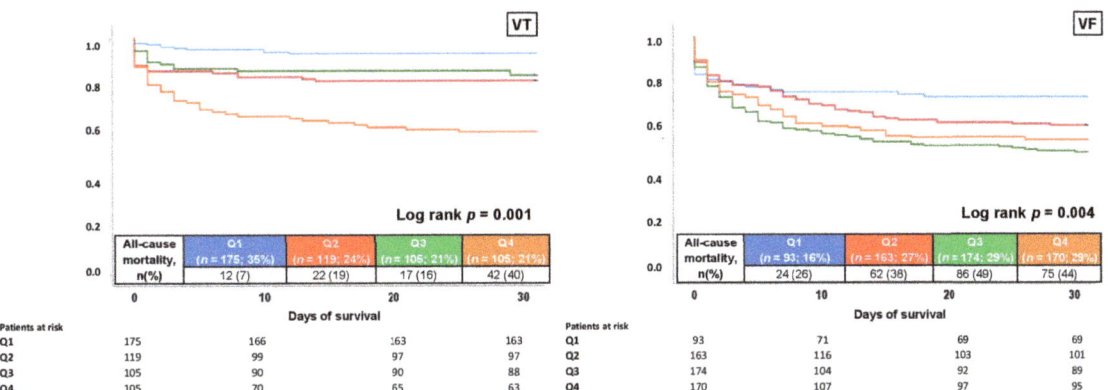

Figure 5. Kaplan–Meier analysis for cTNI with regard to the 30-day all-cause mortality (primary endpoint), stratified by patients with VT (**left** panel) and VF (**right** panel).

When stratified by the presence of AMI, no prognostic impact of cTNI was observed in patients with STEMI (HR = 1.258; 95% CI 0.563–2.813; p = 0.576), whereas patients with NSTEMI (HR = 2.030; 95% CI 1.249–3.300; p = 0.004) and non-AMI (HR = 2.364; 95% CI 1.772–3.152; p = 0.001) had increased risk of 30-day all-cause mortality when presenting with elevated cTNI (Figure 6).

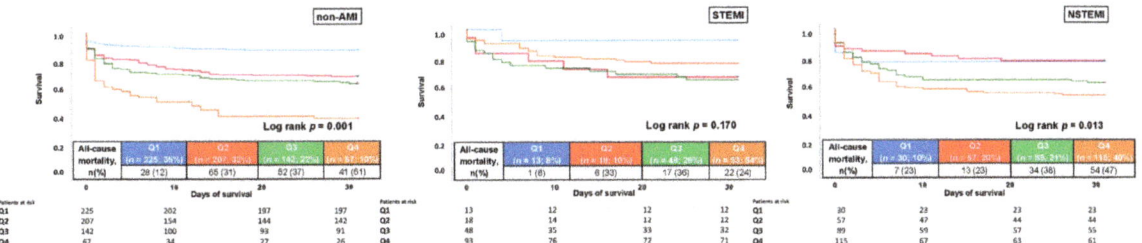

Figure 6. Kaplan–Meier analysis for cTNI with regard to 30-day all-cause mortality (primary endpoint), stratified by the presence or absence of AMI.

Subsequently, prognosis of cTNI was investigated within the subgroup of patients undergoing coronary angiography during index hospitalization. In patients undergoing coronary angiography, high cTNI was associated with increased risk of 30-day mortality in patients with no CAD (HR = 6.421; 95% CI 2.679–15.390; p = 0.001) and CAD (HR = 1.940; 95% CI 1.353–2.783; p = 0.001), and especially in those with MVD (HR = 1.985; 95% CI 1.292–3.048; p = 0.002), CTO (HR = 2.638; 95% CI 1.388–5.016; p = 0.003) and ICMP (HR = 2.106; 95% CI 1.476–3.004; p = 0.001) (Figure 7).

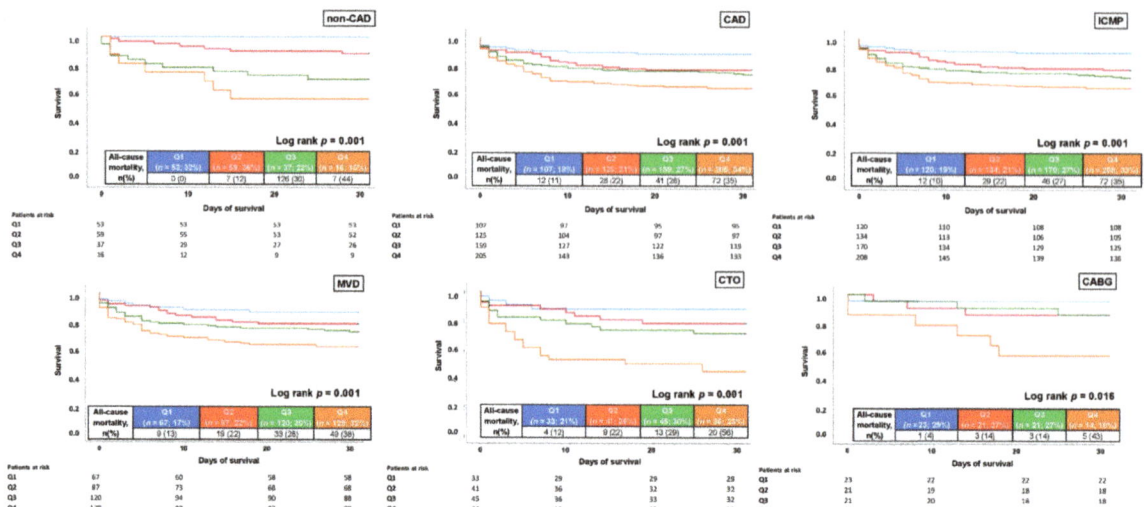

Figure 7. Kaplan–Meier analysis for cTNI with regard to 30-day all-cause mortality (primary endpoint) in different subgroups undergoing coronary angiography.

Finally, high cTNI was not significantly associated with 30-day all-cause mortality in patients with NICMP (HR = 6.299; 95% CI 0.703–56.414; p = 0.100), whereas all-cause mortality was increased in patients with idiopathic VT/VF in the presence of elevated cTNI (HR = 2.674; 95% CI 1.730–4.135; p = 0.001) (Supplemental Figure S1).

3.4. Multivariable Cox Regression Analysis

Even after multivariable adjustment within the entire, unmatched study cohort, high cTNI was associated with increased risk of all-cause mortality at 30 days (HR = 1.541; 95% CI 1.088–2.182; p = 0.0015). Besides cTNI, increased age (HR = 1.141; p = 0.042), chronic kidney disease (HR = 5.786; p = 0.001) and LVEF < 35% (HR = 1.260; p = 0.002) were particularly associated with increased risk of death, whereas the presence of an ICD (HR = 0.096; p = 0.001), electrophysiological examination (HR = 0.261; p = 0.001) and coronary angiography (HR = 0.505; p = 0.001) were associated with favorable outcomes at 30 days (Table 4).

Table 4. Uni- and multivariable Cox regression analysis with regard to 30-day all-cause mortality (primary endpoint).

	Univariable			Multivariable		
	HR	95% CI	p Value	HR	95% CI	p Value
Age	1.030	1.023–1.036	**0.001**	1.014	1.000–1.028	**0.042**
Males	0.843	0.718–0.990	**0.038**	1.232	0.837–1.814	0.291
Diabetes	1.213	1.031–1.428	**0.020**	0.948	0.672–1.336	0.759
Chronic Kidney disease	4.268	3.529–5.161	**0.001**	5.786	3.324–10.073	**0.001**
LVEF < 35%	1.322	1.070–1.633	**0.010**	1.260	1.090–1.458	**0.002**
Nonischemic cardiomyopathy	0.285	0.165–0.494	**0.001**	0.588	0.208–1.660	0.316
Coronary angiography	0.463	0.398–0.538	**0.001**	0.505	0.358–0.713	**0.001**
Electrophysiological examination	0.030	0.015–0.060	**0.001**	0.261	0.063–1.075	0.063
Presence of ICD	0.061	0.042–0.089	**0.001**	0.096	0.049–0.185	**0.001**
Hemoglobin	0.810	0.783–0.838	**0.001**	0.974	0.092–1.052	0.500
Serum potassium	1.481	1.354–1.621	**0.001**	1.130	0.954–1.339	0.157
high cTNI	2.004	1.603–2.505	**0.001**	1.541	1.088–2.182	**0.015**

CI, confidence interval; HR, hazard ratio; ICD, implantable cardioverter defibrillator; LVEF, left ventricular ejection faction. Level of significance is p < 0.05. Bold type indicates statistical significance.

Even when analyzed within important subgroups, both patients with index episodes of VT (HR = 2.333; 95% CI 1.276–4.276; p = 0.006) and VF (HR = 1.708; 95% CI 1.177–2.478; p = 0.005) had increased all-cause mortality at 30 days in the presence of increased cTNI (Table 5). This was still demonstrated in patients with idiopathic ventricular tachyarrhythmias (HR = 2.628; 95% CI 1.223–5.651; p = 0.013) and NICMP (HR = 12.164; 95% CI 0.999–148.093; p = 0.050).

Table 5. Uni- and multivariable hazard ratios for "high cTNI" with regard to 30-day all-cause mortality (primary endpoint) within prespecified subgroups.

	Univariable			Multivariable *		
	HR	95% CI	p Value	HR	95% CI	p Value
Ventricular tachycardia	2.694	1.762–4.121	**0.001**	2.333	1.276–4.267	**0.006**
Ventricular fibrillation	1.496	1.151–1.944	**0.003**	1.708	1.177–2.478	**0.005**
STEMI	1.258	0.563–2.813	0.576	5.047	0.657–38.607	0.120
NSTEMI	2.030	1.249–3.300	**0.004**	2.661	1.126–6.289	**0.026**
No myocardial infarction	2.364	1.772–3.152	**0.001**	1.963	1.331–2.897	**0.001**
Nonischemic cardiomyopathy	6.299	0.703–56.414	0.100	12.164	0.999–148.093	**0.050**
Idiopathic ventricular tachyarrhythmias	2.674	1.730–4.135	**0.001**	2.628	1.223–5.651	**0.013**
Patients with coronary angiography						
Coronary artery disease	1.940	1.353–2.783	**0.001**	1.799	1.093–2.960	**0.021**
No coronary artery disease	6.421	2.679–15.390	**0.001**	5.466	1.725–17.316	**0.004**
Multivessel disease	1.985	1.292–3.048	**0.002**	1.736	0.950–3.171	0.073
Presence of CABG	3.002	0.924–9.752	0.067	2.048	0.473–8.867	0.338
Chronic total occlusion	2.638	1.388–5.016	**0.003**	1.916	0.859–4.272	0.112
Ischemic cardiomyopathy	2.106	1.476–3.004	**0.001**	1.801	1.102–2.942	**0.019**

CI, confidence interval; HR, hazard ratio; CABG, coronary artery bypass grafting; LVEF, left ventricular ejection faction; NSTEMI, non-ST-segment elevation myocardial infarction. * Multivariable models were adjusted for age, sex, diabetes mellitus, chronic kidney disease, LVEF < 35% and nonischemic cardiomyopathies. Level of significance is $p < 0.05$. Bold type indicates statistical significance.

Furthermore, cTNI was associated with adverse outcomes in patients without AMI (HR = 1.963; 95% CI 1.331–2.897; p = 0.001) and NSTMI (HR = 2.661; 95% CI 1.126–6.289; p = 0.026), whereas cTNI had no prognostic impact in patients with STEMI (HR = 5.047; 95% CI 0.657–38.607; p = 0.120). Finally, patients with ischemic cardiomyopathy (HR = 1.801; 95% CI 1.102–2.942; p = 0.019) had especially increased risk of 30-day all-cause mortality when presenting with increased cTNI (Table 5).

3.5. Receiver Operating Characteristic (ROC) Analyses

The ROC analyses were performed within the entire, unmatched study cohort, as well as separately for patients with VT and VF. Despite the different cTNI assays, only cTNI values assessed by the SIEMENS Dimension® Vista 1500™ cTNI assay were included within this analysis. Thus, cTNI showed a moderate predictive value for mortality at 30 days following ventricular tachyarrhythmias (area under the curve (AUC) 0.687; 95% CI 0.595–0.691; p = 0.001) within the entire study cohort. However, cTNI was a more reliable predictive value in patients admitted with VT (AUC 0.734; 95% CI 0.645–0.823; p = 0.001). A cTNI level of 2.3105 ng/mL was determined to be the best cutoff value, with a sensitivity of 55% and a specificity of 85%, respectively. In contrast, cTNI was not predictive in the presence of VF (AUC 0.550; 95% CI 0.483–0.616; p = 0.166) (Figure 8).

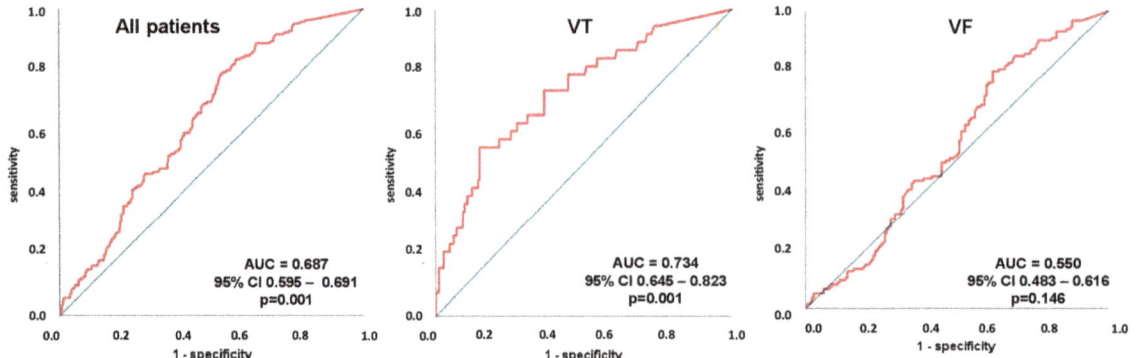

Figure 8. Receiver operator characteristic (ROC) curve analyses of cTNI for the prediction of 30-day all-cause mortality, stratified by patients within the entire study cohort, as well as separated by VT and VF.

Finally, cTNI assessed by the SIEMENS Dimension® Vista 1500™ cTNI assay showed reliable predictions of 30-day all-cause mortality in patients with coronary artery disease (AUC 0.684; 95% CI 0.598–0.769; $p = 0.044$) and NSTEMI (AUC 0.627; 95% CI 0.530–0.724; $p = 0.050$), whereas cTNI was not predictive for all-cause mortality in STEMI patients (AUC 0.559; 95% CI 0.429–0.690; $p = 0.379$) (Supplemental Table S1). Furthermore, cTNI showed good prediction of 30-day all-cause mortality in patients with idiopathic VT/VF (AUC 0.726; 95% CI 0.632–0.820; $p = 0.001$).

4. Discussion

The present study evaluated the prognostic impact of cTNI levels on 30-day all-cause mortality in patients presenting with ventricular tachyarrhythmias on hospital admission. This study suggests that there is increased short-term mortality in patients with increased cTNI, which was seen in patients admitted both with episodes of VT and VF. These findings were consistent, even after multivariable adjustment and propensity score matching. Patients with CAD, ICMP and MVD especially had increased risk of death in the presence of elevated cTNI. Even in VT patients, cTNI demonstrated valuable discrimination of the primary endpoint, with an AUC of 0.734. In contrast, long-term prognostic endpoints (including all-cause mortality and risk of the composite arrhythmic endpoint) were not affected by single cTNI measurements. Surprisingly, risk of cardiac rehospitalization was lower in patients with high cTNI, which was no longer observed after propensity score matching.

Although the identification of patients at high risk for SCD is of major clinical interest, data on the prognostic role of biomarkers in this setting are still limited [31]. Within a large case–control study that included six prospective cohorts and 565 SCD cases (as compared to 1090 matched controls), cTNI, NT-proBNP, high-density lipoprotein cholesterol ratio and high-sensitivity C-reactive protein were especially associated with an increased risk of SCD at 11 years [6]. In line with this finding, a serial increase from baseline cTNI was demonstrated to predict SCD in more than 3000 ambulatory patients who were included in the "Cardiovascular Health Study" [8].

In contrast, to the best of our knowledge, no currently available study has investigated the prognostic impact of cTNI in patients with ventricular tachyarrhythmias on hospital admission. However, some studies have already evaluated the prognostic value of cTNI in patients following CPR with heterogeneous findings. Within a single-center retrospective registry, including 277 patients admitted after out-of-hospital cardiac arrest (OHCA), peak troponin, but not initial troponin was especially associated with an increased risk of PCI. Both initial and peak troponin did not affect the risk of in-hospital death [32]. However, in that study, only 58% of the patients initially had a shockable rhythm, and no further subanalyses were performed with regard to patients with ventricular tachyarrhythmias. On the contrary, a targeted temperature management (TTM) trial substudy composed of 669 OHCA patients suggested that hs-TNT was associated with increased risk of cardiovascular death and multiorgan failure, while the proportion of patients with initial shockable rhythm was higher (79%) [33]. However, the present study has a different point of view, as it included patients with ventricular tachyarrhythmias and only 35% of the patients were admitted to the hospital following OHCA.

Within our study, elevated cTNI levels were associated with increased risk of short-term death, especially in patients with VT, and cTNI was revealed to be a reliable predictor of all-cause deaths. By now, it is well understood that VT occurs particularly in patients with adverse structural remodeling, mainly related to pre-existing CAD, leading to scar-mediated re-entry [34]. Especially due to advances in AMI treatment related to nationwide health-care supply, shorter door-to-balloon times and improved pharmacotherapies following AMI, the number of patients suffering from ischemic heart disease, as well as the number of patients with arrhythmic substrate, have increased [35]. This raises the relevance of improved therapies for VT (such as catheter ablation) and better identification of patients who are at high risk of death. Therefore, this study identifies the cTNI level as an independent predictor of all-cause mortality in patients with VT, with a potentially increased arrhythmic burden. Thus, cTNI was shown to be a good predictor for the need of PCI in patients with CAD, and was found to increase the risk of death in patients with CAD, especially in 3-vessel CAD.

Furthermore, several studies have investigated the prognostic role of cTNI with regard to the occurrence of ventricular tachyarrhythmias. For instance, Liu et al. found that elevated cTNI levels were associated with the occurrence of nonsustained VT in 755 patients with hypertrophic obstructive cardiomyopathy [36]. However, cTNI did not affect the risk of the composite arrhythmic endpoint (i.e., recurrent ventricular tachyarrhythmias, appropriate ICD therapies and SCD) at long-term follow-up. Further studies are necessary to prove the association of cTNI in ventricular tachyarrhythmias, especially focusing on sequential cTNI measurements.

This study has several limitations. Despite the retrospective study design, there may be some confounding due to unmeasured confounding variables, even though we adjusted for potential confounding factors using multivariable Cox regression and propensity score-matching analyses. Patients with ventricular tachyarrhythmias, who were not admitted to our institution due to nonresuscitated OHCA, were beyond the scope of the present study. Although we investigated the prognostic impact of cTNI in different CAD subgroups, important tools to assess the severity of CAD, such as the "Synergy between Percutaneous Coronary Intervention with Taxus and Cardiac Surgery" (SYNTAX) II score, were beyond the scope of the present study. For the present study, risk stratification was performed according to a single cTNI measurement. The cTNI levels during follow-up were only available for a minor portion of the study population, and were therefore beyond the scope of this study. No exact time from arrhythmia-to-cTNI measurement is available for the present study. In 90.6% of the patients, cTNI was assessed at the same day of the index event. Even after investigating the prognostic role of cTNI in patients who had their cTNI assessment on index day, the findings were consistent within both the unmatched and the matched cohorts. Furthermore, minor confounding may be present despite the use of different cTNI assays during the study period. Based on the different types of cTNI assays, ROC analyses were restricted to the SIEMENS Dimension® Vista intelligent lab system for contemporary sensitive cTNI testing. The mode of death was not available in 16% of the patients. Finally, despite the single-center study design, cardiac rehospitalization was assessed only at our institution.

5. Conclusions

In conclusion, in patients admitted with ventricular tachyarrhythmias, cTNI was associated with increased risk of all-cause mortality at 30 days. Especially in patients presenting with index episodes of VT, cTNI was a reliable predictor of all-cause death at 30 days.

Supplementary Materials: The following are available online at https://www.mdpi.com/article/10.3390/jcm11112987/s1, Table S1: Prognostic performance of cTNI for 30-day all-cause mortality in pre-specified subgroups, Figure S1: Prognostic impact of cTNI on 30-day all-cause mortality in patients with NICMP and idiopathic ventricular tachyarrhythmias.

Author Contributions: Conceptualization, T.S., M.B. and I.A.; methodology, T.S., M.A. (Mohammad Abumayyaleh), K.W., J.R., M.A. (Muharrem Akin) and M.K.; software, T.S., T.B. and M.B.; validation, T.S., M.B., J.M., T.B., D.G.M., K.W., J.R. and J.F.; formal analysis, T.S., M.K., M.A. (Muharrem Akin) and J.F.; investigation, T.S., M.B. and I.A.; resources, M.B., T.B., D.G.M. and I.A.; data curation, J.M., K.M., M.K., K.W., J.R., M.A. (Mohammad Abumayyaleh) and J.F.; writing—original draft preparation, I.A. and T.S.; writing—review and editing, T.S., M.B., I.A., K.W., J.R., K.M. and J.M.; visualization, T.S.; supervision, M.B. and I.A.; project administration, M.B. and I.A. All authors have read and agreed to the published version of the manuscript.

Funding: This research received no external funding.

Institutional Review Board Statement: The study was conducted according to the guidelines of the Declaration of Helsinki and approved by the Institutional Ethics Committee of Mannheim (2016-612N-MA).

Informed Consent Statement: Not applicable.

Data Availability Statement: The datasets used and/or analyzed during the current study are available from the corresponding author on reasonable request.

Conflicts of Interest: The authors declare no conflict of interest.

References

1. Burrell, A.J.; Pellegrino, V.A.; Wolfe, R.; Wong, W.K.; Cooper, D.J.; Kaye, D.M.; Pilcher, D.V. Long-term survival of adults with cardiogenic shock after venoarterial extracorporeal membrane oxygenation. *J. Crit. Care* **2015**, *30*, 949–956. [CrossRef] [PubMed]
2. Wong, C.X.; Brown, A.; Lau, D.H.; Chugh, S.S.; Albert, C.M.; Kalman, J.M.; Sanders, P. Epidemiology of Sudden Cardiac Death: Global and Regional Perspectives. *Heart Lung Circ.* **2019**, *28*, 6–14. [CrossRef] [PubMed]
3. Maggioni, A.P.; Anker, S.D.; Dahlström, U.; Filippatos, G.; Ponikowski, P.; Zannad, F.; Amir, O.; Chioncel, O.; Leiro, M.C.; Drozdz, J.; et al. Are hospitalized or ambulatory patients with heart failure treated in accordance with European Society of Cardiology guidelines? Evidence from 12,440 patients of the ESC Heart Failure Long-Term Registry. *Eur. J. Heart Fail.* **2013**, *15*, 1173–1184. [CrossRef]
4. Myerburg, R.J.; Junttila, M.J. Sudden cardiac death caused by coronary heart disease. *Circulation* **2012**, *125*, 1043–1052. [CrossRef] [PubMed]
5. Koplan, B.A.; Stevenson, W.G. Ventricular tachycardia and sudden cardiac death. *Mayo Clin. Proc.* **2009**, *84*, 289–297. [CrossRef] [PubMed]
6. Everett, B.M.; Moorthy, M.V.; Tikkanen, J.T.; Cook, N.R.; Albert, C.M. Markers of Myocardial Stress, Myocardial Injury, and Subclinical Inflammation and the Risk of Sudden Death. *Circulation* **2020**, *142*, 1148–1158. [CrossRef]
7. Priori, S.G.; Blomström-Lundqvist, C.; Mazzanti, A.; Blom, N.; Borggrefe, M.; Camm, J.; Elliott, P.M.; Fitzsimons, D.; Hatala, R.; Hindricks, G.; et al. 2015 ESC Guidelines for the management of patients with ventricular arrhythmias and the prevention of sudden cardiac death: The Task Force for the Management of Patients with Ventricular Arrhythmias and the Prevention of Sudden Cardiac Death of the European Society of Cardiology (ESC)Endorsed by: Association for European Paediatric and Congenital Cardiology (AEPC). *Eur. Heart J.* **2015**, *36*, 2793–2867. [CrossRef]
8. Hussein, A.A.; Gottdiener, J.S.; Bartz, T.M.; Sotoodehnia, N.; deFilippi, C.; Dickfeld, T.; Deo, R.; Siscovick, D.; Stein, P.K.; Lloyd-Jones, D. Cardiomyocyte injury assessed by a highly sensitive troponin assay and sudden cardiac death in the community: The Cardiovascular Health Study. *J. Am. Coll. Cardiol.* **2013**, *62*, 2112–2120. [CrossRef]
9. Patton, K.K.; Sotoodehnia, N.; DeFilippi, C.; Siscovick, D.S.; Gottdiener, J.S.; Kronmal, R.A. N-terminal pro-B-type natriuretic peptide is associated with sudden cardiac death risk: The Cardiovascular Health Study. *Heart Rhythm* **2011**, *8*, 228–233. [CrossRef]
10. Korngold, E.C.; Januzzi, J.L., Jr.; Gantzer, M.L.; Moorthy, M.V.; Cook, N.R.; Albert, C.M. Amino-terminal pro-B-type natriuretic peptide and high-sensitivity C-reactive protein as predictors of sudden cardiac death among women. *Circulation* **2009**, *119*, 2868–2876. [CrossRef]
11. Goldberger, J.J.; Bonow, R.O.; Cuffe, M.; Dyer, A.; Rosenberg, Y.; O'Rourke, R.; Shah, P.K.; Smith, S.C., Jr. beta-Blocker use following myocardial infarction: Low prevalence of evidence-based dosing. *Am. Heart J.* **2010**, *160*, 435–442. [CrossRef]

12. Shah, N.N.; Ayyadurai, P.; Saad, M.; Kosmas, C.E.; Dogar, M.U.; Patel, U.; Vittorio, T.J. Galactin-3 and soluble ST2 as complementary tools to cardiac MRI for sudden cardiac death risk stratification in heart failure: A review. *JRSM Cardiovasc. Dis.* **2020**, *9*, 2048004020957840. [CrossRef] [PubMed]
13. Sutanto, H.; Lyon, A.; Lumens, J.; Schotten, U.; Dobrev, D.; Heijman, J. Cardiomyocyte calcium handling in health and disease: Insights from in vitro and in silico studies. *Prog. Biophys. Mol. Biol.* **2020**, *157*, 54–75. [CrossRef] [PubMed]
14. Katrukha, I.A. Human cardiac troponin complex. Structure and functions. *Biochemistry* **2013**, *78*, 1447–1465. [CrossRef] [PubMed]
15. Chaulin, A.M. Cardiac Troponins Metabolism: From Biochemical Mechanisms to Clinical Practice (Literature Review). *Int. J. Mol. Sci.* **2021**, *22*, 10928. [CrossRef] [PubMed]
16. Shomanova, Z.; Ohnewein, B.; Schernthaner, C.; Höfer, K.; Pogoda, C.A.; Frommeyer, G.; Wernly, B.; Brandt, M.C.; Dieplinger, A.M.; Reinecke, H.; et al. Classic and Novel Biomarkers as Potential Predictors of Ventricular Arrhythmias and Sudden Cardiac Death. *J. Clin. Med.* **2020**, *9*, 578. [CrossRef] [PubMed]
17. Ghersin, I.; Zahran, M.; Azzam, Z.S.; Suleiman, M.; Bahouth, F. Prognostic value of cardiac troponin levels in patients presenting with supraventricular tachycardias. *J. Electrocardiol.* **2020**, *62*, 200–203. [CrossRef]
18. Nakamura, H.; Niwano, S.; Fukaya, H.; Murakami, M.; Kishihara, J.; Satoh, A.; Yoshizawa, T.; Oikawa, J.; Ishizue, N.; Igarashi, T.; et al. Cardiac troponin T as a predictor of cardiac death in patients with left ventricular dysfunction. *J. Arrhythm* **2017**, *33*, 463–468. [CrossRef]
19. Schupp, T.; Behnes, M.; Weiß, C.; Nienaber, C.; Lang, S.; Reiser, L.; Bollow, A.; Taton, G.; Reichelt, T.; Ellguth, D.; et al. Beta-Blockers and ACE Inhibitors Are Associated with Improved Survival Secondary to Ventricular Tachyarrhythmia. *Cardiovasc. Drugs Ther.* **2018**, *32*, 353–363. [CrossRef]
20. Apple, F.S.; Collinson, P.O. Analytical characteristics of high-sensitivity cardiac troponin assays. *Clin. Chem.* **2012**, *58*, 54–61. [CrossRef]
21. Ibanez, B.; James, S.; Agewall, S.; Antunes, M.J.; Bucciarelli-Ducci, C.; Bueno, H.; Caforio, A.L.P.; Crea, F.; Goudevenos, J.A.; Halvorsen, S.; et al. 2017 ESC Guidelines for the management of acute myocardial infarction in patients presenting with ST-segment elevation: The Task Force for the management of acute myocardial infarction in patients presenting with ST-segment elevation of the European Society of Cardiology (ESC). *Eur. Heart J.* **2018**, *39*, 119–177. [CrossRef] [PubMed]
22. Behnes, M.; Mashayekhi, K.; Weiß, C.; Nienaber, C.; Lang, S.; Reiser, L.; Bollow, A.; Taton, G.; Reichelt, T.; Ellguth, D.; et al. Prognostic Impact of Acute Myocardial Infarction in Patients Presenting With Ventricular Tachyarrhythmias and Aborted Cardiac Arrest. *J. Am. Heart Assoc.* **2018**, *7*, e010004. [CrossRef] [PubMed]
23. Elliott, P.; Andersson, B.; Arbustini, E.; Bilinska, Z.; Cecchi, F.; Charron, P.; Dubourg, O.; Kühl, U.; Maisch, B.; McKenna, W.J. Classification of the cardiomyopathies: A position statement from the European Society Of Cardiology Working Group on Myocardial and Pericardial Diseases. *Eur. Heart J.* **2008**, *29*, 270–276. [CrossRef]
24. Elliott, P.M. Classification of cardiomyopathies: Evolution or revolution? *J. Am. Coll. Cardiol.* **2013**, *62*, 2073–2074. [CrossRef] [PubMed]
25. Rapezzi, C.; Arbustini, E.; Caforio, A.L.; Charron, P.; Gimeno-Blanes, J.; Heliö, T.; Linhart, A.; Mogensen, J.; Pinto, Y.; Ristic, A. Diagnostic work-up in cardiomyopathies: Bridging the gap between clinical phenotypes and final diagnosis. A position statement from the ESC Working Group on Myocardial and Pericardial Diseases. *Eur. Heart J.* **2013**, *34*, 1448–1458. [CrossRef] [PubMed]
26. Rusnak, J.; Behnes, M.; Weiß, C.; Nienaber, C.; Reiser, L.; Schupp, T.; Bollow, A.; Taton, G.; Reichelt, T.; Ellguth, D.; et al. Non-ischemic compared to ischemic cardiomyopathy is associated with increasing recurrent ventricular tachyarrhythmias and ICD-related therapies. *J. Electrocardiol.* **2020**, *59*, 174–180. [CrossRef]
27. Behnes, M.; Akin, I.; Kuche, P.; Schupp, T.; Reiser, L.; Bollow, A.; Taton, G.; Reichelt, T.; Ellguth, D.; Engelke, N.; et al. Coronary chronic total occlusions and mortality in patients with ventricular tachyarrhythmias. *EuroIntervention* **2020**, *15*, 1278–1285. [CrossRef]
28. Behnes, M.; Mashayekhi, K.; Kuche, P.; Kim, S.H.; Schupp, T.; von Zworowsky, M.; Reiser, L.; Bollow, A.; Taton, G.; Reichelt, T.; et al. Prognostic impact of coronary chronic total occlusion on recurrences of ventricular tachyarrhythmias and ICD therapies. *Clin. Res. Cardiol.* **2021**, *110*, 281–291. [CrossRef]
29. Yin, J.; Samawi, H.; Linder, D. Improved nonparametric estimation of the optimal diagnostic cut-off point associated with the Youden index under different sampling schemes. *Biom. J.* **2016**, *58*, 915–934. [CrossRef]
30. Yin, J.; Tian, L. Joint confidence region estimation for area under ROC curve and Youden index. *Stat. Med.* **2014**, *33*, 985–1000. [CrossRef]
31. Osman, J.; Tan, S.C.; Lee, P.Y.; Low, T.Y.; Jamal, R. Sudden Cardiac Death (SCD)—Risk stratification and prediction with molecular biomarkers. *J. Biomed. Sci.* **2019**, *26*, 39. [CrossRef] [PubMed]
32. Pearson, D.A.; Wares, C.M.; Mayer, K.A.; Runyon, M.S.; Studnek, J.R.; Ward, S.L.; Kraft, K.M.; Heffner, A.C. Troponin Marker for Acute Coronary Occlusion and Patient Outcome Following Cardiac Arrest. *West J. Emerg. Med.* **2015**, *16*, 1007–1013. [CrossRef] [PubMed]
33. Gilje, P.; Koul, S.; Thomsen, J.H.; Devaux, Y.; Friberg, H.; Kuiper, M.; Horn, J.; Nielsen, N.; Pellis, T.; Stammet, P.; et al. High-sensitivity troponin-T as a prognostic marker after out-of-hospital cardiac arrest—A targeted temperature management (TTM) trial substudy. *Resuscitation* **2016**, *107*, 156–161. [CrossRef] [PubMed]
34. Lopez, E.M.; Malhotra, R. Ventricular Tachycardia in Structural Heart Disease. *J. Innov. Card. Rhythm Manag.* **2019**, *10*, 3762–3773. [CrossRef] [PubMed]

35. Ajijola, O.A.; Tung, R.; Shivkumar, K. Ventricular tachycardia in ischemic heart disease substrates. *Indian Heart J.* **2014**, *66* (Suppl. 1), S24–S34. [CrossRef]
36. Liu, L.; Liu, S.; Shen, L.; Tu, B.; Hu, Z.; Hu, F.; Zheng, L.; Ding, L.; Fan, X.; Yao, Y. Correlations between cardiac troponin I and nonsustained ventricular tachycardia in hypertrophic obstructive cardiomyopathy. *Clin. Cardiol.* **2020**, *43*, 1150–1159. [CrossRef]

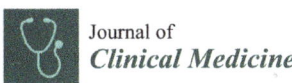

Article

One-Year Follow-Up of Patients Admitted for Emergency Coronary Angiography after Resuscitated Cardiac Arrest

Quentin Delbaere [1,*], Myriam Akodad [1], François Roubille [1], Benoît Lattuca [2], Guillaume Cayla [2] and Florence Leclercq [1]

1. Department of Cardiology, Arnaud de Villeneuve University Hospital, 34295 Montpellier, France; m-akodad@chu-montpellier.fr (M.A.); f-roubille@chu-montpellier.fr (F.R.); f-leclercq@chu-montpellier.fr (F.L.)
2. Department of Cardiology, Caremeau University Hospital, 30900 Nîmes, France; benoit.lattuca@chu-nimes.fr (B.L.); guillaume.cayla@chu-nimes.fr (G.C.)
* Correspondence: q-delbaere@chu-montpellier.fr

Abstract: (1) Background: Despite the improvement of the in-hospital survival rate after aborted sudden cardiac death (SCD), cerebral anoxia may have severe neurologic consequences and may impair long-term outcome and quality of life of surviving patients. The aim of this study was to assess neurological outcomes at one year after resuscitated cardiac arrest; (2) Methods: This prospective, observational, and multicentre study included patients >18 yo admitted in the catheterisation laboratory for coronary angiography after aborted SCD between 1 May 2018 and 31 May 2020. Only patients who were discharged alive from hospital were evaluated. The primary endpoint was survival without neurological sequelae at one-year follow-up defined by a cerebral performance category (CPC) of one or two. Secondary end points included all-cause mortality, New York Heart Association (NYHA) functional class, neurologic evaluation at discharge, three-month and one-year follow-up using the CPC scale, and quality of life at 1 year using the Quality of Life after Brain Injury (QOLIBRI) questionnaire; (3) Results: Among 143 patients admitted for SCD within the study period, 61 (42.7%) were discharged alive from hospital, among whom 55 (90.1%) completed the one-year follow-up. No flow and low flow times were 1.9 ± 2.4 min and 16.5 ± 10.4 min, respectively. For 93.4% of the surviving patients, an initial shockable rhythm ($n = 57$) was observed and acute coronary syndrome was diagnosed in 75.4% of them ($n = 46$). At 1 year, survival rate without neurologic sequelae was 87.2% ($n = 48$). Patients with poor outcome were older (69.3 vs. 57.4 yo; $p = 0.04$) and had lower body mass index (22.4 vs. 26.7; $p = 0.013$) and a lower initial Left Ventricle Ejection Fraction (LVEF) (32.1% vs. 40.3%; $p = 0.046$). During follow-up, neurological status improved in 36.8% of patients presenting sequelae at discharge, and overall quality of life was satisfying for 66.7% of patients according to the QOLIBRI questionnaire; (4) Conclusions: Among patients admitted to the catheterisation laboratory for aborted SCD, mainly related to Acute Coronary Syndrom (ACS), less than a half of them were alive at discharge. However, the one-year survival rate without neurological sequelae was high and overall quality of life was good.

Keywords: sudden cardiac death; coronary angiography; neurological sequelae; quality of life

Citation: Delbaere, Q.; Akodad, M.; Roubille, F.; Lattuca, B.; Cayla, G.; Leclercq, F. One-Year Follow-Up of Patients Admitted for Emergency Coronary Angiography after Resuscitated Cardiac Arrest. *J. Clin. Med.* **2022**, *11*, 3738. https://doi.org/10.3390/jcm11133738

Academic Editors: Michael Behnes and Tobias Schupp

Received: 17 May 2022
Accepted: 17 June 2022
Published: 28 June 2022

Publisher's Note: MDPI stays neutral with regard to jurisdictional claims in published maps and institutional affiliations.

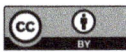

Copyright: © 2022 by the authors. Licensee MDPI, Basel, Switzerland. This article is an open access article distributed under the terms and conditions of the Creative Commons Attribution (CC BY) license (https://creativecommons.org/licenses/by/4.0/).

1. Introduction

Every year, about 350,000 sudden cardiac deaths (SCDs) are reported in the United States and 40,000–50,000 in France, mainly due to acute coronary syndrome (80%) and ventricular fibrillation (VF) [1–3]. Few studies have shown the benefit of immediate coronary angiography (CA) in survivors of out of hospital cardiac arrest (OHCA), especially in the setting of ST-segment elevation myocardial infarction (STEMI) [4,5]. The 2017 European Society of Cardiology Guidelines for the management of patients presenting with STEMI recommended direct admission to the catheterisation laboratory (cathlab) in comatose survivors of OHCA with electrocardiographic criteria for STEMI on the post-resuscitation electrocardiogram (ECG) (Class I, grade B) [6]. In the absence of STEMI criteria, admission to an intensive care unit first is recommended to exclude a non-coronary cause (Class IIa, grade B). Unconscious patients admitted to critical care units after SCD are at high risk for death, and neurologic deficits are common among the survivors [7]. Despite improvement in SCD management, the survival rate remains poor [8]. However, for the past few years, the number of immediate CA in patients with OHCA has increased, and prognosis was much more favourable with an 80% survival rate at discharge in a recent report [9]. During SCD, the brain suffers from temporary blood flow limitation, leading to hypoxic brain injury and cognitive impairment [7]. For survivors, the global anoxia can have severe neurological consequences [10]. While the survival rate seems to be well-known, neurological condition of this group of patients is poorly studied [11]. We therefore aimed to assess long-term neurological prognosis of survivors from SCD initially referred to the cathlab for CA.

2. Materials and Methods

This study was a prospective, observational, and multicentre registry. First, we checked all patients >18 yo who were admitted directly in the cathlab for out of hospital SCD between 1 May 2018 and 31 May 2020 in Montpellier and Nîmes University Hospitals. Then, we excluded patients who presented ventricular arrhythmia with immediate return of normal consciousness, patients without a return of spontaneous rhythm, or patients who died during the in-hospital stay. Therefore, only patients discharged alive from hospital were included for follow-up analysis. Nimes and Montpellier are university hospitals with intensive care units including cardiac monitoring, where appropriate invasive and non-invasive testing can be performed. A cardiovascular team, including interventional cardiology, electrophysiology, and cardiac surgery, are available. Nearly 150 cardiac arrests are admitted directly in the cathlab per year in these two centres.

The primary end point was the survival rate without significant neurological sequelae at one-year follow-up. Neurological outcome was assessed using the cerebral performance categories (CPC) of the Glasgow-Pittsburgh Outcome Categories: Category 1 is conscious and normal; Category 2 is conscious with moderate disability; Category 3 is conscious with severe disability; Category 4 is coma or vegetative state; and Category 5 is death [12–14]. We defined an absence of significant neurological sequelae as conscious, CPC 1 or 2, at one-year follow-up [15]. Secondary end points included total survival and survival without neurological sequelae (CPC 1 or 2) at 3 months, total survival at 1 year, New York Heart Association (NYHA) functional class at 3 months and 1 year, and quality of life at 1 year using the Quality of Life after Brain Injury (QOLIBRI) questionnaire. Quality of life was recorded by phone call or mail for SCD survivors without neurological sequelae at one-year follow-up. The QOLIBRI questionnaire is a novel health-related quality of life (HRQoL) instrument specifically developed for traumatic brain injury providing HRQoL in 6 fields [16,17]. This questionnaire has already been used to evaluate quality of life after an SCD [18]. It consists of 37 items in six scales summarised in Figure 1.

QOLIBRI Scale	Number of items	Content
		"Satisfaction" items
Cognition	7	Cognitive problems such as memory, attention, expressive speech, and decision making
Self	7	Aspects of self, including energy, motivation, physical appearance, and self-esteem
Daily life and autonomy	7	Independence, activities of daily life, and participation in social roles
Social relationships	6	Relationships with friends, family, and partner
		"Bothered" items
Emotions	5	Feelings of depression, anxiety, loneliness, boredom, and anger
Physical problems	5	Physical problems, such as slowness, pain, sensory impairment, or other consequences of injury

Figure 1. QOLIBRI, Quality of Life after Brain Injury.

Patient characteristics, cardiopulmonary resuscitation (CPR) data (time, location, actors, and methods), and intra-hospital progress were collected at inclusion. If available (by phone call or through medical reports), an initial evaluation was performed at 3 months, with survival rate and cardiac and neurological evaluation. The cardiac and neurological status were also collected at one-year follow-up either by using DxCare software or by a phone call. A questionnaire was offered to all patients at one-year follow-up and was obtained by phone or by mail. At this moment, full study information was given and consent was obtained. No additional testing or biological samples were specifically required for the study.

Considering that our active patient file includes 150 cardiac arrests per year, of which 30 are discharged alive per year, we anticipated the inclusion of 60 patients discharged alive from hospital over a two-year period. Based on a previous study [13], we hypothesised that 10% of patients discharged alive from hospital would have severe neurological sequelae at one-year follow-up. Patient characteristics are presented using mean and standard deviation (SD) for continuous variables and frequencies and proportions for categorical variables. The chi-square test or Fisher's exact test was used to compare categorical variables between groups ("good" and "poor" outcome). The Student's *t*-test or the Wilcoxon–Mann–Whitney test was used to compare continuous variables. All analyses were conducted using R software (R Core Team, version 4.0.5, 2021, Vienna, Austria).

3. Results

3.1. Study Population

A flow chart is presented in Figure 2. A total of 143 patients were admitted directly to the cathlab for aborted SCD after return of spontaneous circulation (ROSC) between May 2018 and May 2020. In-hospital mortality was 57.3% (*n* = 82), 61 patients were therefore alive at discharge, with a mean age of 59.4 ± 14.1 yo and 77.0% (*n* = 47) being men. Baseline characteristics are presented in Table 1. Characteristics of six patients lost to follow-up were not different from our baseline population.

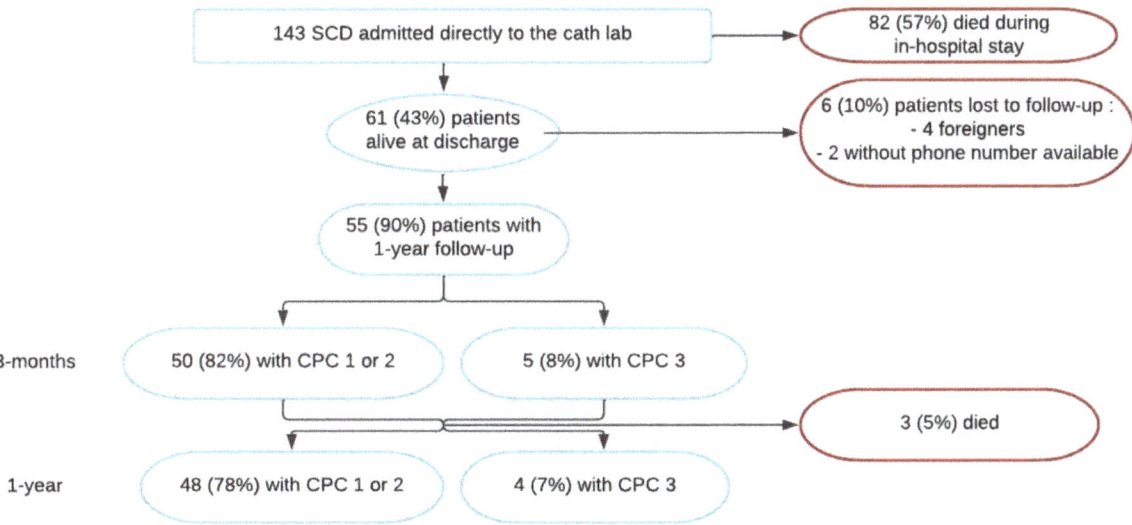

Figure 2. Flow chart. CPC: Cerebral Performance Category; SCD: Sudden Cardiac Death.

Table 1. Patients' study baseline characteristics.

Characteristics n (%)	n = 61
Age (yo)	59.4 ± 14.1
Male sex	47 (77.0)
Current smoking	19 (31.1)
Hypertension	25 (41.0)
Diabetes	5 (8.2)
Dyslipidemia	11 (18.0)
Body mass index, kg/m^2	25.9 ± 4.9
History of ischemic cardiopathy	13 (21.3)
Chronic kidney disease	5 (8.2)
Cardiopulmonary resuscitation:	
>Witness	
Bystander no. (%)	21 (34.4)
Fireman no. (%)	11 (18.0)
Doctor no. (%)	18 (29.5)
Family no. (%)	11 (18.0)
>Location of SCD	
Outdoor no. (%)	25 (41.0)
Home no. (%)	25 (41.0)
Emergency department no. (%)	11 (18.0)
>Timeline	
No-Flow (min)	1.9 ± 2.4
Low-Flow (min)	16.5 ± 10.4
Total (m)	18.3 ± 11.6
Initial shockable rhythm no. (%)	57 (93.4)
Dose of adrenaline (mg)	1.31 ± 2.08
STEMI on ECG after ROSC no. (%)	36 (59.0)
LVEF after ROSC (%)	35.4 ± 16.1
>Main coronary lesion	
Left main coronary no. (%)	1 (1.6)
Left anterior descending no. (%)	25 (41.0)
Left circumflex no. (%)	7 (11.5)
Right coronary no. (%)	13 (21.3)
None	15 (24.6)
>Biology	
hs-cTNT (ng/L)	4818 ± 7342
Creatinin peak (µmol/L)	131 ± 109
K$^+$ (mmol/L)	4.1 ± 0.66
ASAT (UI/L)	280 ± 260
pH	7.34 ± 0.1
Lactate peak (mmol/L)	± 1.9
>Evolution	
Length of ICU stay (d)	7.16 ± 8.32
Length of hospital stay (d)	18.9 ± 11.6
Presence of wall motion abnormalities at entry no. (%)	51 (83.6)
Implantable cardioverter defibrillator no. (%)	19 (31.1)
LVEF > 50% at discharge no. (%)	29 (47.5)
Transfer to rehabilitation centre at discharge no. (%)	18 (29.5)

± Standard Deviation, CA: Cardiac Arrest, ICU: Intensive Cardiac Unit, ROSC: Return of Spontaneous Circulation. LVEF: Left Ventricular Ejection Fraction.

Regarding the cardiovascular risk factors, hypertension was the most frequently observed (n = 25, 40.9%). No-flow duration was 1.9 ± 2.4 min, low-flow duration was 16.5 ± 10.4 min, and an initial shockable rhythm was found in 93.4% of patients (n = 57). Twenty-nine patients (47.5%) of the survival patients at discharge had an SCD in the presence of a witness: for 18 patients (29.5%) in front of a doctor, for 8 patients (13.1%) in the emergency department, and for 3 patients (4.9%), SCD occurred during a hospital stay. The electrocardiogram immediately after the return of spontaneous circulation mostly showed a STEMI (n = 36, 59.0%). The CA found an artery occlusion in 27 patients (44%) and normal status in 15 patients (25%). At discharge, 29 patients (47%) had a left ventricular ejection fraction (LVEF) $\geq$ 50%. Rehabilitation was offered to all patients at discharge: 30% (n = 18), due to medical issues, were directly transferred from hospital to a general rehabilitation centre for neurological improvement, and the others went home to recover before benefiting from cardiac rehabilitation.

Regarding causes of SCD (Figure 3), 75.4% (n = 46) were related to ventricular tachycardia or fibrillation resulting from an acute ischemic syndrome. Of these, 78.2% (n = 36) were due to a STEMI and 21.7% (n = 10) resulted from a severe artery stenosis. Furthermore, 19.7% (n = 12) patients presented with a VT or VF resulting from a non-ischemic cardiopathy, 13.1% (n = 8) with dilated cardiomyopathy, and 6.6% (n = 4) with hypertrophic cardiomyopathy). The last three patients (4.9%) had an initial non-shockable rhythm from an extra-cardiac cause (one stroke, one pulmonary embolism, and one unknown aetiology).

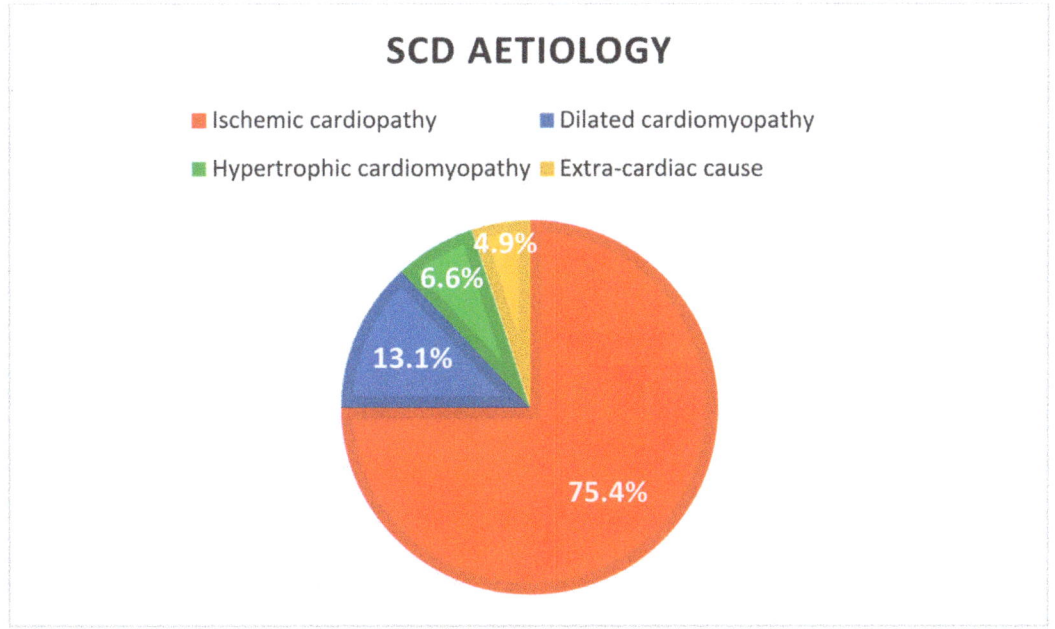

Figure 3. SCD aetiology (n = 61). SCD: Sudden Cardiac Death.

3.2. Primary End Point

At one-year follow-up, clinical information was available for 55 patients (reports, phone call, or mail), representing 90.1% of our cohort. Among them, 48 (87.3%) patients were alive without neurologic sequelae as defined previously. A total of three patients (5.5%) died during follow-up and four (7.3%) had severe neurological sequelae (Category 3 on CPC). These seven patients (12.7%) were therefore classified in the "poor event" group (Figure 4).

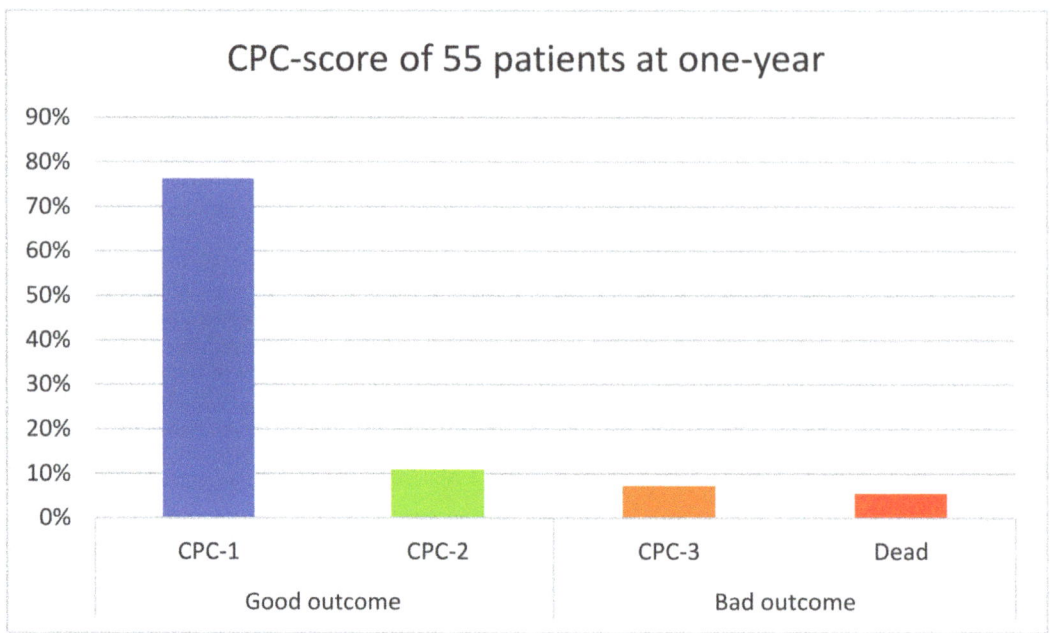

Figure 4. Primary End Point in 55 patients; CPC: Cerebral Performance Category.

In the "good outcome" group, six patients (13%) were classified in CPC 2, meaning mild-to-moderate disabilities.

3.3. Secondary End Points

Secondary end points are listed in Table 2.

Table 2. Secondary end points of 55 patients.

Event	3 Months	1 Year
Total survival no. (%)	55 (100)	52 (94.5)
CPC no. (%)	n = 55	n = 52
1	43 (78.2)	42 (80.7)
2	7 (12.7)	6 (11.5)
3	5 (9.1)	4 (7.7)
Death from cardiac cause no. (%)	0 (0)	0 (0)
NYHA		
1	28 (50.9)	36 (69.2)
2	27 (49.1)	14 (26.9)
3	0 (0)	1 (2)
4	0 (0)	1 (2)
LVEF (%) Mean $\pm$ SD	49 $\pm$ 11	51.5 $\pm$ 9.2

CPC: Cerebral Performance Category, NYHA: New York Heart Association, LVEF: Left Ventricular Ejection Fraction.

All patients were alive at three-month follow-up. Among the three patients who died at one-year follow-up, none died from cardiovascular causes (two died from sepsis and one from stroke). A total of 19 (35%) patients were hospitalised in the year following the SCD. At discharge, $n = 6$ (10%) patients were classified in CPC 3, $n = 13$ (21%) were CPC 2, and $n = 42$ (69%) were CPC 1. Among patients with CPC 2 or 3, $n = 7$ (37%) recovered during the follow-up: one from CPC 3 to CPC 2 and six from CPC 2 to CPC 1.

Cardiac evolution was also favourable with mean LVEF $\geq$ 50% at 1 year (49.1% at 3 months versus 51.5% at 1 year, $p = 0.037$)). Only three patients (5%) experienced a recurrence of VT/FV and two (4%) suffered a new ischemic event. The number of patients with NYHA functional class I increased from 28 (51%) at 3 months to 36 (69%) at 1 year. We therefore compared characteristics between the two groups named "good outcome" and "bad outcome" (Table 3).

Table 3. Univariate analysis.

Characteristic	Good Outcome (n = 48)	Poor Outcome (n = 7)	p Value
Age (y)	57.4 ± 13.6	69.3 ± 9.4	**0.036**
Male sex no. (%)	35 (72.9)	7 (100)	0.18
Body mass index kg/m^2	26.7 ± 5	22.4 ± 2.2	**0.013**
Current smoking no. (%)	14 (29.2)	3 (42.9)	0.66
Hypertension no. (%)	20 (41.7)	4 (57.1)	0.69
Diabetes no. (%)	5 (10.4)	0 (0)	1
Dyslipidemia no. (%)	10 (20.8)	1 (14.3)	1
CKD no. (%)	4 (8.3)	1 (14.3)	0.51
Low flow (min)	16.4 ± 10.7	17 ± 9.3	0.72
No flow (min)	1.9 ± 2.5	2 ± 2.2	0.68
Total CPR (min)	18.3 ± 11.8	19 ± 11	0.65
LAD culprit no. (%)	18 (37.5)	4 (57.1)	0.78
STEMI no. (%)	28 (58.3)	4 (57.1)	0.5
Occlusion no. (%)	20 (41.7)	3 (42.8)	0.88
Outdoor no. (%)	19 (39.6)	4 (57.1)	0.22
Home no. (%)	22 (45.8)	1 (14.3)	0.22
Witness no. (%)	15 (31.3)	4 (57.1)	0.45
Initial shockable no. (%)	44 (91.7)	7 (100)	1
Length of hospital stay (d)	17.6 ± 12.5	31.7 ± 28.6	0.11
Length of reanimation stay (d)	7.5 ± 8.8	7.4 ± 7.7	0.93
ASAT (UI/L)	282 ± 240	356 ± 430	1
K$^+$ (mmol/L)	4 ± 0.6	4.5 ± 0.7	0.16
Lactate peak (mmol/L)	2.8 ± 2	3.5 ± 2	0.23
hs-cTNT (ng/L)	4362 ± 6363	9417 ± 13,903	0.98
Creatinin peak (µmol/L)	140 ± 120	107 ± 29.3	0.88
Initial LVEF (%)	40.3 ± 12	32.1 ± 5.7	**0.046**
LVEF at discharge (%)	48.4 ± 11	41.4 ± 14.1	0.2
LVEF at 3 months (%)	50.1 ± 10.6	42.9 ± 12.5	0.13
LVEF at 1 year (%)	51.9 ± 9.3	46.3 ± 4.7	0.19

CKD: Chronic Kidney Disease (Glomerular Fraction Rate < 50 mL/min/1.73 m^2), CPR: Cardiopulmonary Resuscitation, ICD: Implantable Cardiac Device, LAD: Left Anterior Descending, STEMI: ST-segment Elevation Myocardial Infarction, AST: Aspartate Transaminase, LVEF: Left Ventricular Ejection Fraction. Bold: $p < 0.05$, statistically significant.

In the "poor outcome" group, patients were significantly older (69.3 yo versus 57.4 yo, $p = 0.036$), with lower BMI (22.4 kg/m^2 versus 26.7 kg/m^2, $p = 0.013$), and had lower initial LVEF (32.1 ± 5.7 vs. 40.3 ± 12, $p = 0.046$). Regarding SCD characteristics, there was no difference between the two groups on no-flow or low-flow times and location of initial cardiopulmonary resuscitation (CPR).

3.4. Quality of Life

Among the 48 patients contacted to complete the QOLIBRI questionnaire, 36 (75%) returned the mail or accepted to answer by phone call. Results are represented in Table 4. Scores in "satisfaction items" were quite homogeneous with 23.25 ± 6.34 for cognition, 22.14 ± 5 for self, 23.53 ± 7.2 for daily life activities, and 19.56 ± 3.7 for social relationships.

In "bothered items", scores were also similar with 12 ± 4.6 for emotion and 10.9 ± 4 for physical problems.

Table 4. Mean score for each item of QOLIBRI.

Quality of Life (QOLIBRI)	Mean Score ± SD	Range of the Questionnaire
Part I: Satisfaction	88.5 ± 20	[20-140]
Cognition	23.25 ± 6.3	[5-35]
Self	22.14 ± 5	[5-35]
Daily life activities	23.53 ± 7.2	[5-35]
Social relationships	19.56 ± 3.7	[5-25]
Part II: Problems and complaints	22.9 ± 8.3	[10-40]
Emotion	12 ± 4.6	[5-20]
Physical problems	10.9 ± 4	[5-20]

If we group the answers according to the scale of the questionnaire (from "not at all" to "very"), $n = 18$, 50% of patients were globally satisfied with their quality of life, and $n = 20$, 56% of patients did not report major health problems (Appendix A).

4. Discussion

Our study aimed to evaluate the survival rate and the neurological status of patients discharged alive from hospital after an aborted SCD referred for emergency CA with three main findings: (1) patients discharged alive were relatively young, with few cardiovascular risk factors and with an initial shockable rhythm (97%) mainly related to an ischemic aetiology (75%); (2) the survival rate without neurological sequelae at 1 year was high (87%); (3) younger age, lower BMI, and initial better LVEF were associated with survival with good neurological prognosis. For survivors, neurologic and psychological outcome were the main issues with a moderate impairment of quality of life at one-year follow-up.

Acute ischemic aetiology (with or without coronary occlusion) was identified in 75% of patients, and PCI was performed in most of them. We evaluated the outcome of successfully resuscitated patients who were discharged alive. The survival rate without neurological sequelae at 1 year was 87%, which is very encouraging. We selected patients admitted directly to the cathlab with suspicion of ACS and with hemodynamic success of CPR. According to guidelines, only patients with electrocardiographic criteria in favour of ischemic aetiology on the post-resuscitation electrocardiogram (ECG) may have emergency CA in our centres. As we also excluded patients who died during in-hospital stay (57% of patients), our population was highly selective and was relatively young, with normal BMI and a few cardiovascular risk factors. Moreover, time of no and low flow was relatively short, with the presence of a witness in near half of cases, explaining a sub-normal pH on admission. As we expected, almost all of our patients initially presented a shockable rhythm at the time of the SCD. The cardiac aetiology (ischemic and non-ischemic cardiopathy) of the SCD was predominant in our population and an initial shockable rhythm, observed in 93% of our study population, is a well-known strong factor of good prognosis after a cardiac arrest [19–21]. Therefore, these results are not generalisable to all patients, especially those with an extra-cardiac cause of SCD.

At 1 year, 87% of our patients were alive without neurological sequelae, which is consistent with previous studies [22–24]. In the COACT trial including the population without ST-segment elevation, 64.5% of patients in the immediate CA group were alive at 90 days [25]. An Israelian study found an 85% survival rate at 1 year among patients discharged alive from the intensive cardiology unit [26]. However, beyond mortality, possible anoxic brain injury, mental trauma from surviving a near-death experience, or a new or ongoing cardiac condition can make recovery after SCD difficult. Short-term studies suggest that these complications can lead to an increased physical and psychological burden for both survivors and their relatives [27–29]. The neurologic status of patients discharged with severe sequelae did not improve at 1 year (only one patient switched from CPC 3 to CPC 2). On the contrary, half of the patients with "mild-to-moderate" neurologic disabilities (CPC 2) completely recovered at 1 year (CPC 1), also showing progresses in neuro-cognitive care. On the other hand, despite the absence of neurological disorders, quality of life can be somewhat impaired in survivors of SCD. Most patients reported limitations in cognition, self-behaviour, and daily life activities explained by minor physical problems while others could also experience depression or persistent anxiety due to a post-traumatic state [11]. Rehabilitation has therefore been recommended to improve secondary physical and psychological consequences of SCD, but cooperation between cardiological and neurological rehabilitation teams is needed in case of cognitive consequences [30,31]. Despite many improvements in management, more knowledge is needed regarding expectations of OHCA survivors and their relatives. With a similar protocol in a much larger population and with more self-report outcome measurements, the Danish Cardiac Arrest Survivorship (DANCAS survey) will begin. Results will be used to identify the most prevalent problems suffered by OHCA survivors and their families and those at most risk of suffering them [32].

Characteristics of the two groups (good and poor outcome) were similar, except for age, body mass index (BMI), and initial LVEF. Surprisingly, overweight patients had a better neurologic outcome than normal weight patients. Found in previous studies, this phenomenon has been questioned [33,34]. Several explanations of this apparent paradox have been proposed including that higher BMI may allow for the use of higher doses of cardioprotective medications, such as β-adrenergic blockers, particularly in CAD patients, and conversely, lower BMI is traditionally associated with the increase in bleeding events with antithrombotic therapy required after ACS [35,36]. In a recent prospective trial, however, neurological status was assessed in 605 patients resuscitated from SCD. In this cohort, BMI was not associated with good neurologic and survival outcome at discharge [37].

No death during follow-up was due to cardiovascular cause and LVEF was near normal at 1 year, showing the effectiveness of actual management of ischemic heart disease and the beneficial effect of coronary revascularisation. After ACS, cardiac rehabilitation is known to decrease the mortality related to cardiac disease by 20% with the improvement of heart and lung function, socio-psychological status, and the quality of life. In addition, it delays the progression of atherosclerosis and decreases its severity, focusing on education aimed at a healthy lifestyle and improvement of exercise capacity [38,39]. This rehabilitation is safe and well-tolerated in patients with severe comorbidities, such as after aborted SCD [40]. Therefore, for patients without any neurologic sequelae at discharge, apparition of a new cardiac event or recurrence of initial arrhythmia seems not to be the main issue. In a recent study, Kubota et al. showed that the post-discharge mortality of ACS (STEMI or NSTEMI) patients with OHCA was comparable to that of patients without OHCA [41].

The first limitation of our study, even if we collected all patients discharged alive during the inclusion period, remains the small population evaluated. Multivariate analysis was not achievable due to the small number of patients in each subgroup and low incidence of events in the "poor outcome" group. Results of univariate analysis are thus to be taken with caution as we could not adjust with other parameters. Second, the CPC scale is a validated tool in the assessment of neurological status after SCD but it may not be as discriminant as other neurological tools. A CPC score of one or two is commonly regarded as a 'good outcome' but it includes subjects with 'mild-to-moderate' cognitive impairments, such as dysphasia and permanent memory or mental changes. Furthermore, the CPC seems insensitive to more subtle cognitive impairments. Therefore, the use of a more precise neuropsychological test would be more effective to obtain a precise outcome after SCD [42]. Finally, to assess quality of life, we used the QOLIBRI questionnaire which was initially validated in patients after a traumatic brain injury. Because this work focused on the consequences of neurological sequelae occurring after OHCA, we chose this questionnaire rather than the SF-36 to be more specific. Like others, the accuracy of the statements is uncertain. Moreover, patients' answers can be modified by many events unrelated to the cardiac arrest. Here, the COVID-19 pandemic may have affected our results with perturbation of daily activities and social relationships, impacting the psychological state, whereas quality of life was good in our population.

5. Conclusions

Patients admitted directly to the cathlab after aborted SCD mainly related to ACS had a survival rate of 43% at discharge. For those patients, survival rate without neurological sequelae was excellent at 1 year with 87% of them alive without significant neurological sequelae but with persistent psychological impact in 44% of survivors. These results encourage us to further improve our practices, follow-up methods, and cardiac or multidisciplinary rehabilitation programs.

Author Contributions: Conceptualization, F.L., M.A. and Q.D.; methodology, F.L., M.A. and Q.D.; software, F.L., M.A. and Q.D.; validation, F.L., M.A. and Q.D.; formal analysis, F.L., M.A. and Q.D.; investigation, F.L., M.A., Q.D., G.C., B.L. and F.R.; resources, F.L., M.A. and Q.D.; data curation, Q.D.; writing—original draft preparation, Q.D. and F.L.; writing—review and editing, F.L., M.A. and Q.D.; visualization, F.L., M.A. and Q.D.; supervision, F.L., M.A., Q.D., G.C., B.L. and F.R. All authors have read and agreed to the published version of the manuscript.

Funding: This research received no external funding.

Institutional Review Board Statement: The study was conducted according to the guidelines of the Declaration of Helsinki and approved by the Institutional Review Board (or Ethics Committee) of Montpellier University Hospital (IRB-MTP_2020_05_202000478, 28 May 2020).

Informed Consent Statement: Informed consent was obtained verbally from all subjects involved in the study.

Data Availability Statement: Datas are available in department of cardiology, University of Montpellier, France.

Conflicts of Interest: The authors declare no conflict of interest. The funders had no role in the design of the study; in the collection, analyses, or interpretation of data; in the writing of the manuscript, or in the decision to publish the results.

Appendix A

Table A1. Patients answer of QOLIBRI.

Patient Answer (n = 36)	Satisfaction					Health Problems		
	Cognition	Self	Daily Life	Social Relationships	Total	Emotion	Physical Problems	Total
"Not at all" no. (%)	3 (8.3)	0 (0)	4 (11.1)	1 (2.8)	2 (5.6)	18 (50)	18 (50)	20 (55.6)
"Slightly" no. (%)	7 (19.4)	15 (41.7)	9 (25)	8 (22.2)	10 (27.8)	5 (13.9)	9 (25)	5 (13.9)
"Quite" no. (%)	16 (44.4)	16 (44.4)	5 (13.9)	22 (61.1)	18 (50)	11 (30.6)	9 (25)	11 (30.6)
"Very" no. (%)	10 (27.8)	5 (13.9)	18 (50)	5 (13.9)	6 (16.7)	2 (5.6)	0 (0)	0 (0)

References

1. Luc, G.; Baert, V.; Escutnaire, J.; Genin, M.; Vilhelm, C.; Di Pompéo, C.; El Khoury, C.; Segal, N.; Wiel, E.; Adnet, F.; et al. Epidemiology of out-of-hospital cardiac arrest: A French national incidence and mid-term survival rate study. *Anaesth. Crit. Care Pain Med.* **2019**, *38*, 131–135. [CrossRef] [PubMed]
2. Chugh, S.S.; Reinier, K.; Teodorescu, C.; Evanado, A.; Kehr, E.; Al Samara, M.; Mariani, R.; Gunson, K.; Jui, J. Epidemiology of Sudden Cardiac Death: Clinical and Research Implications. *Prog. Cardiovasc. Dis.* **2008**, *51*, 213–228. [CrossRef] [PubMed]
3. Kuriachan, V.P.; Sumner, G.L.; Mitchell, L.B. Sudden Cardiac Death. *Curr. Probl. Cardiol.* **2015**, *40*, 133–200. [CrossRef] [PubMed]

4. Spaulding, C.M.; Joly, L.-M.; Rosenberg, A.; Monchi, M.; Weber, S.N.; Dhainaut, J.-F.A.; Carli, P. Immediate Coronary Angiography in Survivors of Out-of-Hospital Cardiac Arrest. *N. Engl. J. Med.* **1997**, *336*, 1629–1633. [CrossRef]
5. Leclercq, F.; Lonjon, C.; Marin, G.; Akodad, M.; Roubille, F.; Macia, J.-C.; Cornillet, L.; Gervasoni, R.; Schmutz, L.; Ledermann, B.; et al. Post resuscitation electrocardiogram for coronary angiography indication after out-of-hospital cardiac arrest. *Int. J. Cardiol.* **2020**, *310*, 73–79. [CrossRef]
6. Ibanez, B.; James, S.; Agewall, S.; Antunes, M.J.; Bucciarelli-Ducci, C.; Bueno, H.; Caforio, A.L.P.; Crea, F.; Goudevenos, J.A.; Halvorsen, S.; et al. 2017 ESC Guidelines for the management of acute myocardial infarction in patients presenting with ST-segment elevation: The Task Force for the management of acute myocardial infarction in patients presenting with ST-segment elevation of the European Society of Cardiology (ESC). *Eur. Heart J.* **2018**, *39*, 119–177. [CrossRef]
7. Moulaert, V.R.; Verbunt, J.A.; van Heugten, C.M.; Wade, D.T. Cognitive impairments in survivors of out-of-hospital cardiac arrest: A systematic review. *Resuscitation* **2009**, *80*, 297–305. [CrossRef]
8. Sasson, C.; Rogers, M.A.; Dahl, J.; Kellermann, A.L. Predictors of Survival From Out-of-Hospital Cardiac Arrest: A Systematic Review and Meta-Analysis. *Circ. Cardiovasc. Qual. Outcomes* **2010**, *3*, 63–81. [CrossRef]
9. Patel, N.; Patel, N.J.; Macon, C.J.; Thakkar, B.; Desai, M.; Rengifo-Moreno, P.; Alfonso, C.E.; Myerburg, R.J.; Bhatt, D.L.; Cohen, M. Trends and Outcomes of Coronary Angiography and Percutaneous Coronary Intervention After Out-of-Hospital Cardiac Arrest Associated With Ventricular Fibrillation or Pulseless Ventricular Tachycardia. *JAMA Cardiol.* **2016**, *1*, 890–899. [CrossRef]
10. Daubin, C.; Quentin, C.; Allouche, S.; Etard, O.; Gaillard, C.; Seguin, A.; Valette, X.; Parienti, J.-J.; Prevost, F.; Ramakers, M.; et al. Serum neuron-specific enolase as predictor of outcome in comatose cardiac-arrest survivors: A prospective cohort study. *BMC Cardiovasc. Disord.* **2011**, *11*, 48. [CrossRef]
11. Haydon, G.; Van Der Riet, P.; Inder, K. A systematic review and meta-synthesis of the qualitative literature exploring the experiences and quality of life of survivors of a cardiac arrest. *Eur. J. Cardiovasc. Nurs. J. Work Group Cardiovasc. Nurs. Eur. Soc. Cardiol.* **2017**, *16*, 475–483. [CrossRef] [PubMed]
12. Cummins, R.O.; Chamberlain, D.A.; Abramson, N.S.; Allen, M.; Baskett, P.J.; Becker, L.; Bossaert, L.; Delooz, H.H.; Dick, W.F.; Eisenberg, M.S. Recommended guidelines for uniform reporting of data from out-of-hospital cardiac arrest: The Utstein Style. A statement for health professionals from a task force of the American Heart Association, the European Resuscitation Council, the Heart and Stroke Foundation of Canada, and the Australian Resuscitation Council. *Circulation* **1991**, *84*, 960–975. [CrossRef] [PubMed]
13. Phelps, R.J.; Rea, T.; Maynard, C.; Dumas, F. Cerebral Performance Category and Long-Term Prognosis in Cardiac Arrest Survivors. *Circulation* **2011**, *124* (Suppl. S21), A179. [CrossRef]
14. Edgren, E.; Hedstrand, U.; Kelsey, S.; Sutton-Tyrrell, K.; Safar, P. BRCTI Study Group Assessment of neurological prognosis in comatose survivors of cardiac arrest. *Lancet* **1994**, *343*, 1055–1059. [CrossRef]
15. Martinell, L.; Nielsen, N.; Herlitz, J.; Karlsson, T.; Horn, J.; Wise, M.P.; Undén, J.; Rylander, C. Early predictors of poor outcome after out-of-hospital cardiac arrest. *Crit. Care* **2017**, *21*, 96. [CrossRef]
16. Von Steinbuechel, N.; Wilson, L.; Gibbons, H.; Hawthorne, G.; Höfer, S.; Schmidt, S.; Bullinger, M.; Maas, A.I.; Neugebauer, E.; Powell, J.; et al. Quality of Life after Brain Injury (QOLIBRI): Scale Validity and Correlates of Quality of Life. *J. Neurotrauma* **2010**, *27*, 1157–1165. [CrossRef]
17. Von Steinbüchel, N.; Wilson, L.; Gibbons, H.; Hawthorne, G.; Hofer, S.; Schmidt, S.; Bullinger, M.; Maas, A.I.; Neugebauer, E.; Powell, J.; et al. Quality of Life after Brain Injury (QOLIBRI): Scale Development and Metric Properties. *J. Neurotrauma* **2010**, *27*, 1167–1185. [CrossRef]
18. Middelkamp, W.; Moulaert, V.R.; Verbunt, J.A.; Van Heugten, C.M.; Bakx, W.G.; Wade, D.T. Life after survival: Long-term daily life functioning and quality of life of patients with hypoxic brain injury as a result of a cardiac arrest. *Clin. Rehabil.* **2007**, *21*, 425–431. [CrossRef]
19. Andersen, L.W.; Holmberg, M.J.; Berg, K.M.; Donnino, M.W.; Granfeldt, A. In-Hospital Cardiac Arrest: A Review. *JAMA* **2019**, *321*, 1200–1210. [CrossRef]
20. Nolan, J.P.; Soar, J.; Smith, G.B.; Gwinnutt, C.; Parrott, F.; Power, S.; Harrison, D.; Nixon, E.; Rowan, K. Incidence and outcome of in-hospital cardiac arrest in the United Kingdom National Cardiac Arrest Audit. *Resuscitation* **2014**, *85*, 987–992. [CrossRef]
21. Pasupula, D.K.; Bhat, A.G.; Meera, S.J.; Malleshappa, S.K.S. Influence of comorbidity on survival after out-of-hospital cardiac arrest in the United States. *Resuscitation* **2019**, *145*, 21–25. [CrossRef] [PubMed]
22. Bunch, T.J.; White, R.D.; Gersh, B.J.; Meverden, R.A.; Hodge, D.O.; Ballman, K.V.; Hammill, S.C.; Shen, W.-K.; Packer, D.L. Long-Term Outcomes of Out-of-Hospital Cardiac Arrest after Successful Early Defibrillation. *N. Engl. J. Med.* **2003**, *348*, 2626–2633. [CrossRef] [PubMed]
23. Kalbag, A.; Kotyra, Z.; Richards, M.; Spearpoint, K.; Brett, S. Long-term survival and residual hazard after in-hospital cardiac arrest. *Resuscitation* **2006**, *68*, 79–83. [CrossRef] [PubMed]
24. Pleskot, M.; Hazukova, R.; Parizek, P.; Cermakova, E.; Taceci, I. A seven-year follow-up of discharged patients after out-of-hospital cardiac arrest with respect to ST-segment elevation myocardial infarction. *Signa Vitae J. Intesive Care Emerg. Med.* **2012**, *7*, 33–39.
25. Lemkes, J.S.; Janssens, G.N.; van der Hoeven, N.W.; Jewbali, L.S.; Dubois, E.A.; Meuwissen, M.; Rijpstra, T.A.; Bosker, H.A.; Blans, M.J.; Bleeker, G.B.; et al. Coronary Angiography after Cardiac Arrest without ST-Segment Elevation. *N. Engl. J. Med.* **2019**, *380*, 1397–1407. [CrossRef]

26. Antonelli, D.; Koren, O.; Nahir, M.; Rozner, E.; Freedberg, N.A.; Turgeman, Y. Long-Term Survival of Discharged Patients Admitted to Intensive Coronary Care Unit after Out-of-Hospital Cardiac Arres. *Isr. Med. Assoc. J.* **2017**, *19*, 751–755.
27. Lilja, G.; Nielsen, N.; Bro-Jeppesen, J.; Dunford, H.; Friberg, H.; Hofgren, C.; Horn, J.; Insorsi, A.; Kjaergaard, J.; Nilsson, F.; et al. Return to Work and Participation in Society After Out-of-Hospital Cardiac Arrest. *Circ. Cardiovasc. Qual. Outcomes* **2018**, *11*, e003566. [CrossRef]
28. Van Wijnen, H.G.; Mc Rasquin, S.; Van Heugten, C.M.; Verbunt, J.A.; Moulaert, V.R. The impact of cardiac arrest on the long-term wellbeing and caregiver burden of family caregivers: A prospective cohort study. *Clin. Rehabil.* **2017**, *31*, 1267–1275. [CrossRef]
29. Lilja, G. Follow-Up of Cardiac Arrest Survivors: Why, How, and When? A Practical Approach. *Semin Neurol.* **2017**, *37*, 88–93. [CrossRef]
30. Schaaf, K.P.W.; Artman, L.K.; Peberdy, M.A.; Walker, W.C.; Ornato, J.P.; Gossip, M.R.; Kreutzer, J.S. Anxiety, depression, and PTSD following cardiac arrest: A systematic review of the literature. *Resuscitation* **2013**, *84*, 873–877. [CrossRef]
31. Boyce, L.W.; Goossens, P.H.; Moulaert, V.R.; Pound, G.; Van Heugten, C.M. Out-of-hospital cardiac arrest survivors need both cardiological and neurological rehabilitation! *Curr. Opin. Crit. Care* **2019**, *25*, 240–243. [CrossRef] [PubMed]
32. Joshi, V.L.; Tang, L.H.; Borregaard, B.; Zinckernagel, L.; Mikkelsen, T.B.; Taylor, R.S.; Christiansen, S.R.; Nielsen, J.F.; Zwisler, A.D. Long-term physical and psychological outcomes after out-of-hospital cardiac arrest—protocol for a national cross-sectional survey of survivors and their relatives (the DANCAS survey). *BMJ Open* **2021**, *11*, e045668. [CrossRef] [PubMed]
33. Sakr, Y.; Alhussami, I.; Nanchal, R.; Wunderink, R.G.; Pellis, T.; Wittebole, X.; Martin-Loeches, I.; François, B.; Leone, M.; Vincent, J.-L. Being Overweight Is Associated With Greater Survival in ICU Patients: Results From the Intensive Care Over Nations Audit. *Crit. Care Med.* **2015**, *43*, 2623–2632. [CrossRef] [PubMed]
34. Bunch, T.J.; White, R.D.; Lopez-Jimenez, F.; Thomas, R. Association of body weight with total mortality and with ICD shocks among survivors of ventricular fibrillation in out-of-hospital cardiac arrest. *Resuscitation* **2008**, *77*, 351–355. [CrossRef]
35. Mak, K.-H.; Bhatt, D.L.; Shao, M.; Haffner, S.M.; Hamm, C.W.; Hankey, G.; Johnston, S.C.; Montalescot, G.; Steg, P.G.; Steinhubl, S.R.; et al. The influence of body mass index on mortality and bleeding among patients with or at high-risk of atherothrombotic disease. *Eur. Heart J.* **2009**, *30*, 857–865. [CrossRef]
36. Matinrazm, S.; Ladejobi, A.; Pasupula, D.K.; Javed, A.; Durrani, A.; Ahmad, S.; Munir, M.B.; Adelstein, E.; Jain, S.K.; Saba, S. Effect of body mass index on survival after sudden cardiac arrest. *Clin. Cardiol.* **2018**, *41*, 46–50. [CrossRef]
37. Lee, H.; Oh, J.; Kang, H.; Lim, T.H.; Ko, B.S.; Choi, H.J.; Park, S.M.; Jo, Y.H.; Lee, J.S.; Park, Y.S.; et al. Association between the body mass index and outcomes of patients resuscitated from out-of-hospital cardiac arrest: A prospective multicentre registry study. *Scand. J. Trauma Resusc. Emerg. Med.* **2021**, *29*, 24. [CrossRef]
38. Witt, B.J.; Jacobsen, S.; Weston, S.A.; Killian, J.M.; Meverden, R.A.; Allison, T.G.; Reeder, G.S.; Roger, V.L. Cardiac rehabilitation after myocardial infarction in the community. *J. Am. Coll. Cardiol.* **2004**, *44*, 988–996. [CrossRef]
39. González-Salvado, V.; Rodríguez-Núñez, A.; González-Juanatey, J.R. From Prevention to Rehabilitation: Toward a Comprehensive Approach to Tackling Cardiac Arrest. *Rev. Espanola Cardiol.* **2019**, *72*, 3–6. [CrossRef]
40. Kim, C.; Jung, H.; Choi, H.E.; Kang, S.H. Cardiac Rehabilitation After Acute Myocardial Infarction Resuscitated From Cardiac Arrest. *Ann. Rehabil. Med.* **2014**, *38*, 799–804. [CrossRef]
41. Kubota, T.; Komukai, K.; Miyanaga, S.; Shirasaki, K.; Oki, Y.; Yoshida, R.; Fukushima, K.; Kamba, T.; Okuyama, T.; Maehara, T.; et al. Out-of-Hospital Cardiac Arrest Does Not Affect Post-Discharge Survival in Patients With Acute Myocardial Infarction. *Circ. Rep.* **2021**, *3*, 249–255. [CrossRef] [PubMed]
42. Moulaert, V.R.; Verbunt, J.A.; Van Heugten, C.M.; Bakx, W.G.; Gorgels, A.P.; Bekkers, S.C.; De Krom, M.C.; Wade, D.T. Activity and Life After Survival of a Cardiac Arrest (ALASCA) and the effectiveness of an early intervention service: Design of a randomised controlled trial. *BMC Cardiovasc. Disord.* **2007**, *7*, 26. [CrossRef] [PubMed]

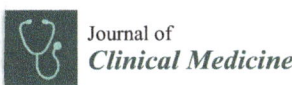

Article

Occurrence and Temporal Variability of Out-of-Hospital Cardiac Arrest during COVID-19 Pandemic in Comparison to the Pre-Pandemic Period in Poland—Observational Analysis of OSCAR-POL Registry

Jakub Ratajczak [1,2,*], Stanisław Szczerbiński [3] and Aldona Kubica [1]

1. Department of Health Promotion, Nicolaus Copernicus University, Collegium Medicum in Bydgoszcz, 85-094 Bydgoszcz, Poland; aldona.kubica@gmail.com
2. Department of Cardiology and Internal Medicine, Nicolaus Copernicus University, Collegium Medicum in Bydgoszcz, 85-094 Bydgoszcz, Poland
3. Emergency Medical Center in Opole, 45-369 Opole, Poland; pielegniarz@tlen.pl
* Correspondence: ratajczak.j.m@gmail.com; Tel.: +48-52-585-40-23; Fax: +48-52-585-40-24

Citation: Ratajczak, J.; Szczerbiński, S.; Kubica, A. Occurrence and Temporal Variability of Out-of-Hospital Cardiac Arrest during COVID-19 Pandemic in Comparison to the Pre-Pandemic Period in Poland—Observational Analysis of OSCAR-POL Registry. *J. Clin. Med.* **2022**, *11*, 4143. https://doi.org/10.3390/jcm11144143

Academic Editors: Michael Behnes and Tobias Schupp

Received: 25 June 2022
Accepted: 15 July 2022
Published: 16 July 2022

Publisher's Note: MDPI stays neutral with regard to jurisdictional claims in published maps and institutional affiliations.

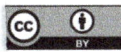

Copyright: © 2022 by the authors. Licensee MDPI, Basel, Switzerland. This article is an open access article distributed under the terms and conditions of the Creative Commons Attribution (CC BY) license (https://creativecommons.org/licenses/by/4.0/).

Abstract: An investigation of the chronobiology of out-of-hospital cardiac arrest (OHCA) during the coronavirus disease 2019 (COVID-19) pandemic and the differences in comparison to the 6-year pre-pandemic period. A retrospective analysis of the dispatch cards from the Emergency Medical Service between January 2014 and December 2020 was performed within the OSCAR-POL registry. The circadian, weekly, monthly, and seasonal variabilities of OHCA were investigated. A comparison of OHCA occurrence between the year 2020 and the 6-year pre-pandemic period was made. A total of 416 OHCAs were reported in 2020 and the median of OHCAs during the pre-pandemic period was 379 (interquartile range 337–407) cases per year. Nighttime was associated with a decreased number of OHCAs (16.6%) in comparison to afternoon (31.5%, $p < 0.001$) and morning (30.0%, $p < 0.001$). A higher occurrence at night was observed in 2020 compared to 2014–2019 (16.6% vs. 11.7%, $p = 0.001$). Monthly and seasonal variabilities were observed in 2020. The months with the highest OHCA occurrence in 2020 were November (13.2%) and October (11.1%) and were significantly higher compared to the same months during the pre-pandemic period (9.1%, $p = 0.002$ and 7.9%, $p = 0.009$, respectively). Autumn was the season with the highest rate of OHCA, which was also higher compared to the pre-pandemic period (30.5% vs. 25.1%, $p = 0.003$). The COVID-19 pandemic was related to a higher occurrence of OHCA. The circadian, monthly, and seasonal variabilities of OHCA occurrence were confirmed. In 2020, the highest occurrence of OHCA was observed in October and November, which coincided with the highest occurrence of COVID-19 infections in Poland.

Keywords: temporal variability; COVID-19; coronavirus; out-of-hospital cardiac arrest (OHCA); sudden cardiac death

1. Introduction

The new coronavirus disease 2019 (COVID-19) pandemic, caused by severe acute respiratory syndrome coronavirus 2 (SARS-CoV-2), became a real challenge for humanity. The World Health Organization reported over 243 million confirmed COVID-19 cases and almost 5 million deaths caused by the disease worldwide as at 24 October 2021 [1]. The first confirmed case of COVID-19 in Poland was recorded on 4 March 2020, with over 3 million diagnosed infections since then [2]. COVID-19 infection, characterized by various stages, might lead to a severe inflammatory response caused by cytokine storm. This could result in acute respiratory insufficiency and multiorgan damage due to shock [3]. Furthermore, there is increasing evidence proving a relationship between COVID-19 and thromboembolic complications, which may result inter alia in myocardial infarction or sudden cardiac death [4].

Out-of-hospital cardiac arrest (OHCA) is a significant health issue worldwide. Despite improvements in treatment, it remains one of the major causes of death characterized by low survival rates [5]. Recently published studies showed lower survival rates in patients with OHCA during the pandemic era in comparison to the pre-pandemic era [6]. It has been proven that one of the basic methods to improve patient survival is to perform cardiopulmonary resuscitation as soon as possible [7]. This became more challenging during the pandemic era due to the risk of infection and the need for the healthcare workers to wear personal protective equipment [8]. The impact of COVID-19 on the incidence and outcome of OHCA was globally investigated in numerous studies; however, only a few compared the pandemic period with a pre-pandemic period that was longer than 1–2 years [6,9–19]. The majority of the studies along with metanalyses revealed an increased number of OHCA cases and a lower survival rate related to increased incidence of COVID-19 [6,15,17]. The Polish experience regarding OHCA and COVID-19 is rather scarce; furthermore, published reports focus predominantly on the early phase of the pandemic [20,21]. The occurrence of cardiac arrest is related to various factors including some environmental factors such as atmospheric conditions [22,23], air pollution [24,25], time variables [26–28]. Temporal variability, especially the circadian variation of OHCA occurrence, is a well-documented phenomenon and has been confirmed in a long-time observation period [27]. However, the temporal variability of OHCA occurrence within the COVID-19 pandemic in Poland remains uncertain.

The aim of the study was to investigate the chronobiology of OHCA during the COVID-19 pandemic and the differences in temporal variability of OHCA occurrence between the year 2020 and the pre-pandemic 6-year period.

2. Materials and Methods

The presented study was designed as a retrospective analysis of dispatch cards from the Emergency Medical Service in Opole, Poland, covering the period from January 2014 to December 2020. The dispatch cards were compatible with the Utstein characteristics. The presented research was a part of the OSCAR-POL registry whose methodology was described in detail in the previous publications [26,27]. Herein, we provide crucial features regarding the methodology. The registry covered an area of Opole district (1683 km^2) with the population of approximately 261,000 inhabitants within the study period. The presumed cardiac etiology in patients over 18 years of age regardless of the initial rhythm, witnessed status or performing of CPR were the inclusion criteria. Late symptoms of death, known non-cardiac etiology, and OHCA in the pediatric population were the exclusion criteria.

OHCA occurrence was analyzed for the year 2020 and compared with the results from the 6-year pre-pandemic period covering the years 2014–2019. The temporal variation of OHCA occurrence was analyzed within the following patterns to stay consistent with previous reports. The circadian rhythm was investigated within 1 h periods as well as four 6 h intervals: "night" (00:00–05:59), "morning" (06:00–11:59), "afternoon" (12:00–17:59), and "evening" (18:00–23:59). Weekly, monthly, and seasonal variability were analyzed between consecutive days of the week, months of the year, and seasons, respectively. Four seasons were defined as spring (from 1 March till 31 May), summer (from 1 June till 31 August), autumn (from 1 September till 30 November), and winter (from 1 December till 28 or 29 February).

The study received the approval of the Ethics Committee of The Nicolaus Copernicus University in Torun, Collegium Medicum in Bydgoszcz (KB 471/2013) and was conducted in accordance with the Declaration of Helsinki and Good Clinical Practice principles.

A two-sided p-value < 0.05 was applied for statistical significance. The Shapiro–Wilk test and the analysis of histograms were performed to determine the data distribution. The differences between variables with non-normal distribution were analyzed using the

Mann–Whitney test for two variables or the Kruskal–Wallis test for three or more variables. When the variables had normal distribution, the differences were tested with the Student t-test or ANOVA adequately to the number of the variables. Categorical variables were presented as absolute values and percentages. Despite the non-normal distribution of time variables in most cases it was decided to present the data as percentages and means with standard deviations (SD), and not medians with interquartile range to better visualize the differences. The statistical analysis was performed with the SPSS Statistic software version 28 (IBM Corp., Armonk, NY, USA).

3. Results

During the analyzed period, 3021 ambulance departures due to OHCA were observed of which 329 cases were excluded (16 cases occurred within the pediatric population and 313 referred to non-cardiac etiology, e.g., trauma or cancer). In the final analysis, 2692 cases were included. The mean age of all patients with OHCA within the study period was 70.2 ± 15.0 years with the majority male (63% vs. 37%, $p < 0.001$). The mean age of patients was 71.1 ± 14.7 in 2020 and 70.0 ± 15.0 ($p = 0.221$) in the years 2014–2019. Both during the pandemic and pre-pandemic periods almost two thirds of patients were male (63.3% vs. 63.0%, $p = 0.903$, respectively).

3.1. Temporal Variability of Out-of-Hospital Cardiac Arrest during 2020

The total number of OHCA cases reported in 2020 was 416. The circadian variability of the OHCA occurrence was observed with regard to division into both 1 h (Figure 1) and 6 h intervals (Figure 2) The highest number of OHCA cases was observed between 09:00 and 09:59 and the lowest between 03:00 and 03:59 (7.2% vs. 1.7%, $p < 0.001$, respectively). The histogram of the circadian distribution of OHCA occurrence presents a trimodal daily peak: between 09:00 and 10:59, between 13:00 and 14:59, and the last between 16:00 and 17:59. In the evening and during early night hours, the number of OHCA cases stayed at a relatively stable level with the nadir between 01:00 and 05:59. The night was associated with decreased number of OHCA cases (16.6%) in comparison to the afternoon (31.5%, $p < 0.001$) and the morning period (30.0%, $p < 0.001$). The difference between the total number of OHCA cases in the evening (21.9%) and in the night was insignificant ($p = 0.127$).

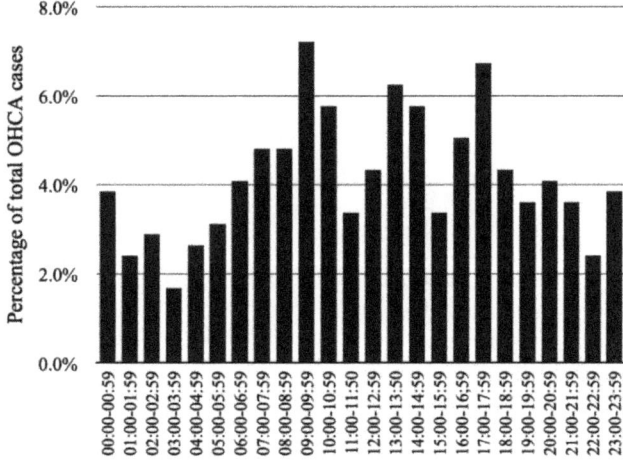

Figure 1. Circadian distribution of out-of-hospital cardiac arrest (OHCA) occurrence divided into 1 h intervals in 2020 ($p < 0.001$).

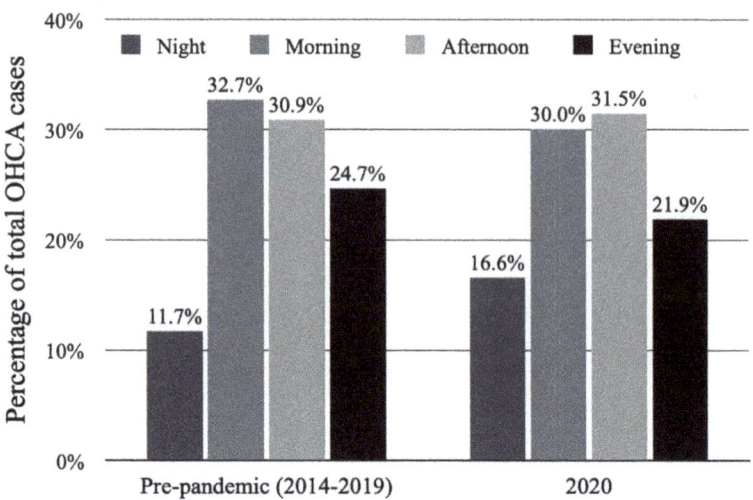

Figure 2. Circadian distribution of out-of-hospital cardiac arrest (OHCA) occurrence in 6 h intervals within 24 h in year 2020 ($p < 0.001$) and during 2014–2019 pre-pandemic period ($p < 0.001$).

The distribution of OHCA occurrence in days of the week is presented in Figure 3. The lowest number of OHCA cases was observed on Monday (10.8%) with a gradually increasing number in the subsequent days reaching the highest value on Friday (16.8%). A slight decrease during the weekend was detected; however, in general the weekly variability did not reach statistical significance ($p = 0.268$).

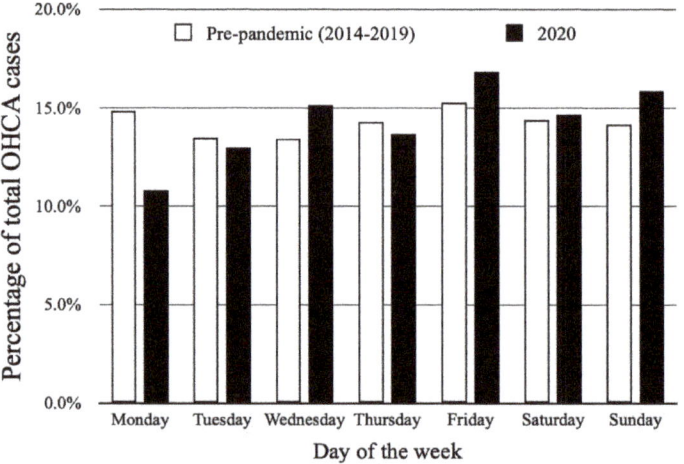

Figure 3. Distribution of out-of-hospital cardiac arrest (OHCA) occurrence in subsequent days of the week in year 2020 ($p = 0.268$) and during 2014–2019 pre-pandemic period ($p = 0.499$).

Monthly ($p = 0.017$) and seasonal ($p = 0.038$) variability was observed during the year 2020. Figure 4 shows the monthly distribution of OHCA cases. The lowest OHCA occurrence was observed in September (6.3%; mean 0.87 ± 0.94) and was significantly lower in comparison to the highest observed in November (13.2%; mean 1.83 ± 1.15, $p < 0.001$) and October (11.1%; mean 1.48 ± 1.12, $p = 0.029$). The season with the highest proportion of OHCA cases (30.5%; mean 1.40 ± 1.13) was autumn, significantly higher compared to summer (21.2%; mean 0.96 ± 1.03, p = 0.031), the season with the lowest OHCA occurrence. The histogram of OHCA seasonal distribution is presented in Figure 5.

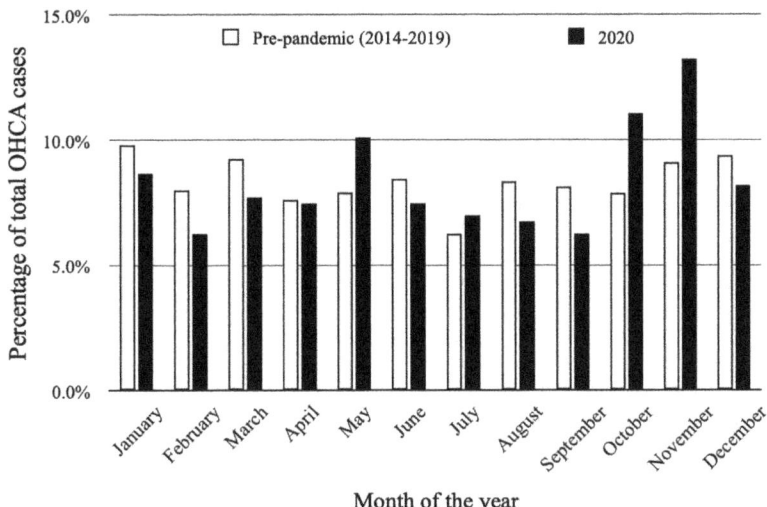

Figure 4. Monthly distribution of out-of-hospital cardiac arrest (OHCA) occurrence in year 2020 (p = 0.017) and during 2014–2019 pre-pandemic period (p = 0.009).

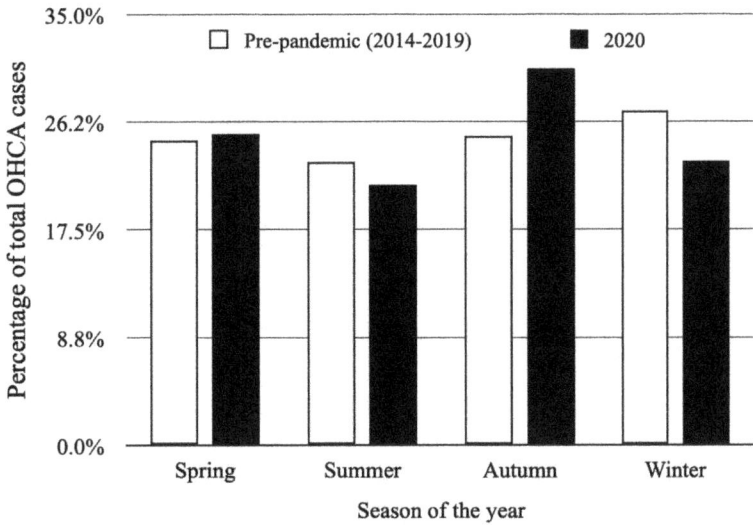

Figure 5. Seasonal distribution of out-of-hospital cardiac arrest (OHCA) occurrence in year 2020 (p = 0.038) and during 2014–2019 pre-pandemic period (p = 0.021).

3.2. Comparison of Temporal Variability between the Year 2020 and 6-Year Pre-Pandemic Period (2014–2019)

The pre-pandemic period was characterized by a lower mean number of OHCA cases (1.04 ± 1.13 vs. 1.14 ± 1.07, p = 0.03). The median value of OHCA per year during that period was 379 with an interquartile range of 337 to 407. Circadian variability was confirmed for the year 2020 (p < 0.001) as well as for the 6-year pre-pandemic period (p = 0.018). Nevertheless, the distribution within a particular time of the day was different between those two time periods (Figure 2). In 2020, the highest percentage of OHCA cases occurred in the afternoon (31.5%); as opposed to the 6-year pre-pandemic period, where the highest percentage of OHCA cases occurred in the morning (32.7%). Higher occurrence during the night was observed in 2020 compared to the 2014–2019 period (16.6%; mean 1.64 ± 1.21 vs. 11.7%; mean 1.06 ± 1.12, $p = 0.001$) with no differences between other time periods during the day (Table 1). Weekly variability was not observed in the pre-pandemic period ($p = 0.499$), similarly to 2020 (Figure 3). OHCA occurred significantly more often on Sundays in 2020 in comparison to the pre-pandemic period. No differences were observed regarding the other days of the week (Table 1). Both analyzed periods were characterized by monthly (Figure 4) and seasonal (Figure 5) variability; however, the distribution of OHCA occurrence was different. In 2020, autumn was the season with the highest percentage of OHCA cases (30.5%) with a significantly higher occurrence of OHCA than in autumn during the pre-pandemic period (25.1%, $p = 0.003$). In the 2014–2019 period, winter was the season with the highest OHCA occurrence (27.2%), while in 2020 it was third, surpassing only summer in regard to the number of OHCA cases (Table 1). The months with the highest OHCA occurrence in 2020 were November (13.2%, mean 1.83 ± 1.15) and October (11.1%, mean 1.48 ± 1.12); the observed values were significantly higher in comparison to the same month during the pre-pandemic period (9.1%, mean 1.15 ± 1.13, $p = 0.002$ and 7.9%, mean 0.96 ± 0.99, $p = 0.009$, respectively). The highest OHCA occurrence in 2020 overlapped with the peak of the COVID-19 pandemic in Poland (Figure 6). No other differences regarding monthly OHCA occurrence were observed between the analyzed time periods (Table 1).

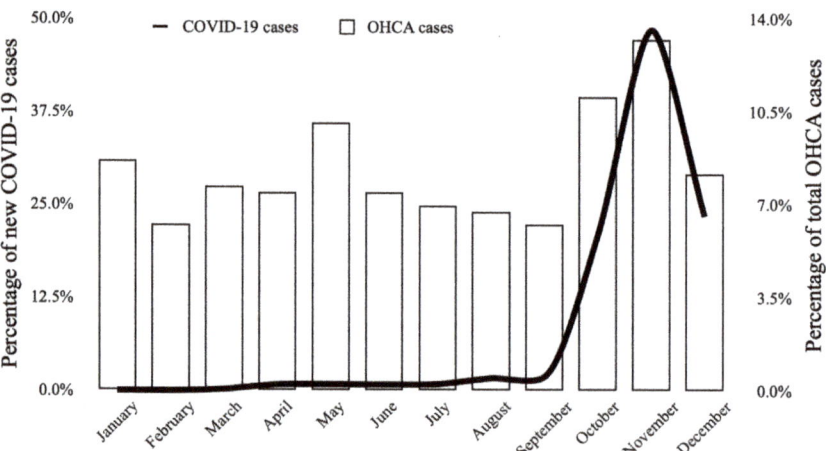

Figure 6. Monthly distribution of out-of-hospital cardiac arrest (OHCA) occurrence and new COVID-19 cases diagnosed in Poland in year 2020. Black line represents the percentage of new COVID-19 cases diagnosed in a particular month (data based on the daily reports of The Ministry of Health of Poland).

Table 1. Comparison of differences in temporal variability of OHCA occurrence between pre-pandemic period and year 2020.

Temporal Variables	2020 Mean ± SD	Pre-Pandemic Period (2014–2019) Mean ± SD	p-Value
Time of the day			
Night	1.06 ± 1.12	1.64 ± 1.21	0.001
Morning	2.96 ± 1.85	2.98 ± 1.70	0.80
Afternoon	2.79 ± 1.67	3.12 ± 1.81	0.35
Evening	2.23 ± 1.68	2.17 ± 1.59	0.96
Day of the week			
Monday	0.87 ± 0.95	1.08 ± 1.12	0.24
Tuesday	1.04 ± 0.99	0.98 ± 1.10	0.47
Wednesday	1.19 ± 1.18	0.98 ± 1.11	0.17
Thursday	1.08 ± 1.11	1.04 ± 1.08	0.85
Friday	1.35 ± 1.12	1.11 ± 1.11	0.12
Saturday	1.17 ± 1.17	1.05 ± 1.22	0.36
Sunday	1.27 ± 0.93	1.03 ± 1.15	0.026
Month of the year			
January	1.16 ± 1.16	1.20 ± 1.21	0.95
February	0.90 ± 0.82	1.08 ± 1.09	0.58
March	1.03 ± 1.11	1.13 ± 1.22	0.81
April	1.03 ± 0.93	0.96 ± 1.03	0.51
May	1.35 ± 1.14	0.97 ± 0.99	0.06
June	1.03 ± 1.03	1.07 ± 1.13	0.99
July	0.94 ± 1.03	0.76 ± 1.06	0.29
August	0.90 ± 1.04	1.02 ± 1.16	0.66
September	0.87 ± 0.94	1.03 ± 1.18	0.65
October	1.48 ± 1.12	0.96 ± 0.99	0.009
November	1.83 ± 1.15	1.15 ± 1.13	0.002
December	1.10 ± 1.04	1.15 ± 1.27	0.89
Season of the year			
Spring	1.14 ± 1.07	1.02 ± 1.08	0.22
Summer	0.96 ± 1.03	0.95 ± 1.12	0.73
Autumn	1.40 ± 1.13	1.05 ± 1.1	0.003
Winter	1.05 ± 1.02	1.14 ± 1.19	0.77

4. Discussion

The presented results showed the circadian, monthly, and seasonal rhythm of OHCA occurrence with no weekly variability in the year 2020 or during the 6-year pre-pandemic period (2014–2019). Nevertheless, the pattern of OHCA occurrence was different in the compared time periods as the mean value of OHCA occurrence was higher during the pandemic year. In 2020, OHCA was observed significantly more often at night, on Sundays, and in autumn, particularly in October and November.

Previous studies delivered evidence of the association between a higher risk of OHCA occurrence and the epidemics of particular infectious diseases such as influenza [29]. The global spread of the SARS-CoV-2 virus is an exceptional challenge for medical staff; hence, its relationship with OHCA occurrence is of great importance. In our study, we observed a higher mean number of OHCA cases during the year 2020 in comparison to the pre-pandemic period. This observation is in line with the majority of previous reports from the United Kingdom [12,30], Lombardy, Italy [10], Singapore [14], the United States [13,17,31,32], and Paris, France [16]. In contrast, studies from Australia [18], Switzerland [33], and Padua, Italy [34] showed no differences in OHCA incidence between pre-pandemic and pandemic eras. Data from Western Australia showed a similar incidence of OHCA cases during the period with the most stringent restrictions due to the COVID-19 pandemic compared to the previous year [18]. However, as underlined by the authors, during that period, a relatively low incidence of COVID-19 was reported (107 cases per 100,000 person-years). The findings indirectly support the observations from other regions with high COVID-19 incidence, where the OHCA occurrence was higher in comparison to the pre-pandemic period. Interestingly, a population-based, observational study from Switzerland showed an increased incidence of OHCA cases in 2020 in Cantons with low COVID-19 morbidity and an opposite situation in Cantons with high COVID-19 incidence [33]. The meta-analysis by Lim et al. [15] included 35,379 OHCA cases from 10 studies, showed a 120% increase in cardiac arrest occurrence regardless of etiology. However, the difference in total OHCA occurrence was predominantly related to a significant increase in arrests caused by trauma (OR 1.69, 95% CI 1.07–2.69, $p = 0.03$), which were excluded from our study. To date, the majority of published studies focused on the OHCA occurrence during the first wave of the COVID19 outbreak and little is known about later developments of the pandemic. Baldi et al. [35] analyzed all OHCA cases in the provinces of Pavia, Lodi, Cremona, Mantua, and Varese in Italy between February and December 2020 and divided this period into two, reflecting the first and second wave of the pandemic. The authors observed a significant positive correlation between increased COVID-19 incidence and the incidence of OHCA cases. Nevertheless, it should be noted, that the correlation was observed only in the provinces most affected by the pandemic and no relationship for provinces with low COVID-19 incidence was found.

In the meta-analysis by Borkowska et al. [6] that included 4210 patients with OHCA, the authors reported lower survival to hospital discharge in the COVID-19 group (OR 0.25, 95% CI 0.12–0.53, $p < 0.001$) along with a lower percentage of shockable rhythms (5.7% vs. 37.4%). The same observation was confirmed in the previously mentioned meta-analysis by Lim et al., which presented a 63% higher chance of achieving the return of spontaneous circulation and a 65% higher chance of survival to hospital discharge before the pandemic [15]. However, some single studies did not show a lower chance of survival during the pandemic. The observational study based on the OHCA registry in Daegu, South Korea, revealed a similar number of OHCA cases of cardiac etiology in the pandemic and pre-pandemic periods (n = 152 vs. n = 142) with no difference in survival to hospital discharge, yet, with a significantly lower rate of patients with a good neurologic outcome (OR 0.23, 95% CI 0.05–0.98) [9]. Results based on a registry from Taiwan also showed a similar rate of survival to discharge between February and April 2020 in comparison to the same period in 2019 (4.98% vs. 5.96%); however, with a significantly lower rate of favorable neurologic outcome (2.09% vs. 4.21%, $p = 0.035$). Potential causes for lower survival could be related to a lower percentage of shockable rhythms, bystander CPR, the longer response time of the emergency medical services, or higher rates of OHCA at home [15,16,36]. The need to wear full personal protective equipment by medical personnel might also be a significant factor for unfavorable outcomes [8].

Polish data regarding the relationship between COVID-19 incidence and OHCA occurrence is scarce. Borkowska et al. [20] performed an observational study of OHCA cases in Masovian Voivodeship between March and April 2020. A total of 527 OHCA cases were analyzed, of which 379 had cardiac etiology. The authors reported OHCA incidence of 0.12/1000 inhabitants during the study period. This result is lower than the incidence reported in previous studies from Poland where it was estimated to be 0.57–1.70 per 1000 inhabitants per year [26,37,38]. It should be noted that the authors analyzed OHCA occurrence within the first two months of the pandemic in Poland, when the total number of COVID-19 infections was very low and strict lockdown restrictions were present. Results from the Polish Registry of Acute Coronary Syndromes showed a decreased number of patients admitted to hospital due to acute coronary syndrome with and without ST-segment elevation during the first wave of the COVID-19 pandemic (March–May 2020) compared to the same period in 2019 [21]. At the same time, the rate of OHCA was higher in 2020 (3.43% vs. 2.75%, $p = 0.049$) in the population of patients with myocardial infarction. The COVID-19 pandemic also affected patients with heart failure.

Kubica et al. [39] showed a reduction in hospital admissions due to acute heart failure by over 23% in the year 2020 with an increase in in-hospital all-cause mortality (6.5% vs. 5.2%, $p < 0.001$).

To the best of our knowledge, this is the first study to focus on the temporal variability of OHCA during the first year of the COVID-19 pandemic. Similar to the results from previous studies, the circadian, monthly, and seasonal variabilities of OHCA occurrence were confirmed in 2020; however, a different pattern was observed [27]. The OHCA rate was significantly higher at night in 2020 compared to the pre-pandemic period. The explanation of this phenomenon requires further study. A potential explanation might be related to the increased number of emergency calls in 2020, especially during the night shift (an increase of almost 80%), which might reflect the general alertness of the population due to new medical threats [40]. In autumn 2020, especially during October and November, the very peak of COVID-19 infections was observed in Poland [41]. This period overlaps with the highest rates of OHCA cases, which were significantly higher compared to the pre-pandemic period. The observation stays in line with the previous studies showing a correlation between increased OHCA cases and increased SARS-CoV-2 infection rates [17,35].

The main limitation of the study is the retrospective design and the lack of detailed data regarding, e.g., patients' medical history or socio-economic status. Secondly, no analysis of witnessed status, initial rhythm, or survival was performed. In the presented study, the year 2020 was considered as the pandemic period, although the first COVID-19 case diagnosed in Poland was diagnosed later than January 2020. A similar approach was also used in previous studies [13]. Therefore, the analysis of seasonal variability of OHCA occurrence in the light of SARS-CoV-2 infections, particularly in the winter, is limited. Still, the main objective of the study was to assess the chronobiology of OHCA occurrence in the year 2020 affected by the COVID-19 pandemic and not to investigate potential influencing factors. The study showed OHCA occurrence in 2020 and the 6-year pre-pandemic period; however, the results reflected the situation on a relatively small territory of Opole district. Due to a relatively low number of cases presented, especially in the year 2020, observed differences should be confirmed on a larger group. Therefore, further national-based studies should be conducted in Poland.

5. Conclusions

The COVID-19 pandemic was related to a higher occurrence of OHCA in comparison to the 6-year pre-pandemic period. The circadian, monthly, and seasonal variabilities of OHCA occurrence were confirmed, both in the year 2020 and in the 2014–2019 period with no differences between the weekdays. A higher number of OHCA cases occurred at night and on Sundays during the pandemic year. In 2020, the highest occurrence of OHCA was observed in autumn, especially in October and November, which coincided with the highest occurrence of COVID-19 infections in Poland during the second wave of the pandemic. Further studies should be performed to explore the long-term impact of SARS-CoV-2 infection on the incidence of OHCA.

Author Contributions: Conceptualization, J.R., S.S. and A.K.; methodology, J.R, S.S. and A.K; formal analysis, J.R.; investigation, J.R., S.S. and A.K.; resources, S.S.; data curation, J.R. and S.S.; writing—original draft preparation, J.R.; writing—review and editing, S.S. and A.K.; visualization, J.R.; supervision, A.K.; project administration, A.K. All authors have read and agreed to the published version of the manuscript.

Funding: This research received no external funding.

Institutional Review Board Statement: The study was conducted in accordance with the Declaration of Helsinki, and approved by the Ethics Committee of The Nicolaus Copernicus University in Torun, Collegium Medicum in Bydgoszcz (KB 471/2013).

Informed Consent Statement: Not applicable.

Data Availability Statement: Data are available upon reasonable request. All data relevant to the study are included in the article. The original data are available from the corresponding author, within the limits of the signed informed consent from the contributors.

Conflicts of Interest: The authors declare no conflict of interest.

References

1. *World Health Organization COVID-19 Weekly Epidemiological Update, Edition 63, 26 October 2021*; World Health Organization: Geneva, Switzerland, 2021.
2. Raport Zakażeń Koronawirusem (SARS-CoV-2)-Koronawirus: Informacje i Zalecenia-Portal Gov.pl. Available online: https://www.gov.pl/web/koronawirus/wykaz-zarazen-koronawirusem-sars-cov-2 (accessed on 21 November 2021).
3. Kubica, J.; Podhajski, P.; Magielski, P.; Kubica, A.; Adamski, P.; Junik, R.; Pinkas, J.; Navarese, E.P. IMPACT of PCSK9 Inhibition on Clinical Outcome in Patients during the Inflammatory Stage of the SARS-COV-2 Infection: Rationale and Protocol of the IMPACT-SIRIO 5 Study. *Cardiol. J.* **2021**, *29*, 140–147. [CrossRef] [PubMed]
4. Gąsecka, A.; Borovac, J.A.; Guerreiro, R.A.; Giustozzi, M.; Parker, W.; Caldeira, D.; Chiva-Blanch, G. Thrombotic Complications in Patients with COVID-19: Pathophysiological Mechanisms, Diagnosis, and Treatment. *Cardiovasc. Drugs Ther.* **2021**, *35*, 215–229. [CrossRef] [PubMed]
5. Hollenberg, J.; Svensson, L.; Rosenqvist, M. Out-of-Hospital Cardiac Arrest: 10 Years of Progress in Research and Treatment. *J. Intern. Med.* **2013**, *273*, 572–583. [CrossRef] [PubMed]
6. Borkowska, M.J.; Jaguszewski, M.J.; Koda, M.; Gasecka, A.; Szarpak, A.; Gilis-Malinowska, N.; Safiejko, K.; Szarpak, L.; Filipiak, K.J.; Smereka, J. Impact of Coronavirus Disease 2019 on Out-of-Hospital Cardiac Arrest Survival Rate: A Systematic Review with Meta-Analysis. *J. Clin. Med.* **2021**, *10*, 1209. [CrossRef]
7. Bruska, M.; Szankin, Z.; Ratajczak, J.; Fabiszak, T. Improvement of the Quality of Cardiopulmonary Resuscitation Performed with Real CPR Help®Device among Medical Students and Medical Workers. *Med. Res. J.* **2021**, *6*, 177–183. [CrossRef]
8. Malysz, M.; Dabrowski, M.; Böttiger, B.W.; Smereka, J.; Kulak, K.; Szarpak, A.; Jaguszewski, M.; Filipiak, K.J.; Ladny, J.R.; Ruetzler, K.; et al. Resuscitation of the Patient with Suspected/Confirmed COVID-19 When Wearing Personal Protective Equipment: A Randomized Multicenter Crossover Simulation Trial. *Cardiol. J.* **2020**, *27*, 497–506. [CrossRef]
9. Ahn, J.Y.; Ryoo, H.W.; Cho, J.W.; Kim, J.H.; Lee, S.-H.; Jang, T.C. Impact of the COVID-19 Outbreak on Adult out-of-Hospital Cardiac Arrest Outcomes in Daegu, South Korea: An Observational Study. *Clin. Exp. Emerg. Med.* **2021**, *8*, 137–144. [CrossRef]
10. Baldi, E.; Sechi, G.M.; Mare, C.; Canevari, F.; Brancaglione, A.; Primi, R.; Klersy, C.; Palo, A.; Contri, E.; Ronchi, V.; et al. COVID-19 Kills at Home: The Close Relationship between the Epidemic and the Increase of out-of-Hospital Cardiac Arrests. *Eur. Heart J.* **2020**, *41*, 3045–3054. [CrossRef]
11. Ball, J.; Nehme, Z.; Bernard, S.; Stub, D.; Stephenson, M.; Smith, K. Collateral Damage: Hidden Impact of the COVID-19 Pandemic on the out-of-Hospital Cardiac Arrest System-of-Care. *Resuscitation* **2020**, *156*, 157–163. [CrossRef]
12. Fothergill, R.T.; Smith, A.L.; Wrigley, F.; Perkins, G.D. Out-of-Hospital Cardiac Arrest in London during the COVID-19 Pandemic. *Resusc. Plus* **2021**, *5*, 100066. [CrossRef]
13. Glober, N.K.; Supples, M.; Faris, G.; Arkins, T.; Christopher, S.; Fulks, T.; Rayburn, D.; Weinstein, E.; Liao, M.; O'Donnell, D.; et al. Out-of-Hospital Cardiac Arrest Volumes and Characteristics during the COVID-19 Pandemic. *Am. J. Emerg. Med.* **2021**, *48*, 191–197. [CrossRef]
14. Lim, S.L.; Shahidah, N.; Saffari, S.E.; Ng, Q.X.; Ho, A.F.W.; Leong, B.S.-H.; Arulanandam, S.; Siddiqui, F.J.; Ong, M.E.H. Impact of COVID-19 on Out-of-Hospital Cardiac Arrest in Singapore. *Int. J. Environ. Res. Public. Health* **2021**, *18*, 3646. [CrossRef]
15. Lim, Z.J.; Ponnapa Reddy, M.; Afroz, A.; Billah, B.; Shekar, K.; Subramaniam, A. Incidence and Outcome of Out-of-Hospital Cardiac Arrests in the COVID-19 Era: A Systematic Review and Meta-Analysis. *Resuscitation* **2020**, *157*, 248–258. [CrossRef]
16. Marijon, E.; Karam, N.; Jost, D.; Perrot, D.; Frattini, B.; Derkenne, C.; Sharifzadehgan, A.; Waldmann, V.; Beganton, F.; Narayanan, K.; et al. Out-of-Hospital Cardiac Arrest during the COVID-19 Pandemic in Paris, France: A Population-Based, Observational Study. *Lancet Public Health* **2020**, *5*, e437–e443. [CrossRef]
17. McVaney, K.E.; Pepe, P.E.; Maloney, L.M.; Bronsky, E.S.; Crowe, R.P.; Augustine, J.J.; Gilliam, S.O.; Asaeda, G.H.; Eckstein, M.; Mattu, A.; et al. The Relationship of Large City Out-of-Hospital Cardiac Arrests and the Prevalence of COVID-19. *EClinicalMedicine* **2021**, *34*, 100815. [CrossRef]
18. Talikowska, M.; Ball, S.; Tohira, H.; Bailey, P.; Rose, D.; Brink, D.; Bray, J.; Finn, J. No Apparent Effect of the COVID-19 Pandemic on out-of-Hospital Cardiac Arrest Incidence and Outcome in Western Australia. *Resusc. Plus* **2021**, *8*, 100183. [CrossRef]
19. Uy-Evanado, A.; Chugh, H.S.; Sargsyan, A.; Nakamura, K.; Mariani, R.; Hadduck, K.; Salvucci, A.; Jui, J.; Chugh, S.S.; Reinier, K. Out-of-Hospital Cardiac Arrest Response and Outcomes during the COVID-19 Pandemic. *JACC Clin. Electrophysiol.* **2021**, *7*, 6–11. [CrossRef]
20. Borkowska, M.J.; Smereka, J.; Safiejko, K.; Nadolny, K.; Maslanka, M.; Filipiak, K.J.; Jaguszewski, M.J.; Szarpak, L. Out-of-Hospital Cardiac Arrest Treated by Emergency Medical Service Teams during COVID-19 Pandemic: A Retrospective Cohort Study. *Cardiol. J.* **2021**, *28*, 15–22. [CrossRef]

21. Hawranek, M.; Grygier, M.; Bujak, K.; Bartuś, S.; Gierlotka, M.; Wojakowski, W.; Legutko, J.; Lesiak, M.; Pączek, P.; Kleinrok, A.; et al. Characteristics of Patients from the Polish Registry of Acute Coronary Syndromes during the COVID-19 Pandemic: The First Report. *Kardiol. Pol.* **2021**, *79*, 192–195. [CrossRef]
22. Ratajczak, J.; Łach, P.; Szczerbiński, S.; Paciorek, P.; Karłowska-Pik, J.; Ziemkiewicz, B.; Jasiewicz, M.; Kubica, A. Atmospheric Conditions and the Occurrence of Out-of-Hospital Cardiac Arrest in Poland—Preliminary Analysis of Poorly Understood Phenomena. *Med. Res. J.* **2018**, *3*, 121–126. [CrossRef]
23. Kubica, A.; Szczerbiński, S.; Kieszkowska, M.; Świątkiewicz, I.; Paciorek, P. Wpływ czynników klimatycznych i chronologicznych na występowanie ostrych incydentów chorobowych. *Folia Cardiol.* **2014**, *9*, 263–266.
24. Kim, J.-H.; Hong, J.; Jung, J.; Im, J.-S. Effect of Meteorological Factors and Air Pollutants on Out-of-Hospital Cardiac Arrests: A Time Series Analysis. *Heart Br. Card. Soc.* **2020**, *106*, 1218–1227. [CrossRef]
25. Gentile, F.R.; Primi, R.; Baldi, E.; Compagnoni, S.; Mare, C.; Contri, E.; Reali, F.; Bussi, D.; Facchin, F.; Currao, A.; et al. Out-of-Hospital Cardiac Arrest and Ambient Air Pollution: A Dose-Effect Relationship and an Association with OHCA Incidence. *PLoS ONE* **2021**, *16*, e0256526. [CrossRef]
26. Szczerbinski, S.; Ratajczak, J.; Lach, P.; Rzeszuto, J.; Paciorek, P.; Karlowska-Pik, J.; Ziemkiewicz, B.; Jasiewicz, M.; Kubica, A. Epidemiology and Chronobiology of Out-of-Hospital Cardiac Arrest in a Subpopulation of Southern Poland: A Two-Year Observation. *Cardiol. J.* **2020**, *27*, 16–24. [CrossRef]
27. Szczerbiński, S.; Ratajczak, J.; Jasiewicz, M.; Kubica, A. Observational AnalysiS of Out-of-Hospital Cardiac Arrest OccurRence and Temporal Variability Patterns in Subpopulation of Southern POLand from 2006 to 2018: OSCAR-POL Registry. *Cardiol. J.* ahead of print. **2021**. [CrossRef]
28. Paciorek, P.; Obońska, K.; Skrzyński, W.; Ratajczak, J. Observational, Retrospective Study Evaluating the Temporal Variability of out-of-Hospital Cardiac Arrests (OHCA) in the District of Bydgoszcz in a 24-Month Period. *Med. Res. J.* **2021**, *6*, 217–223. [CrossRef]
29. Onozuka, D.; Hagihara, A. Extreme Influenza Epidemics and Out-of-Hospital Cardiac Arrest. *Int. J. Cardiol.* **2018**, *263*, 158–162. [CrossRef]
30. Rashid, M.; Gale, C.P.; Curzen, N.; Ludman, P.; De Belder, M.; Timmis, A.; Mohamed, M.O.; Lüscher, T.F.; Hains, J.; Wu, J.; et al. Impact of COVID19 Pandemic on the Incidence and Management of Out of Hospital Cardiac Arrest in Patients Presenting with Acute Myocardial Infarction in England. *J. Am. Heart Assoc.* **2020**, *9*, e018379. [CrossRef]
31. Lai, P.H.; Lancet, E.A.; Weiden, M.D.; Webber, M.P.; Zeig-Owens, R.; Hall, C.B.; Prezant, D.J. Characteristics Associated with Out-of-Hospital Cardiac Arrests and Resuscitations during the Novel Coronavirus Disease 2019 Pandemic in New York City. *JAMA Cardiol.* **2020**, *5*, 1154–1163. [CrossRef]
32. Mathew, S.; Harrison, N.; Chalek, A.D.; Gorelick, D.; Brennan, E.; Wise, S.; Gandolfo, L.; O'Neil, B.; Dunne, R. Effects of the COVID-19 Pandemic on out-of-Hospital Cardiac Arrest Care in Detroit. *Am. J. Emerg. Med.* **2021**, *46*, 90–96. [CrossRef]
33. Baldi, E.; Auricchio, A.; Klersy, C.; Burkart, R.; Benvenuti, C.; Vanetta, C.; Bärtschi, J. SWISSRECA researchers Out-of-Hospital Cardiac Arrests and Mortality in Swiss Cantons with High and Low COVID-19 Incidence: A Nationwide Analysis. *Resusc. Plus* **2021**, *6*, 100105. [CrossRef] [PubMed]
34. Paoli, A.; Brischigliaro, L.; Scquizzato, T.; Favaretto, A.; Spagna, A. Out-of-Hospital Cardiac Arrest during the COVID-19 Pandemic in the Province of Padua, Northeast Italy. *Resuscitation* **2020**, *154*, 47–49. [CrossRef] [PubMed]
35. Baldi, E.; Primi, R.; Bendotti, S.; Currao, A.; Compagnoni, S.; Gentile, F.R.; Sechi, G.M.; Mare, C.; Palo, A.; Contri, E.; et al. Relationship between Out-of-Hospital Cardiac Arrests and COVID-19 during the First and Second Pandemic Wave. The Importance of Monitoring COVID-19 Incidence. *PLoS ONE* **2021**, *16*, e0260275. [CrossRef] [PubMed]
36. Yu, J.-H.; Liu, C.-Y.; Chen, W.-K.; Yu, S.-H.; Huang, F.-W.; Yang, M.-T.; Chen, C.-Y.; Shih, H.-M. Impact of the COVID-19 Pandemic on Emergency Medical Service Response to out-of-Hospital Cardiac Arrests in Taiwan: A Retrospective Observational Study. *Emerg. Med. J.* **2021**, *38*, 679–684. [CrossRef]
37. Nadolny, K.; Zyśko, D.; Obremska, M.; Wierzbik-Strońska, M.; Ładny, J.R.; Podgórski, M.; Gałązkowski, R. Analysis of Out-of-Hospital Cardiac Arrest in Poland in a 1-Year Period: Data from the POL-OHCA Registry. *Kardiol. Pol.* **2020**, *78*, 404–411. [CrossRef]
38. Gach, D.; Nowak, J.U.; Krzych, Ł.J. Epidemiology of Out-of-Hospital Cardiac Arrest in the Bielsko-Biala District: A 12-Month Analysis. *Kardiol. Pol.* **2016**, *74*, 1180–1187. [CrossRef]
39. Kubica, J.; Ostrowska, M.; Stolarek, W.; Kasprzak, M.; Grzelakowska, K.; Kryś, J.; Kubica, A.; Adamski, P.; Podhajski, P.; Navarese, E.P.; et al. Impact of COVID-19 Pandemic on Acute Heart Failure Admissions and Mortality: A Multicentre Study (COV-HF-SIRIO 6 Study). *ESC Heart Fail.* **2021**, *9*, 721–728. [CrossRef]
40. Al-Wathinani, A.; Hertelendy, A.J.; Alhurishi, S.; Mobrad, A.; Alhazmi, R.; Altuwaijri, M.; Alanazi, M.; Alotaibi, R.; Goniewicz, K. Increased Emergency Calls during the COVID-19 Pandemic in Saudi Arabia: A National Retrospective Study. *Healthcare* **2020**, *9*, 14. [CrossRef]
41. Lackowski, P.; Piasecki, M.; Kasprzak, M.; Kryś, J.; Niezgoda, P.; Kubica, J. COVID-19 Pandemic Year in the Cardiology Department. *Med. Res. J.* **2021**, *6*, 40–46. [CrossRef]

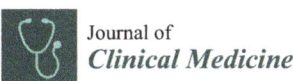

Article

High PEEP Levels during CPR Improve Ventilation without Deleterious Haemodynamic Effects in Pigs

Miriam Renz, Leah Müllejans, Julian Riedel, Katja Mohnke, René Rissel, Alexander Ziebart, Bastian Duenges, Erik Kristoffer Hartmann and Robert Ruemmler *,†

Department of Anaesthesiology, University Medical Center, Johannes Gutenberg University, Langenbeckstrasse 1, 55131 Mainz, Germany
* Correspondence: robert.ruemmler@email.de; Tel.: +49-6131-176755
† Current address: Robert Ruemmler, MD, MBA, Langenbeckstrasse 1, 55131 Mainz, Germany.

Abstract: Background: Invasive ventilation during cardiopulmonary resuscitation (CPR) is very complex due to unique thoracic pressure conditions. Current guidelines do not provide specific recommendations for ventilation during ongoing chest compressions regarding positive end-expiratory pressure (PEEP). This trial examines the cardiopulmonary effects of PEEP application during CPR. Methods: Forty-two German landrace pigs were anaesthetised, instrumented, and randomised into six intervention groups. Three PEEP levels (0, 8, and 16 mbar) were compared in high standard and ultralow tidal volume ventilation. After the induction of ventricular fibrillation, mechanical chest compressions and ventilation were initiated and maintained for thirty minutes. Blood gases, ventilation/perfusion ratio, and electrical impedance tomography loops were taken repeatedly. Ventilation pressures and haemodynamic parameters were measured continuously. Postmortem lung tissue damage was assessed using the diffuse alveolar damage (DAD) score. Statistical analyses were performed using SPSS, and p values <0.05 were considered significant. Results: The driving pressure (P_{drive}) showed significantly lower values when using PEEP 16 mbar than when using PEEP 8 mbar ($p = 0.045$) or PEEP 0 mbar ($p < 0.001$) when adjusted for the ventilation mode. Substantially increased overall lung damage was detected in the PEEP 0 mbar group (vs. PEEP 8 mbar, $p = 0.038$; vs. PEEP 16 mbar, $p = 0.009$). No significant differences in mean arterial pressure could be detected. Conclusion: The use of PEEP during CPR seems beneficial because it optimises ventilation pressures and reduces lung damage without significantly compromising blood pressure. Further studies are needed to examine long-term effects in resuscitated animals.

Keywords: resuscitation; porcine; ventilation; MIGET; EIT

1. Introduction

In regard to the use of ventilation in cardiac arrest and cardiopulmonary resuscitation (CPR), specific recommendations regarding optimal respiratory settings remain elusive [1]. Neither the European Resuscitation Council (ERC) nor the American Heart Association (AHA) provide detailed information on ventilation types or the application of positive end-expiratory pressure (PEEP) [2,3]. Guidelines recommend securing the airway during resuscitation and using an endotracheal tube if trained personnel are present. Once the airway is secured, the guidelines suggest using a ventilation rate of 10 breaths per minute and performing continuous chest compressions [2,3]. However, it is known that using PEEP during resuscitation can have positive effects on survival [4] and oxygenation [5]. When using PEEP during CPR, the improved oxygenation is probably due to the prevention of atelectasis [6,7]. In cases with increased extrathoracic pressures, the use of PEEP can redistribute ventilation to the dorsal lung regions [8,9]. However, the continuous application of PEEP could also lead to increased intrathoracic pressures, which can impair venous blood flow [10,11]. However, previous studies showed no impaired venous return when

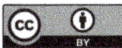

applying continuous PEEP during CPR [4,6,7]. Furthermore, the application of PEEP, in general, aligns with lung-protective ventilation strategies that recommend (among others) the application of a PEEP level greater than 5 cm H_2O [12], although no sufficient data exist to support the clinical relevance during CPR.

In the presented prospective, randomised, large animal trial, three different PEEP levels were compared using standard (intermittent positive pressure ventilation, IPPV) and low tidal (ultralow tidal volume ventilation, ULTVV) ventilation modes during CPR.

The primary aim of the trial was to examine whether the use of high PEEP levels during CPR can improve gas exchange and optimise ventilation pressures by improving lung recruitment. As a secondary aim, we examined the haemodynamic effects of the applied PEEP levels to determine the clinical value of our findings. Thirdly, we assessed lung tissue damage correlated to the interventions.

2. Methods

Anaesthesia and Instrumentation

This animal trial was approved by the State and Institutional Animal Care Committee Rhineland Palatine (approval no. G20-1-065), and all experiments were performed according to the German Animal Protection Law and the ARRIVE guidelines between January and September 2021. The trial was planned as a prospective, randomised trial.

Forty-two German landrace pigs (age: 12–16 weeks, weight: 29–34 kg) were examined. Sedation, transport, and instrumentation were performed as described in detail before [7]. In short, animals were placed under general anaesthesia using iv injections of fentanyl, propofol, and atracurium, followed by endotracheal intubation. Instrumentation was performed placing iv sheaths in femoral arteries and veins into the left and right groin under sonographic guidance. Additionally, an electrode belt was placed circularly around the thorax, approximately 10 cm above the diaphragm, for electrical impedance tomography measurements (EIT, Pulmo Vista 500, Dräger, Lübeck, Germany).

3. Trial Protocol and Data Collection

After induction of anaesthesia and instrumentation, the animals received a fluid bolus of 30 mL/kg balanced electrolyte solution. Six chemically inert gases with different transpulmonary elimination constants (sulphur hexafluoride, krypton, desflurane, enflurane, diethyl ether, acetone) were dissolved in nontoxic doses in saline and given intravenously for the ventilation/perfusion (V/Q) ratio measurements. MIGET was performed after a stabilisation phase of 30 min to reach a steady state.

At the measurement timepoint, baseline healthy (BLH) arterial and central venous blood gases were measured (radiometer, ABL90flex, Copenhagen, Denmark), blood samples for the MIGET measurement (MMIMS-MIGET, Oscillogy LLC, Philadelphia, PA, USA) were taken, and EIT recordings were started. Afterward, the animals received a second dose of atracurium (0.5 mg/kg). The fibrillation catheter was transvenously placed into the right atrium, and continuous ventricular fibrillation was induced with a flicker frequency between 50 and 200 Hertz (Hz). After ECG-confirmed ventricular fibrillation and 5 min of no-flow time, basic life support was started with mechanical chest compressions by the LUCAS 2-System (Stryker, Kalamazoo, MI, USA) with a frequency of 100 compressions/min. Ventilation was performed according to the intervention group. Following the trial protocol, animals were randomised into 6 intervention groups (n = 7 per group, Table 1).

After 30 min of BLS, a rhythm analysis was performed, and guideline-based advanced life support (ALS) was applied if ventricular fibrillation was still detectable. At the CPR measured timepoints of 5 min, 15 min, and 25 min, samples for arterial and central venous blood gas analysis and MIGET measurements were taken. The extended haemodynamic measurements were recorded continuously by using the Datex Ohmeda S5 monitor (GE Healthcare, Munich, Germany). EIT loops were recorded continuously during CPR.

Table 1. Group design and intervention parameters during resuscitation.

Group Parameters	Group 1–3	Group 4–6
Ventilation mode	IPPV	ULTVV
PEEP level	0, 8, 16 mbar (I0, I8, I16)	0, 8, 16 mbar (U0, U8, U16)
Tidal volume (Vt)	9–10 mL/kgBW	2–3 mL/kgBW
Respiratory rate (RR)	10 breaths/min	50 breaths/min
FiO_2	1.0	1.0

Postmortem lung tissue samples were collected from the cranial, caudal, ventral, and dorsal sections of the left and right lung lobes and fixed with formalin 4%. These samples were paraffinised, cut into 2-micrometre-thick slices, and stained with haematoxylin–eosin (HE) by the tissue bank of the University Medical Center Mainz, Mainz, Germany.

Scores and Statistics

The histopathologic lung samples were examined with an Olympus microscope (CX43RF, Olympus Cooperation, Tokyo, Japan) via CellSens Software (CellSens Entry.lnk, creation date 3 December 2018) and scored with the previously established diffuse alveolar damage (DAD) score [13]. All statistical planning and interpretations were performed with the assistance of the Institute of Medical Biometrics and Epidemiology of the Johannes Gutenberg University Mainz. Statistical analyses were performed with SPSS (IBM SPSS Statistics, Version: 23 V5 R, Armonk, NY, USA) by using repeated measurements of ANOVA (RMA) and post hoc analysis with Tukey's test. Statistics of the DAD score were evaluated using linear mixed-effect models. Data in text and graphs are presented as the mean and standard deviation (SD). p values lower than 0.05 were considered statistically significant.

4. Results

In total, 42 experiments were performed, in which no animal achieved a return of spontaneous circulation (ROSC).

The driving pressure (P_{drive}) showed a significant difference between the PEEP groups (RMA $p < 0.001$), when adjusting for the ventilation mode: PEEP 16 mbar had significantly lower values than PEEP 8 mbar (Tukey $p = 0.045$) and PEEP 0 mbar (Tukey $p < 0.001$) during CPR. PEEP 8 mbar also showed lower values than PEEP 0 mbar (Tukey $p = 0.014$). The comparison of the six intervention groups showed analogous findings (Tukey I0 vs. I16, $p = 0.010$; Tukey U0 vs. U16, $p = 0.003$). PEEP 16 displayed a marginal mean P_{drive} of 12.23 mbar ($\pm$ 5.04 mbar), while PEEP 0 mbar showed a marginal mean P_{drive} of 21.06 mbar ($\pm$ 5.91 mbar). The PEEP groups also showed significant differences when observing the P_{mean} (RMA $p < 0.001$) and P_{peak} (RMA $p < 0.001$) during CPR. PEEP 0 and 8 mbar had significantly lower values than PEEP 16 mbar in P_{mean} (Tukey PEEP 0 mbar vs. PEEP 16 mbar, $p < 0.001$; Tukey PEEP 8 mbar vs. PEEP 16 mbar, $p < 0.001$; Tukey PEEP 0 mbar vs. PEEP 8 mbar, $p < 0.001$) and P_{peak} (Tukey PEEP 0 mbar vs. PEEP 16 mbar, $p < 0.001$; Tukey PEEP 8 mbar vs. PEEP 16 mbar, $p = 0.031$). Similar findings may be observed when comparing the P_{mean} of the intervention groups. In P_{peak}, the intervention groups showed a significant difference when comparing I0 vs. I16 (Tukey, $p = 0.011$). PEEP 16 mbar displayed a marginal mean P_{peak} of 28.49 mbar ($\pm$ 5.28 mbar), while PEEP 0 mbar showed a marginal mean P_{peak} of 21.23 mbar ($\pm$ 5.89 mbar). Additionally, significant differences were observed when comparing the ventilation modes, adjusted for the PEEP groups, in the P_{drive} (RMA $p = 0.002$), P_{mean} (RMA $p < 0.001$), and P_{peak} (RMA $p = 0.001$) parameters during CPR, with IPPV leading to significantly higher values than ULTVV (Figure 1).

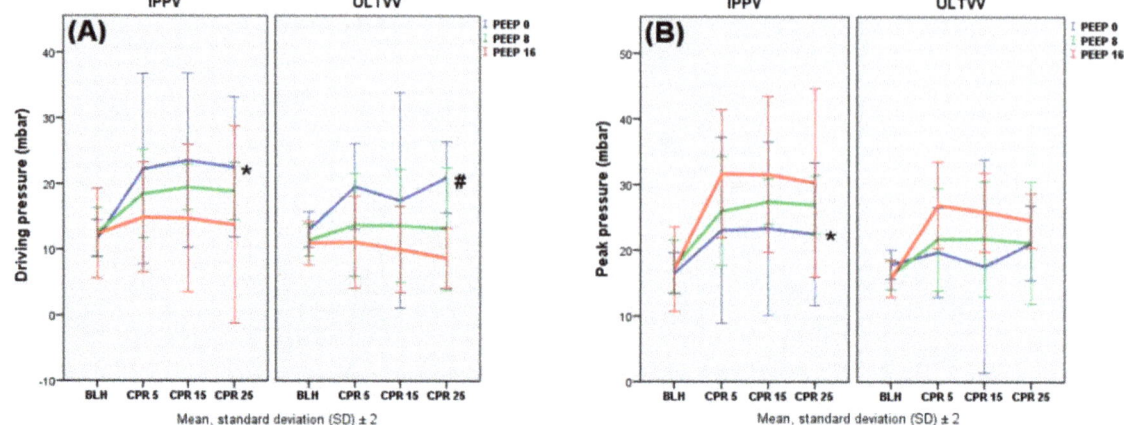

Figure 1. Ventilation: driving pressure (P_{drive}, (**A**)), peak pressure (P_{peak}, (**B**)). Airway pressures were measured in mbar. Data are shown as mean values and standard deviation (SD). Significant differences in P_{drive} (**A**): * vs. I16, $p = 0.010$; # vs. U16, $p = 0.003$ (Tukey). Significant differences in P_{peak} (**B**) * vs. I16, $p = 0.011$ (Tukey).

The ventilation–perfusion ratios (V/Q) were measured via MIGET. The U0 group showed non-significantly higher percentages of shunt and significantly higher percentages of low V/Q (Tukey I0 vs. U0, $p = 0.038$) as well as a non-significantly lower fraction of normal and high V/Q during CPR. The I0 group showed non-significantly increasing normal V/Q as well as high V/Q during the intervention and decreased shunt percentage. Both PEEP 16 mbar groups showed decreasing normal V/Q percentages during the intervention and increasing high and low V/Q as well as shunt percentages. The ULTVV groups showed significantly fewer high V/Q (RMA $p = 0.006$) while having significantly more results of low V/Q (RMA $p = 0.041$), adjusted for the PEEP groups.

The arterial partial pressure of carbon dioxide ($paCO_2$) was significantly higher in the ULTVV mode during the entire intervention (RMA $p = 0.001$), when adjusted for PEEP. At the start of the intervention, the PEEP 0 mbar groups and the U8 group showed high values of $paCO_2$, while, at the end, the groups with PEEP 16 mbar displayed the highest $paCO_2$ values. The significantly lowest arterial partial pressure of oxygen (paO_2) was detected in the PEEP 0 mbar group, adjusted for the ventilation mode (Tukey PEEP 0 mbar vs. PEEP 8 mbar, $p = 0.025$). In all intervention groups, the paO_2 decreased over time (Figure 2).

There were no significant differences in haemodynamic values between the PEEP groups or tidal volume groups. However, U0 mbar showed a non-significantly lower mean arterial pressure (MAP) during CPR than the groups with PEEP (Figure 3). A detailed summary of cardiopulmonary parameters is shown in Table 2.

The lung physiology was monitored via EIT. In the resulting transverse sectional view, the ROIs are numbered 1 to 4 from the ventral thoracic areas (1) to the dorsal areas (4). During CPR, the highest impedances were observed in ROI 2.

In all ROIs, no significant differences were found between the groups during the intervention. In ROI 1, U0 had non-significantly increased impedances compared with the two ULTTV groups with PEEP. In the dorsal thoracic part, the ULTVV mode displayed non-significantly higher impedances than the IPPV mode when adjusted for the PEEP groups. Here, U0 showed high impedances at the beginning of CPR, which then constantly decreased over time. The highest values in the dorsal thoracic part were observed in the PEEP 16 mbar groups (Supplementary Figure S1).

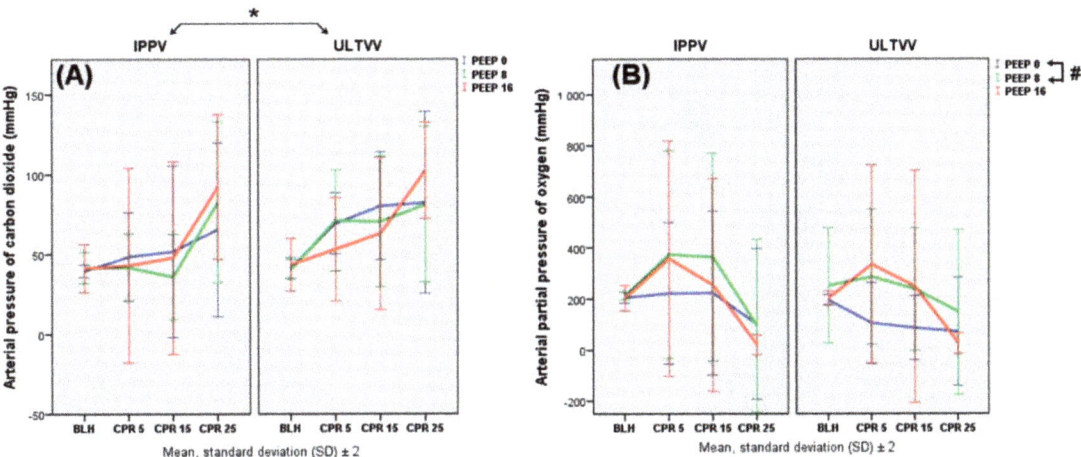

Figure 2. Blood gases: arterial partial pressure of CO_2 (PaCO$_2$, (**A**)), arterial partial pressure of O$_2$ (PaO$_2$, (**B**)). The unit of PaCO$_2$ and PaO$_2$ is mmHg. Data are shown as mean values and standard deviation (SD). Significant differences in paCO$_2$ (**A**): * ULTVV vs. IPPV, when adjusted for PEEP, $p = 0.001$ (RMA). Significant differences in paO$_2$ (**B**): # PEEP 0 mbar vs. PEEP 8 mbar, when adjusted for ventilation mode, $p = 0.025$ (Tukey).

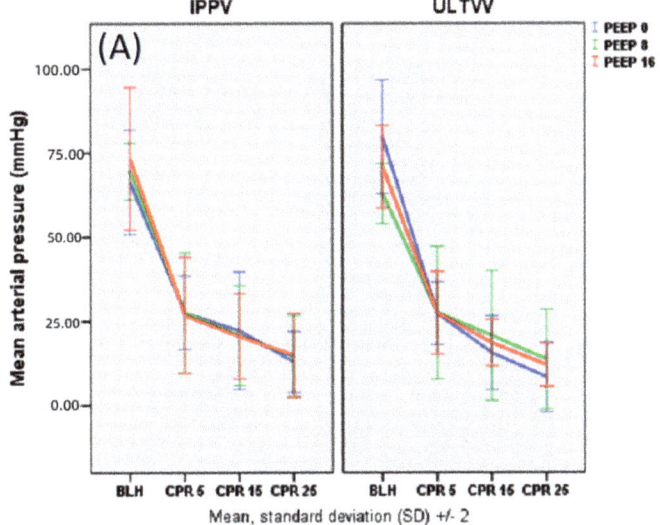

Figure 3. Haemodynamics: mean arterial pressure (MAP, (**A**) The unit of MAP is mmHg. Data are shown as mean values and standard deviation (SD). No significant differences were observed.

Table 2. Overview of relevant ventilation parameters, invasively measured haemodynamic parameters, blood gases, MIGET measurement, DAD score. Standard deviation (SD), driving pressure (P_{drive}), peak pressure (P_{peak}), partial arterial pressure of carbon dioxide ($paCO_2$), partial arterial pressure of oxygen (paO_2), mean arterial pressure (MAP), diffuse alveolar damage (DAD) score, overdistension (overdis.), intermittent positive pressure ventilation (IPPV), ultralow tidal volume ventilation (ULTVV). Statistical analyses were performed using SPSS and p-values < 0.05 were considered significant. Significant statistical differences are shown with the following symbols: *, #, †.

Parameter MEAN (SD)	Intervention Groups	CPR 5 min	CPR 15 min	CPR 25 min	p Values
Pdrive [mbar]	IPPV	18.56 (5.82)	19.27 (6.08)	18.40 (6.35)	* vs. IPPV, 0.002
	ULTVV *	14.82 (4.96)	13.73 (6.21)	14.31 (6.10)	
	PEEP 0 mbar	20.93 (5.57)	20.51 (7.82)	21.77 (4.14)	* vs. PEEP 0, 0.014
	PEEP 8 mbar *	16.12 (4.28)	16.58 (4.37)	16.05 (4.57)	# vs. PEEP 0, 0.000; † vs. PEEP 8, 0.045
	PEEP 16 mbar #,†	13.02 (4.20)	12.40 (5.04)	11.25 (5.93)	
Ppeak [mbar]	IPPV	26.92 (6.38)	27.46 (6.03)	26.58 (6.03)	* vs. IPPV, 0.001
	ULTVV *	22.79 (4.57)	21.74 (6.33)	22.29 (3.59)	
	PEEP 0 mbar	21.39 (5.60)	20.48 (7.70)	21.80 (4.21)	
	PEEP 8 mbar	23.86 (4.45)	24.61 (4.35)	24.07 (4.61)	# vs. PEEP 0, 0.000; † vs. PEEP 8, 0.031
	PEEP 16 mbar #,†	29.31 (4.70)	28.71 (5.41)	27.44 (5.87)	
shunt [%]	IPPV	19.60 (21.67)	17.42 (14.99)	19.00 (19.85)	
	ULTVV	15.80 (13.56)	17.99 (12.00)	23.06 (11.48)	
	PEEP 0 mbar	29.06 (26.04)	21.59 (12.47)	19.08 (10.87)	
	PEEP 8 mbar	8.78 (4.11)	19.47 (15.43)	14.54 (7.92)	
	PEEP 16 mbar	15.94 (10.95)	12.05 (10.94)	29.47 (22.70)	
$paCO_2$ [mmHg]	IPPV	44.60 (19.45)	45.32 (24.26)	80.27 (26.36)	* vs. IPPV, 0.001
	ULTVV *	64.70 (15.80)	71.43 (20.84)	88.80 (24.27)	
	PEEP 0 mbar	59.05 (15.75)	66.18 (26.13)	74.02 (28.09)	
	PEEP 8 mbar	56.60 (19.96)	53.35 (24.48)	82.00 (23.79)	
	PEEP 16 mbar	48.30 (24.03)	55.60 (27.22)	97.57 (19.22)	
paO_2 [mmHg]	IPPV	318.38 (197.12)	281.12 (192.31)	72.85 (129.10)	
	ULTVV	242.60 (169.22)	191.30 (163.44)	82.73 (118.34)	
	PEEP 0 mbar	164.26 (123.97)	155.42 (136.91)	87.27 (124.16)	# vs. PEEP 0, 0.025
	PEEP 8 mbar #	330.57 (170.61)	301.68 (173.26)	122.38 (161.54)	
	PEEP 16 mbar	346.63 (205.03)	251.53 (209.41)	23.71 (19.15)	
MAP [mmHg]	IPPV	27.38 (7.42)	21.22 (7.17)	14.19 (5.45)	
	ULTVV	27.46 (6.82)	18.38 (6.70)	11.43 (5.69)	
	PEEP 0 mbar	27.48 (4.84)	18.99 (7.77)	10.73 (5.21)	
	PEEP 8 mbar	27.62 (9.02)	20.79 (8.22)	14.20 (6.51)	
	PEEP 16 mbar	27.17 (7.18)	19.62 (4.98)	13.49 (5.01)	
Post mortem					
DAD. atelectasis [points]	IPPV	1.95 (1.04)			* vs. IPPV, 0.000
	ULTVV *	2.59 (1.10)			
	PEEP 0 mbar	2.45 (1.40)			# vs. PEEP 0, 0.047
	PEEP 8 mbar #	2.29 (1.06)			
	PEEP 16 mbar	2.06 (0.77)			
DAD. overdistens. [points]	IPPV	1.51 (0.98)			# vs. IPPV, 0.001
	ULTVV *	1.03 (0.91)			
	PEEP 0 mbar	0.99 (0.97)			
	PEEP 8 mbar	1.14 (0.91)			# vs. PEEP 0, 0.000; † vs. PEEP 8, 0.012
	PEEP 16 mbar #,†	1.68 (0.92)			

Lung histology was evaluated with the DAD score. There was significantly higher lung damage in the sum total category in the PEEP 0 mbar group (all DAD-score-associated significances were evaluated by linear mixed-effect models) (vs. PEEP 8 mbar, $p = 0.038$; vs. PEEP 16 mbar, $p = 0.009$), which could also be observed when comparing the IPPV intervention groups (I0 vs. I8, $p = 0.012$; I0 vs. I16, $p = 0.040$). Nonetheless, the IPPV group showed lower values than the ULTVV group (IPPV vs. ULTVV, $p = 0.012$), which was also observed in an intervention group comparison (I8 vs. U8, $p = 0.003$). Regarding the individual items of the DAD score, the ULTVV mode, adjusted for the PEEP groups, showed greater microatelectrauma (vs. IPPV, $p < 0.001$), while the IPPV group showed more overdistension (vs. ULTVV, $p = 0.001$). In examining the PEEP groups, both PEEP 16 mbar groups showed the greatest overdistension within their ventilation mode (U16 vs. U0, $p < 0.001$; U16 vs. U8, $p = 0.001$). The PEEP 0 mbar groups showed the most microatelectatic tissue in their ventilation mode (I0 vs. I8, $p = 0.016$; U0 vs. U16, $p = 0.013$) as well as haemorrhage (I0 vs. I8, $p = 0.049$; U0 vs. U8, $p = 0.013$, U0 vs. U16, $p < 0.001$) (Figure 4, Supplementary Figure S2).

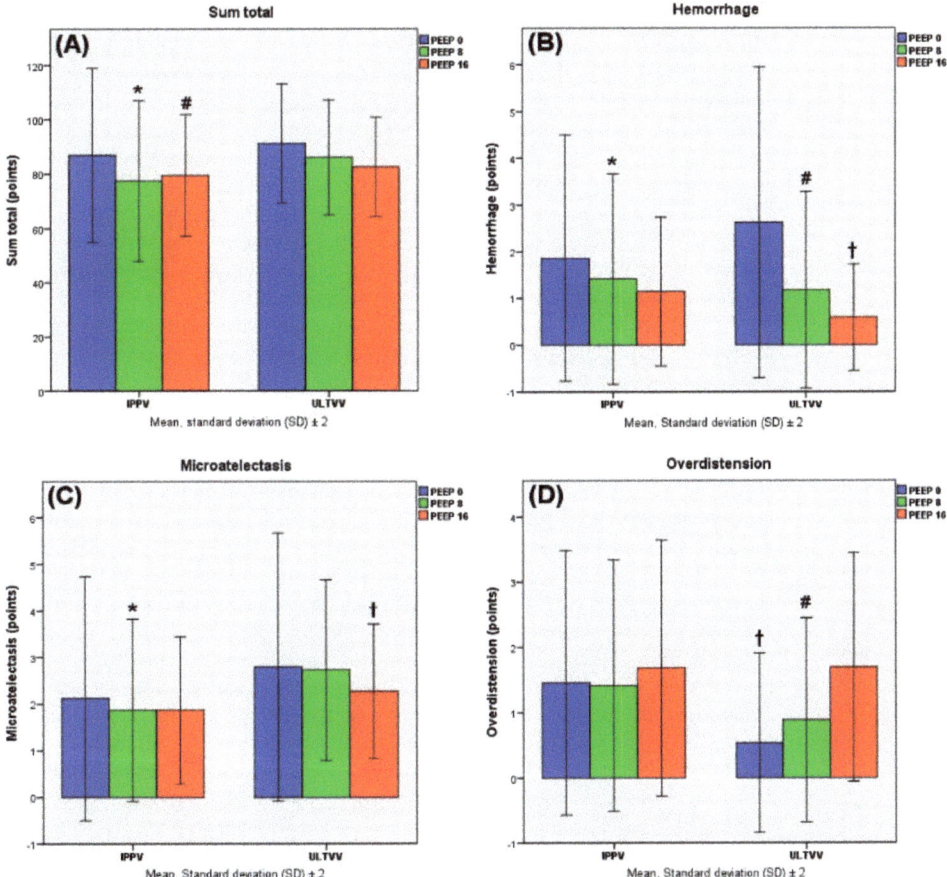

Figure 4. Lung histology evaluated with the DAD score. Categories were scored in points. Data are shown as mean values and standard deviation (SD). Significant differences in sum total (**A**): * vs. I0, $p = 0.012$; # vs. I0, $p = 0.040$ (linear mixed-effect models). Significant differences in haemorrhage (**B**): * vs. I0, $p = 0.049$; # vs. U0, $p = 0.013$; † vs. U0, $p < 0.001$ (linear mixed-effect models). Significant differences in microatelectasis (**C**): * vs. I0, $p = 0.016$; † vs. U0, $p = 0.013$ (linear mixed-effect models). Significant differences in overdistension (**D**): † vs. U16, $p < 0.001$; # vs. U16, $p = 0.001$ (linear mixed-effect models).

5. Discussion

In this prospective, randomised, controlled animal trial, we examined three different PEEP levels in a standard and low tidal volume ventilation mode during CPR. We discovered that the application of higher PEEP values significantly decreased driving pressures, when adjusted for the ventilation mode. Additionally, we showed that increased PEEP levels did not substantially impair mean arterial blood pressure levels during CPR, suggesting general feasibility while resuscitation efforts via chest compressions are ongoing. EIT and MIGET measurements supported the hypothesis that higher PEEP provides improved recruitment of dependent lung areas, whereas 0 mbar PEEP showed higher histologic damage values with increased atelectrauma.

Ventilation during resuscitation is challenging due to extreme thoracic pressure variances due to chest compressions. The concept of lung-protective ventilation recommends using PEEP greater than 5 cm H_2O, maintaining P_{peak} below 30 cm H_2O, and aiming for a low P_{drive}, limiting it to 15 cm H_2O or less [12,14]. In this trial, the intervention groups with PEEP showed significantly lower P_{drive} values during CPR compared to PEEP 0 mbar. When comparing IPPV versus ULTVV, the latter showed significantly lower peak and driving pressures in the respective PEEP groups. This was expected considering that the volume-controlled ventilation mode was set to substantially lower volumes initially. Lower tidal volume strategies lead to less alveolar pressure and thus can avoid overdistention [15]. The reduction in high ventilation pressures can lower the risk of overdistension, which can cause harmful lung damage and may lead to barotrauma [11,12,15].

The histologic examination of both the PEEP 16 mbar groups and all three IPPV groups revealed more overdistended lung tissue, suggesting overinflation and increased stress caused by the increased ventilation pressures necessary to achieve the set tidal volumes. However, the overall lung damage was substantial in the ULTVV mode and the PEEP 0 mbar group, which was mainly driven by significantly higher ratios of bleeding and microatelectasis. This leads to the question of which type of tissue damage—if any—is more crucial for post-ROSC oxygenation and overall outcome. To the best of our knowledge, no concise data are available on this correlation. Using PEEP in general can be beneficial because it leads to better oxygenation and lung recruitment as well as less atelectatic tissue [16]. The paO_2 values decreased in all six intervention groups during the intervention. However, when using PEEP, increased oxygenation could be observed in this trial. A study that investigated whether different PEEP levels could optimise carbon dioxide clearance during CPR showed that higher PEEP levels lead to significantly decreased $paCO_2$ levels and increased minute volume because of a higher fraction of gas oscillations generated by chest compressions [17]. However, this study intentionally did not adhere to resuscitation guidelines regarding respiratory rates, partially explaining these results and potentially reducing their clinical relevance. In our trial, at early resuscitation timepoints, the $paCO_2$ was high in the groups without PEEP and the U8 group. The results of the MIGET measurements support the observation of impaired gas exchange when not using PEEP. Especially in the U0 group, overall global hypoventilation with higher shunt perfusion was found. Determinations of high, normal, and low V/Q ratios and shunt volumes were achieved by analysing gas elimination during lung perfusion using a mass spectrometer. The use of MIGET technology during CPR was validated in previous trials [7,18] and can provide additional information about (impaired) circulation and ventilation during CPR. In the IPPV group, a distinct increase in high V/Q volume was observed compared to ULTVV when adjusted for PEEP, which supports an increase in hyperinflated lung areas and is in accordance with previous studies [7]. When using PEEP, lower shunt fractions could be detected, particularly in early resuscitation, suggesting improved recruitment and optimised ventilation. This aligns with studies that showed that using PEEP during resuscitation can prevent airway closure and ensure alveolar ventilation [19,20] and has positive effects on systemic oxygenation [4,5,21]. In our trial, oxygenation was improved when using PEEP, especially in early resuscitation. The ameliorated oxygenation could result from the prevention of atelectasis [4,6,7], thus decreasing shunt perfusion, improving lung recruitment, and preventing airway closure [19,20]. EIT measurements during CPR have not yet been systematically performed and can only yield supportive data, even though general feasibility has been shown previously [22]. Generally, EIT can support the titration of PEEP to avoid atelectasis and prevent regional hyperinflation [23–26]. In a direct comparison of not using PEEP versus using PEEP, the use of PEEP led to the redistribution of ventilation from the ventral to the dorsal lung regions [8], which could also be suspected in our recordings during CPR, especially in the PEEP 16 groups. Further experimental assessment is needed to validate the method during CPR.

In terms of prolonged CPR, all PEEP groups showed decreasing paO$_2$ with an increase in shunt perfusion and lower normal V/Q values. These effects were less pronounced in the PEEP 8 groups, which could emphasise the beneficial effects of moderate PEEP for longer use of CPR.

Interestingly, even when using high PEEP levels, we found no differences in the haemodynamic values, although, theoretically, the continuous application of PEEP and a consecutive high P_{peak} and P_{mean} could lead to increased intrathoracic pressure, which could cause impaired venous return and, consequently, cardiac output (CO) [10,11,21]. A study evaluating the effects of PEEP on CO during CPR suggested a PEEP of 5 mbar as the optimal level in their model [21]. However, the detected decreases—albeit statistically significant—were marginal in absolute values, showing a CO decrease of 0.3 L/min when comparing a PEEP of 0 mbar with 20 mbar, thus determining that the clinical relevance in resuscitation is uncertain. This also aligns with the findings of the present study concerning the MAP, where no significant differences could be detected, which is in line with previous studies focusing on the ULTVV and IPPV modes [7,27], even if only a PEEP of 5 mbar was used in these studies. However, one limitation of our approach is the lack of coronary perfusion pressure measurements (CPP), which is defined as aortic diastolic pressure minus left ventricular end-diastolic pressure and has been linked to positive outcomes and ROSC [28]. Since the primary goal of this study was to evaluate the respiratory effects of higher PEEP during resuscitations, and due to the technical restrictions of our model, these measurements could not be acquired.

In our experiments, no animal achieved ROSC. Since we expanded the uninterrupted chest compression time to 30 min without any drug treatment or defibrillation, this is not surprising, since survival and achievement of ROSC are highly dependent on short intervals leading to first adrenaline dose and shock [29,30].

The use of adrenaline has been shown to increase the rates of survival to hospital admission and long-term survival, although there were no significant differences in cases in which a favourable neurologic outcome was observed [2,31,32]. However, because our trial did not have the specific goal of ROSC, no vasopressors were used during CPR before the 30 min mark, as recommended by the guidelines [2,3]. While there were no differences in MAP when using PEEP, potential effects on survival, neurological outcome, and pulmonary function should be examined in further studies with a focus on shorter resuscitation times, early application of advanced life support algorithms, and post-ROSC monitoring.

6. Conclusions

This prospective, randomised, controlled animal trial showed that the use of PEEP during CPR ventilation seems beneficial. It leads to a ventilation pattern with lower driving pressures, optimised ventilation–perfusion ratios, lower shunt perfusion, as well as less atelectatic lung tissue and less overall lung damage. Additionally, no detrimental haemodynamic effects were observed even with high PEEP levels, emphasising the potential benefits of oxygenation without compromising organ perfusion. Further studies are needed to confirm these results and to examine potential long-term effects in resuscitated animals.

Supplementary Materials: The following supporting information can be downloaded at: https://www.mdpi.com/article/10.3390/jcm11164921/s1, Figure S1: Lung physiology via Electrical impedance tomography (EIT): the picture shows EIT loops during CPR at the intervention timepoint CPR 5 min. A = ULTVV PEEP 0 mbar, B = IPPV PEEP 0 mbar, C = ULTVV PEEP 16 mbar, D = IPPV

PEEP 16 mbar. Global EIT recordings and recordings of ROI (region of interest) 1 to ROI 4 are pictured. There were no significant differences detected. Figure S2: Microphotographs of histologic lung samples with the 7 aspects of the DAD-Score used.

Author Contributions: E.K.H., M.R. and R.R. (Robert Ruemmler) designed and planned the study, M.R., L.M., J.R., K.M., B.D. and R.R. (René Rissel) performed the experiments, M.R., A.Z., B.D. and R.R. (Robert Ruemmler) analysed the data, L.M. performed histologic analyses, M.R., R.R. (Robert Ruemmler) and E.K.H. drafted the manuscript. All authors have read and agreed to the published version of the manuscript.

Funding: This study was partially funded by a personal grant of the German Research Foundation to Robert Ruemmler (DFG grant no.: RU 2371/1-1). No additional external funding was used. The LUCAS-2 device was provided by the manufacturer unconditionally.

Institutional Review Board Statement: This animal trial was approved by the State and Institutional Animal Care Committee Rhineland Palatine (approval no. G20-1-065), and all experiments were performed according to the German Animal Protection Law and the ARRIVE guidelines.

Informed Consent Statement: Not applicable.

Data Availability Statement: All data analysed for this study are provided in the manuscript and the Supplementary Materials.

Acknowledgments: This trial will be part of the doctoral thesis at the Johannes Gutenberg-University Mainz, written by Leah Müllejans. We would like to thank D. Dirvonskis for her committed and active support during the entire trial. The LUCAS 2-system and the EIT device were provided unconditionally by the manufacturers for animal research purposes only. Tissue samples were provided by the tissue bank of the University Medical Center Mainz in accordance with the regulations of the tissue biobank and the approval of the ethics committee of the University Medical Center Mainz.

Conflicts of Interest: The authors declare no conflict of interest.

References

1. Newell, C.; Grier, S.; Soar, J. Airway and ventilation management during cardiopulmonary resuscitation and after successful resuscitation. *Crit. Care* **2018**, *22*, 190. [CrossRef] [PubMed]
2. Soar, J.; Böttiger, B.W.; Carli, P.; Couper, K.; Deakin, C.D.; Djärv, T.; Lott, C.; Olasveengen, T.; Paal, P.; Pellis, T.; et al. European resuscitation council guidelines 2021: Adult advanced life support. *Resuscitation* **2021**, *161*, 115–151. [CrossRef] [PubMed]
3. Panchal, A.R.; Bartos, J.A.; Cabañas, J.G.; Donnino, M.W.; Drennan, I.R.; Hirsch, K.G.; Kudenchuk, P.J.; Kurz, M.C.; Lavonas, E.J.; Morley, P.T.; et al. Part 3 adult basic and advanced life support: 2020 American Heart Association guidelines for cardiopulmonary resuscitation and emergency cardiovascular care. *Circulation* **2020**, *142* (Suppl. S2), S366–S468. [CrossRef] [PubMed]
4. McCaul, C.; Kornecki, A.; Engelberts, D.; McNamara, P.; Kavanagh, B.P. Positive end-expiratory pressure improves survival in a rodent model of cardiopulmonary resuscitation using high-dose epinephrine. *Anesth. Analg.* **2009**, *109*, 1202–1208. [CrossRef]
5. Hodgkin, B.C.; Lambrew, C.T.; Lawrence, F.H., III; Angelakos, E.T. Effects of PEEP and of increased frequency of ventilation during CPR. *Crit. Care Med.* **1980**, *8*, 123–126. [CrossRef]
6. Kill, C.; Hahn, O.; Dietz, F.; Neuhaus, C.; Schwarz, S.; Mahling, R.; Wallot, P.; Jerrentrup, A.; Steinfeldt, T.; Wulf, H.; et al. Mechanical ventilation during cardiopulmonary resuscitation with intermittent positive-pressure ventilation, bilevel ventilation, or chest compression synchronized ventilation in a pig model. *Crit. Care Med.* **2014**, *42*, e89–e95. [CrossRef]
7. Ruemmler, R.; Ziebart, A.; Moellmann, C.; Garcia-Bardon, A.; Kamuf, J.; Kuropka, F.; Duenges, B.; Hartmann, E.K. Ultra-low tidal volume ventilation—A novel and effective ventilation strategy during experimental cardiopulmonary resuscitation. *Resuscitation* **2018**, *132*, 56–62. [CrossRef]
8. Frerichs, I.; Schmitz, G.; Pulletz, S.; Schädler, D.; Zick, G.; Scholz, J.; Weiler, N. Reproducibility of regional lung ventilation distribution determined by electrical impedance tomography during mechanical ventilation. *Physiol. Meas.* **2007**, *28*, S261–S267. [CrossRef]
9. Shono, A.; Katayama, N.; Fujihara, T.; Böhm, S.H.; Waldmann, A.D.; Ugata, K.; Nikai, T.; Saito, Y. Positive end-expiratory pressure and distribution of ventilation in pneumoperitoneum combined with steep trendelenburg position. *Anesthesiology* **2020**, *132*, 476–490. [CrossRef]
10. Richard, J.C.M.; Lefebvre, J.C.; Tassaux, D.; Brochard, L. Update in mechanical ventilation 2010. *Am. J. Respir. Crit. Care Med.* **2011**, *184*, 32–36. [CrossRef]
11. Pinsky, M.R.; Summer, W.R.; Wise, R.A.; Permutt, S.; Bromberger-Barnea, B. Augmentation of cardiac function by elevation of intrathoracic pressure. *J. Appl. Physiol. Respir. Environ. Exerc. Physiol.* **1983**, *54*, 950–955. [CrossRef]

12. Fichtner, F.; Moerer, O.; Weber-Carstens, S.; Nothacker, M.; Kaisers, U.; Laudi, S.; Guideline Group. Clinical guideline for treating acute respiratory insufficiency with invasive ventilation and extracorporeal membrane oxygenation: Evidence-based recommendations for choosing modes and setting parameters of mechanical ventilation. *Respiration* **2019**, *98*, 357–372. [CrossRef]
13. Ziebart, A.; Hartmann, E.K.; Thomas, R.; Liu, T.; Duenges, B.; Schad, A.; Bodenstein, M.; Thal, S.C.; David, M. Low tidal volume pressure support versus controlled ventilation in early experimental sepsis in pigs. *Respir. Res.* **2014**, *15*, 101. [CrossRef]
14. Amato, M.B.; Meade, M.O.; Slutsky, A.S.; Brochard, L.; Costa, E.L.; Schoenfeld, D.A.; Stewart, T.E.; Briel, M.; Talmor, D.; Mercat, A.; et al. Driving pressure and survival in the acute respiratory distress syndrome. *N. Engl. J. Med.* **2015**, *372*, 747–755. [CrossRef]
15. Cheifetz, I.M.; Craig, D.M.; Quick, G.; McGovern, J.J.; Cannon, M.L.; Ungerleider, R.M.; Smith, P.K.; Meliones, J.N. Increasing tidal volumes and pulmonary overdistention adversely affect pulmonary vascular mechanics and cardiac output in a pediatric swine model. *Crit. Care Med.* **1998**, *26*, 710–716. [CrossRef]
16. Acosta, P.; Santisbon, E.; Varon, J. The use of positive end-expiratory pressure in mechanical ventilation. *Crit. Care Clin.* **2007**, *23*, 251–261. [CrossRef]
17. Levenbrown, Y.; Hossain, M.J.; Keith, J.P.; Burr, K.; Hesek, A.; Shaffer, T.H. Effect of positive end-expiratory pressure on additional passive ventilation generated by CPR compressions in a porcine model. *Intensive Care Med. Exp.* **2021**, *9*, 37. [CrossRef]
18. Hartmann, E.K.; Duenges, B.; Boehme, S.; Szczyrba, M.; Liu, T.; Klein, K.U.; Baumgardner, J.E.; Markstaller, K.; David, M. Ventilation/perfusion ratios measured by multiple inert gas elimination during experimental cardiopulmonary resuscitation. *Acta Anaesthesiol. Scand.* **2014**, *58*, 1032–1039. [CrossRef]
19. Charbonney, E.; Grieco, D.L.; Cordioli, R.L.; Badat, B.; Savary, D.; Richard, J.C.M. Ventilation during cardiopulmonary resuscitation: What have we learned from models? *Respir. Care* **2019**, *64*, 1132–1138. [CrossRef]
20. Cordioli, R.L.; Grieco, D.L.; Charbonney, E.; Richard, J.C.; Savary, D. New physiological insights in ventilation during cardiopulmonary resuscitation. *Curr. Opin. Crit. Care* **2019**, *25*, 37–44. [CrossRef]
21. Levenbrown, Y.; Hossain, M.J.; Keith, J.P.; Burr, K.; Hesek, A.; Shaffer, T. The effect of positive end-expiratory pressure on cardiac output and oxygen delivery during cardiopulmonary resuscitation. *Intensive Care Med. Exp.* **2020**, *8*, 36. [CrossRef]
22. Kamuf, J.; Garcia-Bardon, A.; Duenges, B.; Liu, T.; Jahn-Eimermacher, A.; Heid, F.; David, M.; Hartmann, E.K. Endexpiratory lung volume measurement correlates with the ventilation/perfusion mismatch in lung injured pigs. *Respir. Res.* **2017**, *18*, 101. [CrossRef]
23. Bodenstein, M.; David, M.; Markstaller, K. Principles of electrical impedance tomography and its clinical application. *Crit. Care Med.* **2009**, *37*, 713–724. [CrossRef]
24. Muders, T.; Luepschen, H.; Putensen, C. Impedance tomography as a new monitoring technique. *Curr. Opin. Crit. Care* **2010**, *16*, 269–275. [CrossRef]
25. Luepschen, H.; Meier, T.; Grossherr, M.; Leibecke, T.; Karsten, J.; Leonhardt, S. Protective ventilation using electrical impedance tomography. *Physiol. Meas.* **2007**, *28*, S247–S260. [CrossRef]
26. Walsh, B.K.; Smallwood, C.D. Electrical impedance tomography during mechanical ventilation. *Respir. Care* **2016**, *61*, 1417–1424. [CrossRef]
27. Ruemmler, R.; Ziebart, A.; Kuropka, F.; Duenges, B.; Kamuf, J.; Garcia-Bardon, A.; Hartmann, E.K. Bi-Level ventilation decreases pulmonary shunt and modulates neuroinflammation in a cardiopulmonary resuscitation model. *PeerJ* **2020**, *8*, e9072. [CrossRef] [PubMed]
28. Reynolds, J.C.; Salcido, D.D.; Menegazzi, J.J. Coronary perfusion pressure and return of spontaneous circulation after prolonged cardiac arrest. *Prehosp. Emerg. Care* **2010**, *14*, 78–84. [CrossRef] [PubMed]
29. Hüpfl, M.; Selig, H.F.; Nagele, P. Chest-compression-only versus standard cardiopulmonary resuscitation: A meta-analysis. *Lancet* **2010**, *376*, 1552–1557. [CrossRef]
30. Kiguchi, T.; Okubo, M.; Nishiyama, C.; Maconochie, I.; Ong, M.E.H.; Kern, K.B.; Wyckoff, M.H.; McNally, B.; Christensen, E.F.; Tjelmeland, I.; et al. Out-of-hospital cardiac arrest across the World: First report from the international liaison committee on resuscitation (ILCOR). *Resuscitation* **2020**, *152*, 39–49. [CrossRef] [PubMed]
31. Perkins, G.D.; Ji, C.; Deakin, C.D.; Quinn, T.; Nolan, J.P.; Scomparin, C.; Regan, S.; Long, J.; Slowther, A.; Pocock, H.; et al. A randomized trial of epinephrine in out-of-hospital cardiac arrest. *N. Engl. J. Med.* **2018**, *379*, 711–721. [CrossRef]
32. Panchal, A.R.; Berg, K.M.; Hirsch, K.G.; Kudenchuk, P.J.; Del Rios, M.; Cabañas, J.G.; Link, M.S.; Kurz, M.C.; Chan, P.S.; Morley, P.T.; et al. 2019 American heart association focused update on advanced cardiovascular life support: Use of advanced airways, vasopressors, and extracorporeal cardiopulmonary resuscitation during cardiac arrest: An update to the american heart association guidelines for cardiopulmonary resuscitation and emergency cardiovascular care. *Circulation* **2019**, *140*, e881–e894. [CrossRef]

Systematic Review

Tracheal Intubation during Advanced Life Support Using Direct Laryngoscopy versus Glidescope® Videolaryngoscopy by Clinicians with Limited Intubation Experience: A Systematic Review and Meta-Analysis

Hans van Schuppen [†], Kamil Wojciechowicz [†], Markus W. Hollmann [*] and Benedikt Preckel

Department of Anesthesiology, Amsterdam UMC location University of Amsterdam, Meibergdreef 9, 1105 AZ Amsterdam, The Netherlands
* Correspondence: m.w.hollmann@amsterdamumc.nl
† These authors contributed equally to this work.

Abstract: The use of the Glidescope® videolaryngoscope might improve tracheal intubation performance in clinicians with limited intubation experience, especially during cardiopulmonary resuscitation (CPR). The objective of this systematic review and meta-analysis is to compare direct laryngoscopy to Glidescope® videolaryngoscopy by these clinicians. PubMed/Medline and Embase were searched from their inception to 7 July 2020 for randomized controlled trials, including simulation studies. Studies on adult patients or adult-sized manikins were included when direct laryngoscopy was compared to Glidescope® videolaryngoscopy by clinicians with limited experience in tracheal intubation (<10 intubations per year). The primary outcome was the intubation first-pass success rate. Secondary outcomes were time to successful intubation and chest compression interruption duration during intubation. The risk of bias was assessed with the Cochrane risk of bias tool. Certainty of evidence was assessed using the Grading of Recommendations Assessment, Development and Evaluation (GRADE). We included 4 clinical trials with 525 patients and 20 manikin trials with 2547 intubations. Meta-analyses favored Glidescope® videolaryngoscopy over direct laryngoscopy regarding first-pass success (clinical trials: risk ratio [RR] = 1.61; 95% confidence interval [CI]: 1.16–2.23; manikin trials: RR = 1.17; 95% CI: 1.09–1.25). Clinical trials showed a shorter time to achieve successful intubation when using the Glidescope® (mean difference = 17.04 s; 95% CI: 8.51–25.57 s). Chest compression interruption duration was decreased when using the Glidescope® videolaryngoscope. The certainty of evidence ranged from very low to moderate. When clinicians with limited intubation experience have to perform tracheal intubation during advanced life support, the use of the Glidescope® videolaryngoscope improves intubation and CPR performance compared to direct laryngoscopy.

Keywords: airway management; cardiopulmonary resuscitation; advanced life support; emergency medical service; tracheal intubation; videolaryngoscopy

1. Introduction

Airway management is an essential part of advanced life support to facilitate ventilation of the lungs. During cardiopulmonary resuscitation (CPR), many professionals still favor tracheal intubation, although supraglottic airway devices (SAD) are increasingly used as the primary advanced airway technique. However, when SADs fail to facilitate oxygenation in situations such as aspiration, drowning, or trauma, tracheal intubation is still indicated. In addition, in the current COVID-19 pandemic tracheal intubation is regarded as the best airway technique during CPR to minimize aerosol generation by chest compressions [1,2].

The challenge with tracheal intubation during CPR is to achieve first-pass success, while fast, safe, and without interruption of chest compressions. More experienced clinicians have a higher intubation success rate but gaining and maintaining sufficient experience in tracheal intubation is challenging, especially for EMS organizations [3–5]. It takes a minimum of 50 tracheal intubations to achieve an intubation success rate of 90% within two attempts, under optimal (non-emergency) conditions [6]. More than 240 tracheal intubations are needed to perform tracheal intubation during CPR with a 90% success rate and high-quality standards [7]. EMS clinicians often perform less than 10 tracheal intubations per year [8,9]. Getting a clinician with sufficient intubation experience on the scene within an acceptable time is often a challenge and sometimes not possible, such as in remote and military settings. There are several risks when tracheal intubation is performed by personnel with limited experience, including oropharyngeal injury, significant interruption of chest compressions, and incorrect tube placement with consecutive hypoxia [10–12].

Videolaryngoscopy has the potential to increase the tracheal intubation success rate when clinicians with limited experience are confronted with a patient with an indication for tracheal intubation. Furthermore, videolaryngoscopy may decrease interruptions in chest compressions during CPR. The Glidescope® was the first commercially available videolaryngoscope. The hyperangulated blade includes a camera, connected to a video screen, which improves visualization of the larynx (Figure 1). The tracheal tube can then be inserted into the airway by using a rigid stylet (Gliderite® Stylet).

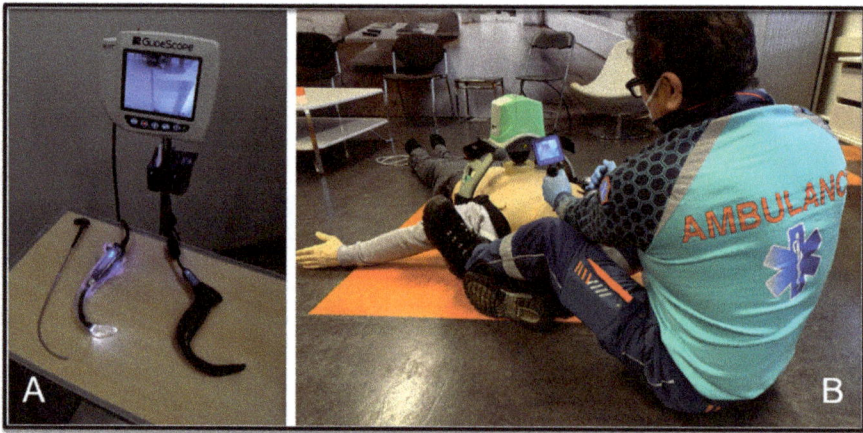

Figure 1. (**A**) The Glidescope® videolaryngoscope with the former GVL blade (**left**) and recent LoPro blade (**right**), and the Gliderite® rigid stylet. (**B**) The portable GlidescopeGo®, used by an EMS clinician in a simulated prehospital advanced life support setting.

The objective of this study was to perform a systematic review and meta-analysis on the use of the hyperangulated Glidescope® videolaryngoscope for tracheal intubation by clinicians with limited intubation experience regarding first-pass success rate and time to intubation when compared to direct laryngoscopy. The secondary aim was to determine differences in chest compression interruptions during CPR. As the Glidescope® videolaryngoscope is one of the most widely used videolaryngoscopes and prehospital care clinicians often have an annual tracheal intubation exposure of <10 tracheal intubations we searched for studies comparing direct laryngoscopy to Glidescope® videolaryngoscopy in oral tracheal intubation by clinicians with limited experience in tracheal intubation. With this study we aimed to provide an answer to the question; should clinicians with limited intubation experience use the Glidescope® for tracheal intubation?

2. Materials and Methods

The protocol of this systematic review and meta-analysis has been registered in the international prospective register of systematic reviews PROSPERO (review record CRD42018096251) and is included in Supplementary Materials 1. This review followed the

Preferred Reporting Items for Systematic Reviews and Meta-Analyses (PRISMA) guidelines, see Supplementary Materials 2 for the PRISMA checklist [13]. Primary outcome is first-pass success rate of tracheal intubation, secondary outcomes are time needed for successful intubation and duration of chest compression interruption for CPR.

2.1. Eligibility Criteria

Studies were included if they met all of the following criteria:

1. Comparison of direct laryngoscopy to Glidescope® videolaryngoscopy (either conventional Glidescope® or Glidescope® Ranger) for tracheal intubation
2. Randomized and quasi-randomized controlled trials
3. Clinicians had limited experience in tracheal intubation, defined as less than 10 intubations per year
4. Adult patients or adult-sized manikins
5. Contained any outcome of interest (first-pass success rate, and/or time to intubation, and/or hands-off time during CPR)

Studies on nasotracheal intubation were excluded.

2.2. Information Sources and Search Strategy

MEDLINE/PubMed and Embase were systematically searched (1966 to 7 July 2020) for randomized trials comparing tracheal intubation using direct laryngoscopy versus Glidescope® videolaryngoscopy. The following search terms were used in MEDLINE/PubMed: (Glidescope®) OR (video laryngoscop* [tiab]). In Embase the search term (Glidescope® or video laryngoscop*).ti,ab,kw was used. Bibliographies of selected manuscripts were hand-searched for additional relevant studies.

2.3. Study Selection

The first author (KW) performed the search. In duplicate and independently, the first two authors (K.W., H.S.) performed the bibliographic review of the search results. Disagreement was resolved by discussion and arbitrated if necessary, by a third independent researcher (BP).

2.4. Data Collection and Data Items

Two reviewers extracted data including the year of publication, country of origin, sample size, operator background, operator training, whether intubation was performed on a real patient or manikin, in which setting the intubation was performed, rate of successful intubation at first attempt, time required to intubate, and hands-off time during CPR. We contacted investigators for missing data if necessary.

2.5. Risk of Bias in Individual Studies

Risk of bias in the individual studies was independently reviewed by two investigators. The Cochrane risk of bias tool was used to determine selection bias, performance bias, detection bias, attrition bias, reporting bias, and other biases in the included studies [14].

2.6. Data Synthesis and Analysis

Because the setting of actual patient care and differences in design of simulation studies can influence the results, the analysis was divided into three subgroups. The three main groups are:

1. Intubations performed in the clinical setting
2. Intubations performed in a simulation setting, using manikins
3. Intubations performed in a simulation setting, using manikins with a difficult airway scenario

Differences in first-pass intubation success rate are expressed in risk ratio (RR) and differences in time to intubate and hands-off time during CPR are expressed in mean difference (MD) in seconds. Interquartile ranges were converted into standard deviations. The random effects method of Mantel–Haenszel was used to generate a pooled RR or

MD across studies. We assessed statistical heterogeneity using Cochrane's Q statistic (with $p < 0.05$ considered significant) and expressed the quantity using the I2 statistic and 95% confidence interval (CI). We followed the Cochrane handbook classification for importance of I2. To explore heterogeneity, subgroup analyses were performed for specific clinical scenarios (normal airway, difficult airway, etc.). Statistical analyses as well as forest plots were made using Review Manager (RevMan) [Computer program], Version 5.2. Copenhagen: The Nordic Cochrane Centre, The Cochrane Collaboration, 2012. The overall certainty of evidence was assessed using the Grading of Recommendations Assessment, Development and Evaluation (GRADE) method [15]. The GRADE tables were made with the GRADEpro GDT online software [GRADEpro GDT: GRADEpro Guideline Development Tool [Software]. McMaster University and Evidence Prime, 2021. Available from gradepro.org, accessed on 31 January 2022].

3. Results

3.1. Study Selection

The literature search was performed on 7 July 2020. A total of 1022 citations were identified from Medline (PubMed) and Embase (Ovid). We excluded 943 citations on the initial screening of the title and abstract of the article and 13 on the screening of the full article. Of the remaining articles, 42 articles were excluded because there was no data on the primary or secondary endpoint, it regarded only pediatric patients, it regarded nasal intubation, there was no comparison between direct laryngoscopy and Glidescope®, or intubation was performed by experienced clinicians. The references of the 55 excluded articles are included in Supplementary Materials 3. Three articles were included after discussion by the first two authors. This resulted in 24 inclusions and 997 exclusions (Figure 2).

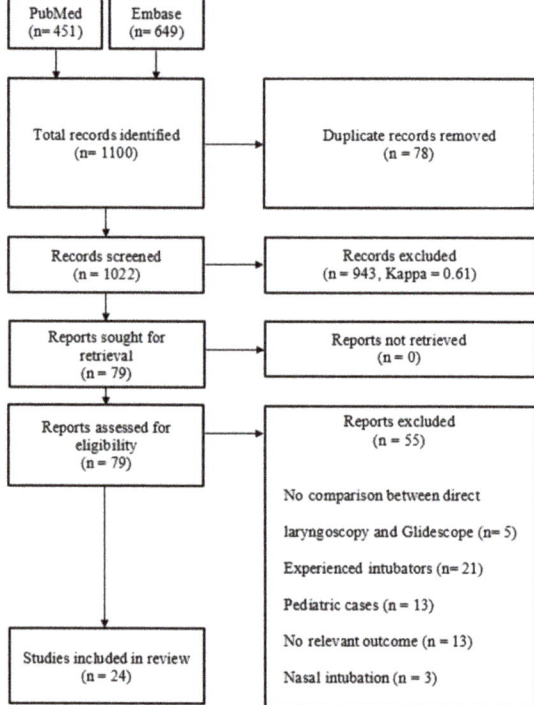

Figure 2. PRISMA diagram.

3.2. Study Characteristics

We identified four randomized trials in which patients were intubated in the clinical setting and 20 randomized trials in which the intubation was performed on a manikin [16–39]. See Table 1 for the study characteristics. A total of 525 clinical intubations were included as well as 2547 manikin intubations. Of the clinical studies, three were performed on patients in the operating room (OR) and one was performed during CPR. The patients included in the OR setting were ASA 1 and 2 patients in elective situations, without a known or anticipated difficult airway.

Of the manikin studies, nine studies had a protocol with only a normal airway, eleven studies included a protocol with a manikin with a normal airway as well as a difficult airway, and one study solely included a protocol with a manikin with a difficult airway. Difficult airway protocols included cervical spine immobilization, intubation during chest compressions, tongue edema or pharyngeal obstruction, a Cormack–Lehane grade 3 view, intubation on the floor, or a combination of two or more of these circumstances. When a study allowed participants to run the same scenario more than once, the data of the first scenario was included for meta-analysis.

In the trials using a manikin, all participants used both intubation techniques. In all trials except one, the operators had no prior intubation experience. In the trial in which the operators had prior intubation experience, all operators had performed less than 10 intubations in their careers [25].

Table 1. Study characteristics of clinical and manikin trials. (*) The number of intubations in this table includes only the first scenario with normal airway. (ASA = American Society of Anesthesiologists, CL = Cormack–Lehane, CPR = cardiopulmonary resuscitation, DL = direct laryngoscopy, GS = Glidescope® videolaryngoscopy, USA = United States of America).

			Clinical studies			
First author, year	Country of origin	Number of patients	Randomized per group	Operators	Training	Patients
Nouruzi, 2009 [38]	Essen, Germany	200	DL: 100 GS: 100	Students (paramedic, nurse & medical)	Manikin training	ASA 1–2 predicted non difficult airway
Ayoub, 2010 [36]	Beirut, Lebanon	42	DL: 21 GS: 21	Medical students	Manikin training	ASA 1–2 predicted non difficult airway
Hirabayashi, 2010 [37]	Shimotsuke, Japan	200	DL: 100 GS: 100	Non-anaesthesia residents	Short demonstration and 5–6 practices on a manikin	ASA 1–2 predicted non difficult airway
Park, 2015 [39]	Seoul, Republic of Korea	83	DL: 34 GS: 49	Inexperienced emergency physicians	Airway session of 8 h	CPR patients
4		525	DL: 255 GS: 270			
			Manikin studies			
First author, year	Country of origin	Number of intubations	Randomized per group	Operators	Training	Scenario
Lim, 2004 [16]	Singapore	80	DL: 20 GS: 20	Medical students	Instructions and 3 min practice	Normal airway CL grade 3
You, 2009 [20]	Ulsan, Korea	41	DL: 20 GS: 21	Medical students	Lecture of 30 min	Normal airway
Lin, 2009 [17]	Hualien, Taiwan	164	DL: 41 GS: 41	Medical students	Instructions and 5 attempts with both devices	Normal airway CL grade 3
Malik, 2009 [18]	Galway, Ireland	318	DL: 53 * GS: 53 *	Medical students	Instruction of 5 min and 5 attempts	Normal airway Cervical immobilisation Pharyngeal obstruction

Table 1. Cont.

				Manikin studies		
First author, year	Country of origin	Number of intubations	Randomized per group	Operators	Training	Scenario
Powell, 2009 [19]	Sheffield, UK	42	DL: 21 GS: 21	Non-anaesthesists	Individual standard demonstration	Normal airway
Cinar, 2011 [21]	Ankara, Turkey	242	DL: 121 GS: 121	Paramedic students	Lecture and demonstration	Normal airway
Kaki, 2011 [22]	Jeddah, Saudi Arabia	100	DL: 50 GS: 50	Non-anaesthesists	Standardized instruction and practice	Normal airway
Kim, 2011 [23]	Seoul, Republic of Korea	80	DL: 20 GS: 20	Paramedic students	Training of one hour	Normal airway CPR on the floor
Shin, 2011 [25]	Seoul, Republic of Korea	128	DL: 32 GS: 32	Interns with <10 tracheal intubations	Instruction of 20 min and 3 intubations on a manikin	Normal airway Chest compressions
Stroumpoulis, 2011 [26]	Athens, Greece	88	DL: 44 GS: 44	ACLS providers	Brief presentation and 5 min of practice	Normal airway
Wass, 2011 [24]	Rochester, USA	100	DL: 25 GS: 25	Medical students	Tutorial of 5–10 min	Normal airway Pharyngeal obstruction
Xanthos, 2011 [27]	Athens, Greece	180	DL: 45 GS: 45	Doctors inexperienced in airway management	Instruction of 20 min and practice on manikin	Normal airway Chest compressions
Xanthos, 2012 [28]	Athens, Greece	192	DL: 96 GS: 96	Medical and nursing graduates	Instruction of 20 min and practice on manikin	Normal airway
Biermann, 2013 [29]	Amsterdam, the Netherlands	78	DL: 39 GS: 39	Unexperienced registrars in internal medicine	Explanation and demonstration	Normal airway
Tung, 2013 [30]	Vancouver, Canada	68	DL: 34 GS: 34	Medical students	Standardized video instruction and 10 min of practice	Normal airway
Wang, 2013 [31]	Hualien, Taiwan	120	DL: 20 GS: 20	Medical students	Demonstration of 3–5 min and practice 1–3 times on bodies	Normal airway On the floor Cervical immobilisation Cervical immobilisation on the floor
Ambrosio, 2014 [32]	San Diego, USA	40	DL: 19 GS: 21	First-year non anaesthesia residents	Manikin training, ended upon 1 successfull intubation with both DL and Glidescope®	CL grade 3 + cervical immobilisation
Kim, 2014 [33]	Seoul, Republic of Korea	156	DL: 39 GS: 39	Medical students	5 intubations	Normal airway Cervical immobilisation
Bahhatiq, 2016 [34]	Makkah Mukarramah, Saudi Arabia	200	DL: 50 GS: 50	Paramedic students	Lecture of one hour, demonstration of 10 min and practice one time	Normal airway Cervical immobilisation
Pieters, 2016 [35]	Nijmegen, the Netherlands	130	DL: 65 GS: 65	Medical students	Demonstration of 5 min, no practice	Normal airway
20		2547	DL: 1273 GS: 1274			

3.3. Certainty of Evidence across Studies

The evidence was rated as low to moderate certainty regarding first-pass success rate and as very low to moderate certainty regarding time to intubation when using Glidescope® videolaryngoscopy versus direct laryngoscopy. See Supplementary Materials 4 for the GRADE table. Only one study reported chest compression interruptions [39].

3.4. Risk of Bias within Studies

The risk of bias within all included studies (both clinical and manikin studies) is illustrated in Figures 3 and 4 [14]. The performance bias attributes to the blinding of participants and personnel. As it is impossible to blind participants and observers for the device used, all included studies score a high risk of bias in this domain.

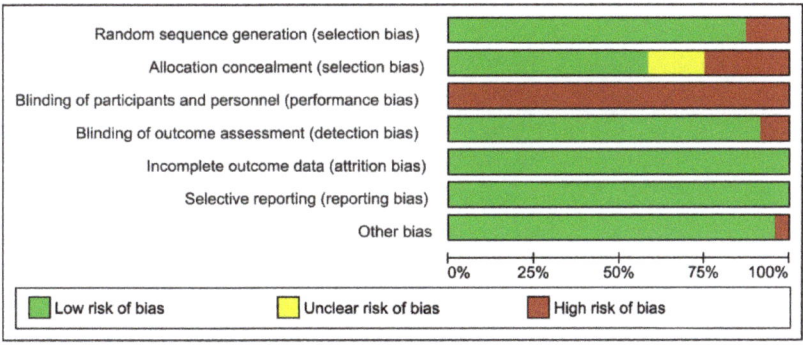

Figure 3. Risk of bias graph.

3.5. Outcomes

3.5.1. Intubation First-Pass Success Rate

All included trials presented data on intubation success and time needed for intubation (Table 2). The pooled RR for first-pass success across the clinical studies was 1.61 (95% CI 1.16, 2.23; $p = 0.004$) (Figure 5). The level of certainty of the evidence was moderate.

The pooled RR for first-pass success in the manikin studies was 1.17 (95% CI 1.09, 1.25; $p < 0.0001$) (Figure 6). There was substantial between-study heterogeneity. All three subgroup analyses revealed a significant effect in favor of the Glidescope® videolaryngoscope. The overall certainty of the evidence was rated as low for these trials, see Supplementary Materials 4 for the GRADE table.

3.5.2. Time to Intubation

The time required to intubate was available in all included studies (Table 2). The forest plots in Figures 7 and 8 represent the clinical and manikin trials, respectively. The pooled MD across the clinical trials favors the Glidescope® videolaryngoscope (MD 17.04 s, 95% CI 8.51, 25.57 s; $p < 0.0001$). There was substantial between-study heterogeneity, and the overall certainty of the evidence was graded as moderate. Of the manikin trials, only the subgroup analyses with the difficult airway scenarios showed a significant difference in mean intubation time in favor of the Glidescope® videolaryngoscope (MD 12.51 s, 95% CI 1.46, 23.56 s; $p = 0.03$). There was considerable between-study heterogeneity. The other subgroups showed no significant difference in intubation times. The overall certainty of the evidence was rated as very low for the manikin trials, because of inconsistency and indirectness (see Supplementary Materials 4 for GRADE table).

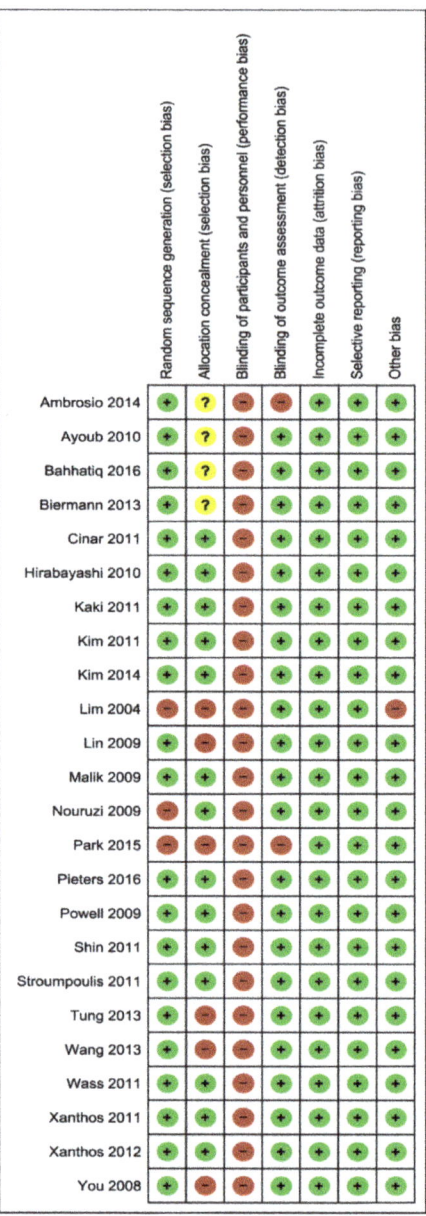

Figure 4. Risk of bias summary. Ambrosio, 2014 [32]; Ayoub, 2010 [36]; Bahhatiq, 2016 [34]; Biermann, 2013 [29]; Cinar, 2011 [21]; Hirabayashi, 2010 [37]; Kaki, 2011 [22]; Kim, 2011 [23]; Kim, 2014 [33]; Lim, 2004 [16]; Lin, 2009 [17]; Malik, 2009 [18]; Nouruzi, 2009 [38]; Park, 2015 [39]; Pieters, 2016 [35]; Powell, 2009 [19]; Shin, 2011 [25]; Stroumpoulis, 2011 [26]; Tung, 2013 [30]; Wang, 2013 [31]; Wass, 2011 [24]; Xanthos, 2011 [27]; Xanthos, 2012 [28]; You, 2009 [20]. Green +: low risk of bias, Red -: high risk of bias, Yellow ?: unclear risk of bias.

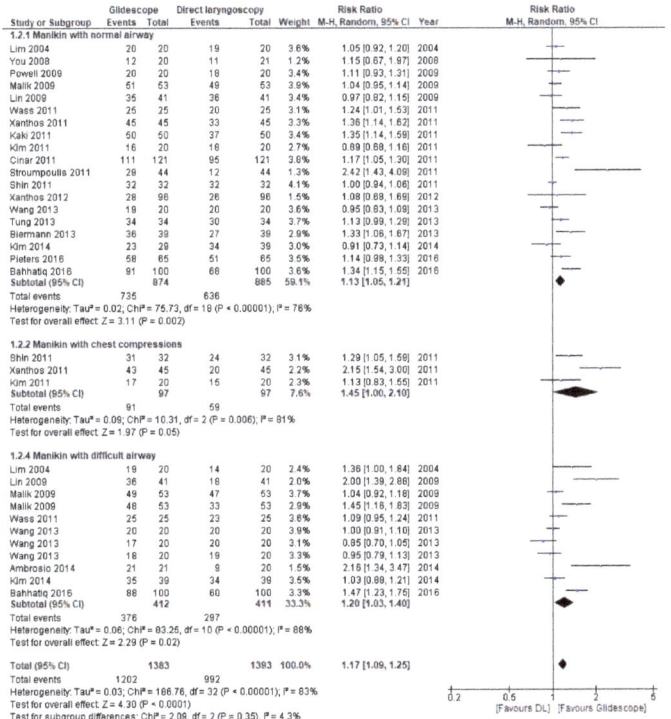

Figure 5. Risk ratios (RR) of successful first-attempt intubation in clinical trials comparing Glidescope® videolaryngoscopy to direct laryngoscopy. The pooled estimate (rhombus) was derived using the DerSimonian and Laird random effects method. The squares depict individual study point estimates of the RR. Horizontal lines display the 95% CI of the point estimate. The vertical line represents an RR of 1.00 indicating no difference between Glidescope® videolaryngoscopy and direct laryngoscopy; (DL = direct laryngoscopy). Nouruzi, 2009 [38]; Ayoub, 2010 [36]; Hirabayashi, 2010 [37]; Park, 2015 [39].

Figure 6. Risk ratios (RR) of successful first-attempt intubation in manikin trials comparing Glidescope® videolaryngoscopy to direct laryngoscopy. The pooled estimate (rhombus) was derived using the DerSimonian and Laird random effects method. The squares depict individual study point estimates of the RR. Horizontal lines display the 95% CI of the point estimate. The vertical line represents an RR of 1.00 indicating no difference between Glidescope® videolaryngoscopy and direct laryngoscopy; DL = direct laryngoscopy, GS = Glidescope® videolaryngoscopy). Ambrosio, 2014 [32]; Bahhatiq, 2016 [34]; Biermann, 2013 [29]; Cinar, 2011 [21]; Kaki, 2011 [22]; Kim, 2011 [23]; Kim, 2014 [33]; Lim, 2004 [16]; Lin, 2009 [17]; Malik, 2009 [18]; Pieters, 2016 [35]; Powell, 2009 [19]; Shin, 2011 [25]; Stroumpoulis, 2011 [26]; Tung, 2013 [30]; Wang, 2013 [31]; Wass, 2011 [24]; Xanthos, 2011 [27]; Xanthos, 2012 [28]; You, 2009 [20].

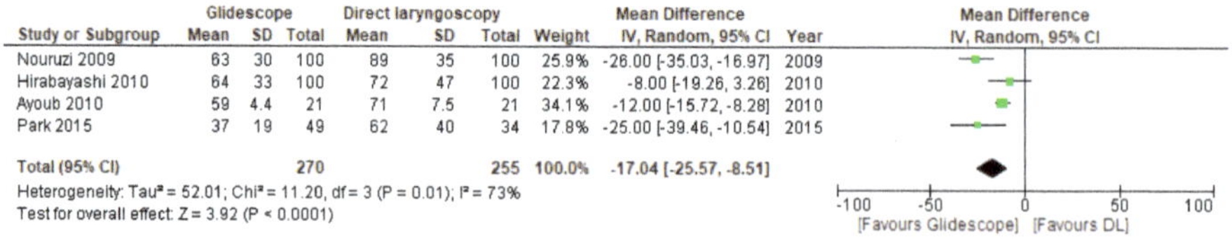

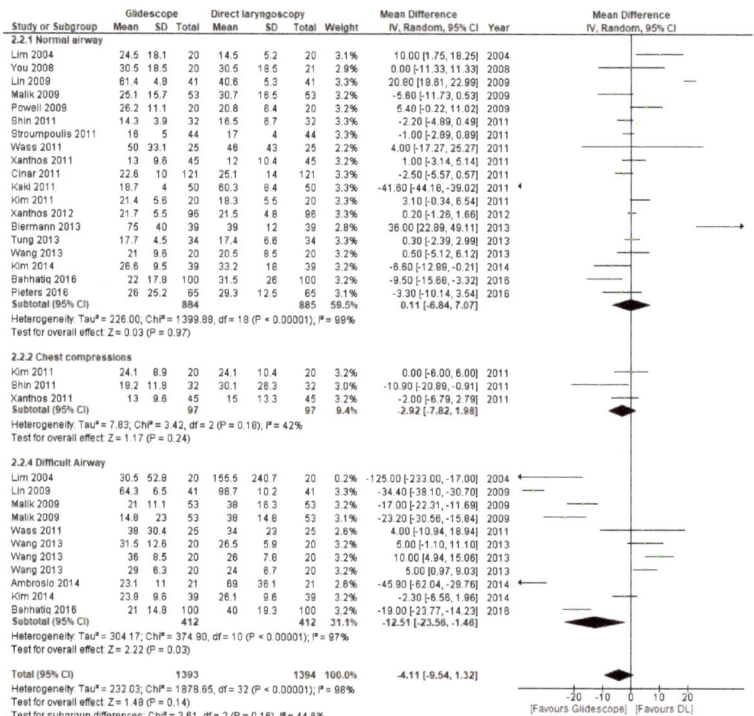

Figure 7. Mean difference (MD) in time to intubation (in seconds) in clinical trials comparing Glidescope® videolaryngoscope to direct laryngoscopy. The pooled estimate (rhombus) was derived using the DerSimonian and Laird random effects method. The squares depict an individual study point estimate of the mean difference. Solid horizontal lines display the 95% CI of the point estimate. The vertical line represents an MD of 0, indicating no difference between Glidescope® videolaryngoscopy and direct laryngoscopy. (DL = direct laryngoscopy). Nouruzi, 2009 [38]; Ayoub, 2010 [36]; Hirabayashi, 2010 [37]; Park, 2015 [39].

Figure 8. Mean difference (MD) in time to intubation (in seconds) in manikin trials comparing Glidescope® videolaryngoscope to direct laryngoscopy. The pooled estimate (rhombus) was derived using the DerSimonian and Laird random effects method. The squares depict an individual study point estimate of the mean difference. Solid horizontal lines display the 95% CI of the point estimate. The vertical line represents an MD of 0, indicating no difference between Glidescope® videolaryngoscopy and direct laryngoscopy. (DL = direct laryngoscopy). Ambrosio, 2014 [32]; Bahhatiq, 2016 [34]; Biermann, 2013 [29]; Cinar, 2011 [21]; Kaki, 2011 [22]; Kim, 2011 [23]; Kim, 2014 [33]; Lim, 2004 [16]; Lin, 2009 [17]; Malik, 2009 [18]; Pieters, 2016 [35]; Powell, 2009 [19]; Shin, 2011 [25]; Stroumpoulis, 2011 [26]; Tung, 2013 [30]; Wang, 2013 [31]; Wass, 2011 [24]; Xanthos, 2011 [27]; Xanthos, 2012 [28]; You, 2009 [20].

Table 2. Outcomes of clinical and manikin trials comparing Glidescope® videolaryngoscope to direct laryngoscopy. We created separate rows in the table for several studies as they used different scenarios in the same study. (*) The data in this row include only the first scenario with normal airways in this study. (CL = Cormack–Lehane, sec. = seconds, SD = standard deviation).

First Author, Year	Successful First Intubation Attempt			Time to Intubation (sec.) +/- SD		
	Direct Laryngoscopy	Glidescope®	P	Direct Laryngoscopy	Glidescope®	P
Clinical studies						
Nouruzi, 2009 [38]	51/100 (51.0%)	93/100 (93.0%)	$p < 0.001$	89.0 +/- 35.0	63.0 +/- 30.0	$p < 0.01$
Ayoub, 2010 [36]	3/21 (14.3%)	10/21 (47.6%)	$p = 0.04$	70.7 +/- 7.50	59.3 +/- 4.4	$p = 0.006$
Hirabayashi, 2010 [37]	77/100 (77.0%)	94/100 (94.0%)	$p = 0.03$	72.0 +/- 47.0	64.0 +/- 33.0	$p = 0.13$
Park, 2015 [39]	19/34 (55.9%)	45/49 (91.8%)	$p < 0.001$	62.0 +/- 40.0	37.0 +/- 19.3	$p < 0.001$
Manikin with normal airway						
Lim, 2004 [16]	19/20 (95.0%)	20/20 (100%)	$p = 1$	14.5 +/- 5.20	24.5 +/- 18.1	$p = 0.02$
You, 2009 [20]	11/21 (55.0%)	12/20 (57.0%)	$p > 0.05$	30.5 +/- 18.5	26.6 +/- 14.3	$p = 0.35$
Lin, 2009 [17]	36/41 (87.8%)	35/41 (85.3%)	$p = 1$	40.6 +/- 5.30	61.4 +/- 4.80	$p < 0.001$
Malik, 2009 * [18]	49/53 (92.4%)	51/53 (96.2%)	$p = 0.68$	30.7 +/- 16.5	25.1 +/- 15.7	$p = 0.08$
Powell, 2009 [19]	18/20 (90.0%)	20/20 (100%)	$p = 0.49$	20.8 +/- 6.40	26.2 +/- 11.1	$p = 0.07$
Cinar, 2011 [21]	95/121 (78.5%)	111/121 (91.7%)	$p = 0.006$	25.1 +/- 14.0	22.6 +/- 10.0	$p = 0.11$
Kaki, 2011 [22]	37/50 (74.0%)	50/50 (100%)	$p < 0.001$	60.3 +/- 8.40	18.7 +/- 0.40	$p < 0.001$
Kim, 2011 [23]	18/20 (90.0%)	16/20 (80.0%)	$p = 0.15$	18.3 +/- 5.50	21.4 +/- 5.60	$p = 0.24$
Shin, 2011 [25]	31/32 (96.9%)	32/32 (100%)	$p = 0.36$	16.5 +/- 6.70	14.3 +/- 3.90	$p = 0.03$
Stroumpoulis, 2011 [26]	12/44 (27.3%)	29/44 (65.9%)	$p < 0.001$	17.0 +/- 4.00	16.0 +/- 5.00	$p > 0.05$
Wass, 2011 [24]	20/25 (80.0%)	25/25 (100%)	$p = 0.05$	46.0 +/- 43.0	50.0 +/- 33.1	$p = 0.71$
Xanthos, 2011 [27]	33/45 (73.3%)	45/45 (100%)	$p = 0.001$	12.0 +/- 10.4	13.0 +/- 9.60	$p = 0.64$
Xanthos, 2012 [28]	26/96 (27.1%)	28/96 (29.1%)	$p = 0.87$	21.5 +/- 4.80	21.7 +/- 5.50	$p = 0.79$
Biermann, 2013 [29]	27/39 (69.2%)	36/39 (92.3%)	$p = 0.02$	39.0 +/- 12.0	75.0 +/- 40.0	$p < 0.001$
Tung, 2013 [30]	30/34 (88.2%)	34/34 (100%)	$p = 0.11$	17.4 +/- 6.60	17.7 +/- 4.50	$p = 0.45$
Wang, 2013 [31]	20/20 (100%)	19/20 (95.0%)	$p = 1$	20.5 +/- 8.50	21.0 +/- 9.60	$p = 0.86$
Kim, 2014 [33]	34/39 (87.1%)	23/29 (58.9%)	$p = 0.008$	33.2 +/-18.0	26.6 +/- 9.50	$p = 0.18$
Bahhatiq, 2016 [34]	68/100 (68.0%)	91/100 (91.0%)	$p < 0.001$	31.5 +/- 26.0	22.0 +/- 17.8	$p < 0.001$
Pieters, 2016 [35]	51/65 (78.4%)	58/65 (89.2%)	$p = 0.1$	29.3 +/- 12.5	26.0 +/- 25.2	$p = 0.35$
Manikin with chest compressions						
Shin, 2011 [25]	24/32 (75.0%)	31/32 (96.9%)	$p = 0.01$	30.1 +/- 26.3	19.2 +/- 11.8	$p = 0.006$
Xanthos, 2011 [27]	20/45 (44.4%)	43/45 (95.6%)	$p < 0.001$	15.0 +/- 13.3	13.0 +/- 9.60	$p = 0.42$
Manikin with chest compressions on the floor						
Kim, 2011 [23]	15/20 (75.0%)	17/20 (85.0%)	$p = 0.69$	24.1 +/- 10.4	24.1 +/- 8.90	$p = 0.99$
Manikin with CL grade 3						
Lim, 2004 [16]	14/20 (70.0%)	19/20 (95.0%)	$p = 0.09$	156 +/- 241	30.5 +/- 52.8	$p < 0.001$
Lin, 2009 [17]	18/41 (43.9%)	36/41 (87.8%)	$p < 0.001$	98.7 +/- 10.2	64.3 +/- 6.50	$p < 0.001$

Table 2. Cont.

First Author, Year	Successful First Intubation Attempt			Time to Intubation (sec.) +/- SD		
	Direct Laryngoscopy	Glidescope®	P	Direct Laryngoscopy	Glidescope®	P
Manikin with cervical immobilisation						
Malik, 2009 [18]	47/53 (88.7%)	49/53 (92.5%)	p = 0.74	38.0 +/- 14.8	23.0 +/- 14.8	p < 0.001
Wang, 2013 [31]	20/20 (100%)	17/20 (85.0%)	p = 0.23	26.5 +/- 5.90	31.5 +/- 12.6	p = 0.12
Kim, 2014 [33]	34/39 (87.1%)	35/39 (89.7%)	p = 0.72	26.1 +/- 9.60	23.8 +/- 9.60	p = 0.49
Bahhatiq, 2016 [34]	60/100 (60.0%)	88/100 (88.0%)	p < 0.001	40.0 +/- 19.3	21.0 +/- 14.8	p < 0.001
Manikin with cervical immobilisation on the floor						
Wang, 2013 [31]	19/20 (95.0%)	18/20 (90.0%)	p = 1	26.0 +/- 7.80	36.0 +/- 8.50	p < 0.001
Manikin with cervical immobilisation and CL grade 3						
Ambrosio, 2014 [32]	9/19 (47.7%)	21/21 (100%)	p < 0.001	69.0 +/- 36.1	23.1 +/- 11.0	p < 0.001
Manikin with pharyngeal obstruction						
Malik, 2009 [18]	33/53 (62.3%)	48/53 (90.6%)	p = 0.001	38.0 +/- 16.3	21.0 +/- 11.1	p < 0.001
Wass, 2011 [24]	23/25 (92.0%)	25/25 (100%)	p = 0.49	34.0 +/- 23.0	38.0 +/- 30.4	p = 0.60
Manikin on the floor						
Wang, 2013 [31]	20/20 (100%)	20/20 (100%)	p = 1	24.0 +/- 6.70	29.0 +/- 6.30	p = 0.05

3.5.3. Intubation during Cardiopulmonary Resuscitation

We included one clinical study performed on patients during cardiac arrest [39]. The first-pass success rate of the Glidescope® group was higher than that of the DL group (91.8% versus 55.9%, $p < 0.001$). It took less time to complete tracheal intubation with Glidescope® than with DL (median time 37 vs. 62 s; $p < 0.001$). The median duration of chest compression interruptions during CPR was reduced from seven seconds (IQR 3–16 s) with direct laryngoscopy to zero seconds (IQR 0–0 s) with Glidescope® videolaryngoscopy.

Three manikin studies reported on tracheal intubation during chest compressions [23,25,27]. The RR of successful intubation with the Glidescope® was 1.45 (95% CI 1.00, 2.10; $p = 0.05$). There was substantial between-study heterogeneity. The time required for intubation was not significantly different. All three manikin studies used scenarios with uninterrupted chest compressions, so the difference in duration of chest compression interruptions was not an applicable outcome measure.

4. Discussion

This systematic review and meta-analysis of the literature on tracheal intubation using direct laryngoscopy versus videolaryngoscopy with the Glidescope® videolaryngoscope by clinicians with limited intubation experience showed a significant improvement in first-pass success rate in both clinical and manikin randomized trials, a shorter time needed for intubation in clinical trials as well as in manikin trials with difficult airway scenarios. The only clinical trial in the CPR setting showed a positive effect on first-pass success rate and a reduction in chest compression interruptions when using the Glidescope® videolaryngoscope [39]. The positive effect on first-pass success was also seen in manikin studies with a CPR setting, although in lesser amounts. The time needed for intubation during CPR was no longer for the Glidescope® videolaryngoscope in these manikin trials [23,25,27].

Many of the analyzed groups showed significant between-study heterogeneity. This could be a limitation for the interpretation of our results. Differences in the definition of successful and failed intubation existed in the included studies. Failed intubation was defined as intervention by senior staff and/or actual misplacement of the tube. Another explanation could be the difference in initial skill training in the clinicians. Nearly all studies used different approaches to train tracheal intubation clinicians. All manikin studies used training varying from five minutes to one hour, and the clinical studies a training of ten minutes to eight hours. This could also explain differences in success rates between studies and thus significant between-study heterogeneity.

Several limitations of our systematic review should be highlighted. First of all, the number of clinical studies is limited. Furthermore, in our analysis of the manikin studies, subgroups with different scenarios were included. Except for the manikin with a normal airway, all subgroups consisted of no more than three studies. To overcome the small number of studies in each subgroup, we pooled the manikin studies employing difficult airway scenarios as an entire group. Random effects model was employed. As a result, the pooled estimates are more conservative when significant between-study heterogeneity exists [40]. Our systematic review included both clinical and simulation trials with the use of manikins. A manikin can simulate reality only to a limited degree. Despite the resemblances, even the most advanced high-fidelity simulation manikins are unable to fully recreate the feel and finer aspects of human airway anatomy [41]. Especially for clinicians with limited experience, intubation during prehospital resuscitation in an out-of-hospital cardiac arrest airway management can be far more challenging than in manikins. This might explain why clinical trials show a stronger effect in favor of the Glidescope® videolaryngoscopy. More (randomized) clinical studies are needed to confirm the effects, especially in the setting of prehospital CPR. Finally, our approach to focus on one type of videolaryngoscope lead to uncertainty about whether or not the results are generalizable to other types of videolaryngoscopes.

Our findings provide specific insight into tracheal intubation with the Glidescope® videolaryngoscopy by clinicians with limited experience. Previous reviews often include a mix of experience levels and multiple types of videolaryngoscopes [42,43]. Griesdale et al. [43] published a systematic review comparing direct laryngoscopy with Glidescope® videolaryngoscopy. However, the authors included all studies, regardless of the level of experience of the clinicians. The increased success rate with the Glidescope® found in our review is not seen among experienced intubators in the systematic review by Griesdale et al. [43]. In their systematic review, two studies focused on inexperienced personnel; one of those is also included in our systematic review [38], and the other employed nasotracheal intubation which was one of the exclusion criteria in our study [44]. Videolaryngoscopy was also shown to improve the first-pass success rate in emergency intubations in less experienced clinicians in a recent systematic review by Arulkumaran et al. [42]. However, various types of videolaryngoscopes and different operator experience levels for tracheal intubation were included in this review.

The guidelines by the International Liaison Committee on Resuscitation and European Resuscitation Council recommend that tracheal intubation should only be performed by rescuers with a high intubation success rate [45,46]. However, clinicians with limited intubation experience can still be confronted with patients in whom bag-valve-mask ventilation and supraglottic airway device placement are not successful. Especially in the prehospital, remote, or military setting, experienced airway clinicians may take an unacceptably long time to get to the patient. Tracheal intubation is a complex and high-risk procedure, especially when performed by clinicians with limited experience. Large studies on airway management during out-of-hospital cardiac arrest (OHCA) show first-pass success rates of 60–70% [47,48]. Multiple intubation attempts can distract EMS clinicians from ensuring high-quality chest compressions and treating the cause of the arrest. This might be the explanation for a recent study showing that multiple intubation attempts are associated with a decrease in survival [49]. It, therefore, seems important that efforts should be made to improve the tracheal intubation first-pass success rate. When clinicians with limited intubation experience are confronted with a patient requiring tracheal intubation, the use of the Glidescope helps to improve the first-pass success rate, time to intubation, and CPR quality. Videolaryngoscopy is also the intubation technique to be considered in (suspected) COVID-19 patients requiring tracheal intubation [1]. The current European Resuscitation Council Guidelines state that the rescuers' choice of the use of videolaryngoscopy during CPR should be guided by local protocols and rescuer experience [46]. With our review, we hope to provide the evidence needed to consider the use of the Glidescope® videolaryngoscope, particularly during CPR.

5. Conclusions

Tracheal intubation performed by clinicians with limited intubation experience (<10 intubations per year) using the Glidescope® videolaryngoscope has a higher first-pass success rate and shorter time to intubation when compared to direct laryngoscopy. Furthermore, intubation using the Glidescope® videolaryngoscope helps to minimize chest compression interruption during CPR. Although the number of clinical studies is limited, the use of the Glidescope® videolaryngoscope by clinicians with limited experience in tracheal intubation has important advantages when other initial airway techniques have failed. In particular, in the setting of prehospital advanced life support, further clinical studies are needed to confirm these findings and determine the effects on outcomes in out-of-hospital cardiac arrest.

Supplementary Materials: The following supporting information can be downloaded at: https://www.mdpi.com/article/10.3390/jcm11216291/s1, Supplementary Materials 1: PROSPERO Protocol, Supplementary Materials 2: PRISMA Checklist, Supplementary Materials 3: References of Excluded Articles, Supplementary Materials 4: GRADE Table.

Author Contributions: H.v.S., K.W.: Conceptualization, methodology, software, validation, formal analysis, investigation, resources, writing—original draft, writing—review and editing, visualization. M.W.H.: validation, writing—review and editing, supervision, project administration. B.P.: conceptualization, methodology, validation, writing—original draft, writing—review and editing, supervision, project administration. All authors have read and agreed to the published version of the manuscript.

Funding: This research received no external funding.

Institutional Review Board Statement: Not applicable.

Informed Consent Statement: Patient consent was waved due to this study is based on published literature.

Data Availability Statement: Data can be requested via the corresponding author.

Acknowledgments: We would like to thank Faridi van Etten-Jamaludin at the Medical Library of the Academic Medical Center, Amsterdam for her help in the development of the search strategy.

Conflicts of Interest: Hans van Schuppen is the Chair of the Medical Board of the Dutch Resuscitation Council and reports grants to his institution from the AMC Foundation, the Zoll Foundation, and Stryker Emergency Care, all outside the submitted work. Kamil Wojciechowicz reports no conflicts of interest. Markus Hollmann is the Executive Section Editor of Pharmacology for Anesthesia & Analgesia, Section Editor of Anesthesiology of the Journal of Clinical Medicine and Editor for Frontiers in Physiology, and reports grants to his institution from ZonMW, EACTA, and ESA, and consulting fees to his institution from CSL Behring, IDD Pharma and MSD, all outside the submitted work. Benedikt Preckel reports grants to his institution from ZonMW, EACTA, and ESA, and consulting fees to his institution from Sensium Healthcare UK, all outside the submitted work. None of the authors have any relationship with Glidescope® or Verathon Inc.

References

1. International Liaison Committee on Resuscitation (ILCOR). COVID-19—Practical Guidance for Implementation. Available online: https://www.ilcor.org/covid-19 (accessed on 31 January 2022).
2. Somri, M.; Gaitini, L.; Gat, M.; Sonallah, M.; Paz, A.; Gómez-Ríos, M. Cardiopulmonary Resuscitation during the COVID-19 pandemic. Do supraglottic airways protect against aerosol-generation? *Resuscitation* **2020**, *157*, 123–125. [CrossRef] [PubMed]
3. Pepe, P.E.; Roppolo, L.P.; Fowler, R.L. Prehospital endotracheal intubation: Elemental or detrimental? *Crit. Care* **2015**, *19*, 121. [CrossRef] [PubMed]
4. Crewdson, K.; Lockey, D.J.; Røislien, J.; Lossius, H.M.; Rehn, M. The success of pre-hospital tracheal intubation by different pre-hospital providers: A systematic literature review and meta-analysis. *Crit. Care* **2017**, *21*, 31. [CrossRef] [PubMed]

5. Pilbery, R. How do paramedics learn and maintain the skill of tracheal intubation? A rapid evidence review. *Br. Paramed. J.* **2018**, *3*, 7–21. [CrossRef]
6. Buis, M.L.; Maissan, I.M.; Hoeks, S.E.; Klimek, M.; Stolker, R.J. Defining the learning curve for endotracheal intubation using direct laryngoscopy: A systematic review. *Resuscitation* **2016**, *99*, 63–71. [CrossRef]
7. Kim, S.Y.; Park, S.O.; Kim, J.W.; Sung, J.; Lee, K.R.; Lee, Y.H.; Hong, D.Y.; Baek, K.J. How much experience do rescuers require to achieve successful tracheal intubation during cardiopulmonary resuscitation? *Resuscitation* **2018**, *133*, 187–192. [CrossRef]
8. Deakin, C.D.; King, P.; Thompson, F. Prehospital advanced airway management by ambulance technicians and paramedics: Is clinical practice sufficient to maintain skills? *Emerg. Med. J.* **2009**, *26*, 888–891. [CrossRef]
9. Dyson, K.; Bray, J.E.; Smith, K.; Bernard, S.; Straney, L.; Nair, R.; Finn, J. Paramedic Intubation Experience Is Associated With Successful Tube Placement but Not Cardiac Arrest Survival. *Ann. Emerg. Med.* **2017**, *70*, 382–390.e1. [CrossRef]
10. Mort, T.C. Emergency tracheal intubation: Complications associated with repeated laryngoscopic attempts. *Anesth. Analg.* **2004**, *99*, 607–613. [CrossRef]
11. Chrimes, N.; Higgs, A.; Hagberg, C.A.; Baker, P.A.; Cooper, R.M.; Greif, R.; Kovacs, G.; Law, J.A.; Marshall, S.D.; Myatra, S.N.; et al. Preventing unrecognised oesophageal intubation: A consensus guideline from the Project for Universal Management of Airways and international airway societies. *Anaesthesia* **2022**. [online ahead of print]. [CrossRef]
12. Wang, H.E.; Simeone, S.J.; Weaver, M.D.; Callaway, C.W. Interruptions in cardiopulmonary resuscitation from paramedic endotracheal intubation. *Ann. Emerg. Med.* **2009**, *54*, 645–652.e1. [CrossRef] [PubMed]
13. Page, M.J.; McKenzie, J.E.; Bossuyt, P.M.; Boutron, I.; Hoffmann, T.C.; Mulrow, C.D.; Shamseer, L.; Tetzlaff, J.M.; Akl, E.A.; Brennan, S.E.; et al. The PRISMA 2020 statement: An updated guideline for reporting systematic reviews. *BMJ* **2021**, *372*, n71. [CrossRef] [PubMed]
14. Higgins, J.P.; Altman, D.G.; Gøtzsche, P.C.; Jüni, P.; Moher, D.; Oxman, A.D.; Savovic, J.; Schulz, K.F.; Weeks, L.; Sterne, J.A. The Cochrane Collaboration's tool for assessing risk of bias in randomised trials. *BMJ* **2011**, *343*, d5928. [CrossRef] [PubMed]
15. Schünemann, H.; Brożek, J.; Guyatt, G.; Oxman, A. (Eds.) *GRADE Handbook for Grading Quality of Evidence and Strength of Recommendations*; Updated October 2013; The GRADE Working Group: Singapore, 2013.
16. Lim, Y.; Lim, T.J.; Liu, E.H.C. Ease of intubation with the GlideScope or Macintosh laryngoscope by inexperienced operators in simulated difficult airways. *Can. J. Anesth.* **2004**, *51*, 641–642. [CrossRef]
17. Lin, P.C.; Ong, J.; Lee, C.-L.; Chen, T.-Y.; Lee, Y.; Lai, H.-Y. Comparisons of the GlideScope and Macintosh laryngoscope in tracheal intubation by medical students on fresh human cadavers. *Tzu Chi Med. J.* **2009**, *21*, 147–150. [CrossRef]
18. Malik, M.A.; Hassett, P.; Carney, J.; Higgins, B.D.; Harte, B.H.; Laffey, J.G. A comparison of the Glidescope, Pentax AWS, and Macintosh laryngoscopes when used by novice personnel: A manikin study. *Can. J. Anaesth.* **2009**, *56*, 802–811. [CrossRef]
19. Powell, L.; Andrzejowski, J.; Taylor, R.; Turnbull, D. Comparison of the performance of four laryngoscopes in a high-fidelity simulator using normal and difficult airway. *Br. J. Anaesth.* **2009**, *103*, 755–760. [CrossRef]
20. You, J.S.; Park, S.; Chung, S.P.; Park, Y.S.; Park, J.W. The usefulness of the GlideScope video laryngoscope in the education of conventional tracheal intubation for the novice. *Emerg. Med. J.* **2009**, *26*, 109–111. [CrossRef]
21. Cinar, O.; Cevik, E.; Yildirim, A.O.; Yasar, M.; Kilic, E.; Comert, B. Comparison of GlideScope video laryngoscope and intubating laryngeal mask airway with direct laryngoscopy for endotracheal intubation. *Eur J. Emerg. Med.* **2011**, *18*, 117–120. [CrossRef]
22. Kaki, A.M.; Almarakbi, W.A.; Fawzi, H.M.; Boker, A.M. Use of Airtraq, C-Mac, and Glidescope laryngoscope is better than Macintosh in novice medical students' hands: A manikin study. *Saudi J. Anaesth.* **2011**, *5*, 376–381. [CrossRef]
23. Kim, Y.M.; Kang, H.G.; Kim, J.H.; Chung, H.S.; Yim, H.W.; Jeong, S.H. Direct versus video laryngoscopic intubation by novice prehospital intubators with and without chest compressions: A pilot manikin study. *Prehosp. Emerg. Care* **2011**, *15*, 98–103. [CrossRef] [PubMed]
24. Wass, T.C.; Jacob, A.K.; Kopp, S.L.; Torscher, L.C. A prospective randomized high fidelity simulation center based side-by-side comparison analyzing the success and ease of conventional versus new generation video laryngoscope technology by inexperienced laryngoscopists. *Signa Vitae J. Intesive Care Emerg. Med.* **2011**, *6*, 36–45.
25. Shin, D.H.; Choi, P.C.; Han, S.K. Tracheal intubation during chest compressions using Pentax-AWS (®), GlideScope (®), and Macintosh laryngoscope: A randomized crossover trial using a mannequin. *Can. J. Anaesth.* **2011**, *58*, 733–739. [CrossRef] [PubMed]
26. Stroumpoulis, K.; Xanthos, T.; Bassiakou, E.; Iacovidou, N.; Koudouna, E.; Michaloliakou, C.; Papadimitriou, L. Macintosh and Glidescope®performance by Advanced Cardiac Life Support providers: A manikin study. *Minerva Anestesiol.* **2011**, *77*, 11–16. [PubMed]
27. Xanthos, T.; Stroumpoulis, K.; Bassiakou, E.; Koudouna, E.; Pantazopoulos, I.; Mazarakis, A.; Demestiha, T.; Iacovidou, N. Glidescope(®) videolaryngoscope improves intubation success rate in cardiac arrest scenarios without chest compressions interruption: A randomized cross-over manikin study. *Resuscitation* **2011**, *82*, 464–467. [CrossRef] [PubMed]
28. Xanthos, T.; Bassiakou, E.; Koudouna, E.; Stroumpoulis, K.; Vlachos, I.; Johnson, E.O.; Vasileiou, P.; Papalois, A.; Iacovidou, N. Inexperienced nurses and doctors are equally efficient in managing the airway in a manikin model. *Heart Lung* **2012**, *41*, 161–166. [CrossRef]
29. Biermann, H.; van der Heiden, E.; Beishuizen, A.; Girbes, A.R.J.; de Waard, M.C. Endotracheal intubation by inexperienced registrars in internal medicine: A comparison of video-laryngoscopy versus direct laryngoscopy. *Neth. J. Crit. Care* **2013**, *17*, 7–9.

30. Tung, A.; Griesdale, D.E. Comparing the novel GlideScope Groove videolaryngoscope with conventional videolaryngoscopy: A randomized mannequin study of novice providers. *J. Clin. Anesth.* **2013**, *25*, 644–650. [CrossRef]
31. Wang, P.K.; Huang, C.C.; Lee, Y.; Chen, T.Y.; Lai, H.Y. Comparison of 3 video laryngoscopes with the Macintosh in a manikin with easy and difficult simulated airways. *Am. J. Emerg. Med.* **2013**, *31*, 330–338. [CrossRef]
32. Ambrosio, A.; Pfannenstiel, T.; Bach, K.; Cornelissen, C.; Gaconnet, C.; Brigger, M.T. Difficult airway management for novice physicians: A randomized trial comparing direct and video-assisted laryngoscopy. *Otolaryngol. Head Neck Surg.* **2014**, *150*, 775–778. [CrossRef]
33. Kim, W.; Choi, H.J.; Lim, T.; Kang, B.S. Can the new McGrath laryngoscope rival the GlideScope Ranger portable video laryngoscope? A randomized manikin study. *Am. J. Emerg. Med.* **2014**, *32*, 1225–1229. [CrossRef] [PubMed]
34. Bahathiq, A.O.; Abdelmontaleb, T.H.; Newigy, M.K. Learning and performance of endotracheal intubation by paramedical students: Comparison of GlideScope (®) and intubating laryngeal mask airway with direct laryngoscopy in manikins. *Indian J. Anaesth.* **2016**, *60*, 337–342. [CrossRef] [PubMed]
35. Pieters, B.M.; Wilbers, N.E.; Huijzer, M.; Winkens, B.; van Zundert, A.A. Comparison of seven videolaryngoscopes with the Macintosh laryngoscope in manikins by experienced and novice personnel. *Anaesthesia* **2016**, *71*, 556–564. [CrossRef] [PubMed]
36. Ayoub, C.M.; Kanazi, G.E.; Al Alami, A.; Rameh, C.; El-Khatib, M.F. Tracheal intubation following training with the GlideScope compared to direct laryngoscopy. *Anaesthesia* **2010**, *65*, 674–678. [CrossRef] [PubMed]
37. Hirabayashi, Y.; Otsuka, Y.; Seo, N. GlideScope videolaryngoscope reduces the incidence of erroneous esophageal intubation by novice laryngoscopists. *J. Anesth.* **2010**, *24*, 303–305. [CrossRef] [PubMed]
38. Nouruzi-Sedeh, P.; Schumann, M.; Groeben, H. Laryngoscopy via Macintosh blade versus GlideScope: Success rate and time for endotracheal intubation in untrained medical personnel. *Anesthesiology* **2009**, *110*, 32–37. [CrossRef]
39. Park, S.O.; Kim, J.W.; Na, J.H.; Lee, K.H.; Lee, K.R.; Hong, D.Y.; Baek, K.J. Video laryngoscopy improves the first-attempt success in endotracheal intubation during cardiopulmonary resuscitation among novice physicians. *Resuscitation* **2015**, *89*, 188–194. [CrossRef]
40. Reade, M.C.; Delaney, A.; Bailey, M.J.; Angus, D.C. Bench-to-bedside review: Avoiding pitfalls in critical care meta-analysis–funnel plots, risk estimates, types of heterogeneity, baseline risk and the ecologic fallacy. *Crit. Care* **2008**, *12*, 220. [CrossRef]
41. Rai, M.R.; Popat, M.T. Evaluation of airway equipment: Man or manikin? *Anaesthesia* **2011**, *66*, 529. [CrossRef]
42. Arulkumaran, N.; Lowe, J.; Ions, R.; Mendoza, M.; Bennett, V.; Dunser, M.W. Videolaryngoscopy versus direct laryngoscopy for emergency orotracheal intubation outside the operating room: A systematic review and meta-analysis. *Br. J. Anaesth.* **2018**, *120*, 712–724. [CrossRef]
43. Griesdale, D.E.; Liu, D.; McKinney, J.; Choi, P.T. Glidescope®video-laryngoscopy versus direct laryngoscopy for endotracheal intubation: A systematic review and meta-analysis. *Can. J. Anaesth.* **2012**, *59*, 41–52. [CrossRef] [PubMed]
44. Shimada, N.; Hirabayashi, Y.; Otsuka, Y.; Urayama, M.; Yokotsuka, C.; Yamanaka, T.; Takeuchi, M. GlideScope Ranger: Clinical assessment of the performance in 100 patients. *Masui* **2011**, *60*, 1314–1316.
45. Soar, J.; Berg, K.M.; Andersen, L.W.; Böttiger, B.W.; Cacciola, S.; Callaway, C.W.; Couper, K.; Cronberg, T.; D'Arrigo, S.; Deakin, C.D.; et al. Adult Advanced Life Support: 2020 International Consensus on Cardiopulmonary Resuscitation and Emergency Cardiovascular Care Science with Treatment Recommendations. *Resuscitation* **2020**, *156*, A80–A119. [CrossRef]
46. Soar, J.; Böttiger, B.W.; Carli, P.; Couper, K.; Deakin, C.D.; Djärv, T.; Lott, C.; Olasveengen, T.; Paal, P.; Pellis, T.; et al. European Resuscitation Council Guidelines 2021: Adult advanced life support. *Resuscitation* **2021**, *161*, 115–151. [CrossRef] [PubMed]
47. Wang, H.E.; Yealy, D.M. How many attempts are required to accomplish out-of-hospital endotracheal intubation? *Acad. Emerg. Med.* **2006**, *13*, 372–377. [CrossRef] [PubMed]
48. Benger, J.R.; Kirby, K.; Black, S.; Brett, S.J.; Clout, M.; Lazaroo, M.J.; Nolan, J.P.; Reeves, B.C.; Robinson, M.; Scott, L.J.; et al. Effect of a Strategy of a Supraglottic Airway Device vs Tracheal Intubation During Out-of-Hospital Cardiac Arrest on Functional Outcome: The AIRWAYS-2 Randomized Clinical Trial. *JAMA* **2018**, *320*, 779–791. [CrossRef]
49. Murphy, D.L.; Bulger, N.E.; Harrington, B.M.; Skerchak, J.A.; Counts, C.R.; Latimer, A.J.; Yang, B.Y.; Maynard, C.; Rea, T.D.; Sayre, M.R. Fewer tracheal intubation attempts are associated with improved neurologically intact survival following out-of-hospital cardiac arrest. *Resuscitation* **2021**, *167*, 289–296. [CrossRef]

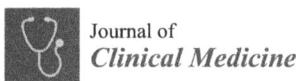

Article

Strategies of Advanced Airway Management in Out-of-Hospital Cardiac Arrest during Intra-Arrest Hypothermia: Insights from the PRINCESS Trial

Jonathan Tjerkaski [1], Thomas Hermansson [1], Emelie Dillenbeck [1], Fabio Silvio Taccone [2], Anatolij Truhlar [3,4], Sune Forsberg [1], Jacob Hollenberg [1], Mattias Ringh [1], Martin Jonsson [1], Leif Svensson [5] and Per Nordberg [1,6,*]

[1] Department of Clinical Science and Education, Södersjukhuset, Center for Resuscitation Science, Karolinska Institute, 11883 Stockholm, Sweden
[2] Department of Intensive Care, Hôpital Universitaire de Bruxelles (HUB), Université Libre de Bruxelles (ULB), 1070 Brussels, Belgium
[3] Emergency Medical Services of the Hradec Kralove Region, 500 05 Hradec Kralove, Czech Republic
[4] Department of Anaesthesiology and Intensive Care Medicine, Charles University in Prague, University Hospital Hradec Kralove, 500 05 Hradec Kralove, Czech Republic
[5] Department of Medicine, Karolinska Institute, 17176 Solna, Sweden
[6] Function Perioperative Medicine and Intensive Care, Karolinska University Hospital, 17176 Stockholm, Sweden
* Correspondence: per.nordberg@ki.se

Abstract: Background: Trans-nasal evaporative cooling is an effective method to induce intra-arrest therapeutic hypothermia in out-of-hospital cardiac arrest (OHCA). The use of supraglottic airway devices (SGA) instead of endotracheal intubation may enable shorter time intervals to induce cooling. We aimed to study the outcomes in OHCA patients receiving endotracheal intubation (ETI) or a SGA during intra-arrest trans-nasal evaporative cooling. Methods: This is a pre-specified sub-study of the PRINCESS trial (NCT01400373) that included witnessed OHCA patients randomized during resuscitation to trans-nasal intra-arrest cooling vs. standard care followed by temperature control at 33 °C for 24 h. For this study, patients randomized to intra-arrest cooling were stratified according to the use of ETI vs. SGA prior to the induction of cooling. SGA was placed by paramedics in the first-tier ambulance or by physicians or anesthetic nurses in the second tier while ETI was performed only after the arrival of the second tier. Propensity score matching was used to adjust for differences at the baseline between the two groups. The primary outcome was survival with good neurological outcome, defined as cerebral performance category (CPC) 1–2 at 90 days. Secondary outcomes included time to place airway, overall survival at 90 days, survival with complete neurologic recovery (CPC 1) at 90 days and sustained return of spontaneous circulation (ROSC). Results: Of the 343 patients randomized to the intervention arm (median age 64 years, 24% were women), 328 received intra-arrest cooling and had data on the airway method ($n = 259$ with ETI vs. $n = 69$ with SGA). Median time from the arrival of the first-tier ambulance to successful airway management was 8 min for ETI performed by second tier and 4 min for SGA performed by the first or second tier ($p = 0.001$). No significant differences in the probability of good neurological outcome (OR 1.43, 95% CI 0.64–3.01), overall survival (OR 1.26, 95% CI 0.57–2.55), full neurological recovery (OR 1.17, 95% CI 0.52–2.73) or sustained ROSC (OR 0.88, 95% CI 0.50–1.52) were observed between ETI and SGA. Conclusions: Among the OHCA patients treated with trans-nasal evaporative intra-arrest cooling, the use of SGA was associated with a significantly shorter time to airway management and with similar outcomes compared to ETI.

Keywords: cardiac arrest; intra-arrest hypothermia; airway management

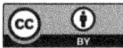

1. Introduction

Out-of-hospital cardiac arrest (OHCA) is a major public health concern, affecting approximately 275,000 individuals each year in Europe [1]. The overall OHCA mortality rate is approximately 90%, with lifelong disabilities being common among the survivors [2]. Airway management and ventilation is an important element of the advanced cardiac life support (ACLS) protocol, which has been formulated in order to improve outcomes for OHCA victims [3]. Currently, most patients receive advanced airway management during resuscitation, either using endotracheal intubation (ETI) or a supraglottic airway (SGA) [4].

ETI has been used by emergency medical services (EMS) since the 1970s [5]. However, several studies have questioned the safety and effectiveness of ETI performed by EMS in the pre-hospital setting [6,7]. The potential harms of pre-hospital ETI include unrecognized tube misplacement or dislodgement, iatrogenic hyperventilation and chest compression interruptions during placement [8–10]. SGA insertion is most often simpler and faster to insert than ETI [11], which results in higher success rates and fewer interruptions in the administration of chest compressions [12–14]. Despite the supposed benefits of SGA, several observational studies have suggested that ETI may be associated with better outcomes than SGA [15]. However, recent randomized controlled trials have raised some controversies on this issue [13,14]. Thus, the optimal strategy for airway management in OHCA remains unclear.

Targeted temperature management remains an important intervention that may influence survival with good neurological function among cardiac arrest patients [16]. In particular, intra-arrest cooling using trans-nasal evaporative cooling may provide some benefits on neurologic recovery in patients with initial shockable rhythms (i.e., ventricular fibrillation or pulseless ventricular tachycardia) [17–19]. Trans-nasal evaporative intra-arrest cooling has emerged as a promising therapeutic strategy in OHCA [18,20,21]. The use of SGA in these cases has the potential to shorten the time to successful airway management and thereby enable a shorter time to start cooling. However, as SGA may be associated with an increased risk for aspiration, it is important to examine the safety of advanced airway management in the setting of trans-nasal evaporative intra-arrest cooling therapy.

In this sub-study of the PRINCESS trial, we aimed to compare the effect on neurologic outcome among OHCA patients that had received airway management with ETI versus SGA prior to trans-nasal evaporative intra-arrest cooling.

2. Methods

2.1. Study Design

We performed a post hoc sub-analysis of data from the PRINCESS trial, which is a multicenter randomized clinical trial that compared trans-nasal evaporative intra-arrest cooling to the standard ACLS in a bystander-witnessed OHCA (Trial registration: NCT01400373) [20]. Ethics and institutional committees in each of the participating countries approved the study protocol [22]. Written informed consent was obtained from the next of kin or a legal representative after hospital admission and from each study participant who regained mental capacity. In this sub-analysis, the patients in the intervention arm in PRINCESS were the primary study population that was subsequently divided into two groups depending on the strategy for airway management.

2.2. Study Participants

We included bystander witnessed OHCA randomized to the intervention arm in the PRINCESS trial. The exclusion criteria were age ≥80 years; an etiology of cardiac arrest due to trauma, head trauma, severe bleeding, drug overdose, cerebrovascular accident, drowning, smoke inhalation, electrocution, or hanging; hypothermia at the time of evaluation; an anatomical barrier preventing the insertion of intra-nasal catheters; an existing do-not-attempt resuscitation order; known terminal illness; known or clinically apparent pregnancy; known coagulopathy (except when therapeutically induced); need for supplemental oxygen; ROSC prior to randomization; and EMS response time (i.e., from collapse to EMS arrival) greater than 15 min. In this sub-study of the PRINCESS trial, we also excluded study participants who were randomized to the control group as well as study participants who were initially randomized to the intervention group but did not receive intra-arrest cooling. Patients were divided into two different treatment groups depending on the airway management technique used prior to trans-nasal evaporative cooling (i.e., those receiving ETI versus those receiving SGA).

2.3. Emergency Medical Services

All study sites had two-tiered EMS systems where the first vehicle used bag mask ventilation only or SGA with bag-valve ventilation connected to the SGA prior to the arrival of the second tier. The second tier was manned by physicians or anesthetic nurses, trained in advance airway management including placing an SGA and endotracheal intubation. In addition, the intra-arrest cooling equipment was carried by the second tier. Thus, patients could have had the SGA placed by paramedics from the first vehicle and subsequently, cooling was started after randomization and application of trans-nasal evaporative cooling by the crew in the second tier. Among patients receiving bag mask ventilation by the paramedics, ETI was performed after the arrival of the second tier. The use of SGA could also be due to ETI being difficult to perform in the field. No data were collected on the number of intubation attempts or change in airway strategy. The confirmation of the tube was undertaken with end tidal CO_2, but this was only recorded in a limited number of patients and not presented in this analysis.

2.4. Exposure

The exposure of interest was defined as the type of airway management technique used prior to cooling. All of the study participants included in the PRINCESS trial were treated with advanced airway management prior to randomization using either ETI or an SGA [22]; patients were therefore divided into two different treatment groups depending on the airway management technique used prior to trans-nasal evaporative cooling.

2.5. Treatment

The RhinoChill™ device delivers a mixture of air or oxygen and a chemically inert cooling liquid (perfluorohexane) via nasal catheters directly into the nasal cavity, with the goal of primarily cooling the brain [20,21,23]. Trans-nasal evaporative cooling is maintained until hospital arrival, and whenever possible until systemic cooling is initiated. The study participants received standard post-resuscitation care upon admission to the intensive care unit (ICU). Intravenous sedation, analgesia, and neuromuscular blockade were used according to the institutional cooling protocols. The targets for respiratory management, blood pressure, and glucose control have been previously described [22]. The study participants were treated with targeted temperature management at 32–34 °C for 24 h.

2.6. Outcome

Neurological outcome assessment was performed at 90 days via a structured telephone interview or during a follow-up appointment using the cerebral performance categories (CPC) scale [24]. The primary outcome of this study was survival with good neurologic outcome (CPC 1–2) at 90 days. The secondary outcomes were overall survival at 90 days, survival with complete neurologic recovery (CPC 1) at 90 days, and hospital admission with the sustained return of spontaneous circulation (ROSC) (defined as ROSC >20 min). Additional safety parameters that were investigated included the time until successful airway management, the time until the initiation of intra-arrest cooling, arterial blood gas parameters, and the prevalence of pneumonia. The time until successful airway management was defined as the time interval that elapsed between EMS arrival at the site of the arrest and the time of successful airway device placement. Similarly, we defined the time until the initiation of trans-nasal evaporative cooling as the time duration between EMS arrival and the initiation of intra-arrest cooling.

2.7. Statistical Analysis

Continuous variables were presented as means and standard deviations (SD) if normally distributed, or as medians and interquartile ranges (IQR) if not normally distributed.

Categorical variables were reported as counts and percentages. We assessed the group differences in continuous variables using either the Mann–Whitney U-test or Student's T-test, as appropriate. Group-wise differences in categorical variables were assessed using Pearson's chi-squared test.

A range of factors may influence the decision of EMS personnel to use one advanced airway device or strategy over any other form of airway management. Therefore, we used propensity score matching to balance known confounding variables across the two treatment groups, in a manner reminiscent of that conducted in the work of Hasegawa et al. and McMullan et al. [4,7]. Propensity scores were calculated using a logistic regression model with the following independent variables: EMS response time, age, sex, bystander CPR, initial rhythm, etiology, and body mass index (BMI). Propensity score matching (1:2) was carried out using the nearest neighbor method with a caliper width of 0.2. We used the standardized mean difference (SMD) to examine group differences in the covariates before and after matching. We fit a series of conditional logistic regression models to evaluate the association between each outcome variable and airway management strategy. We calculated bootstrapped 95% confidence intervals for the odds ratios using 1000 bootstrapped datasets.

We used multiple imputation by chained equations (mice) to impute missing data, generating five imputed datasets [25]. The analysis described above was separately performed in each of the imputed datasets. The resulting regression coefficients and test statistics were subsequently pooled across all imputed datasets [25,26].

3. Results

3.1. Study Population

Of the 343 patients who were allocated to intra-arrest cooling in the PRINCESS trial, six did not receive the assigned intervention, and data on airway management were missing for nine study participants (Figure 1). Thus, the study cohort consisted of 328 patients; 259 (79%) received orotracheal intubation (ETI group), while in the SGA group, six were treated using a laryngeal tube and the others (n = 63) with a laryngeal mask airway. Patients who were treated with SGA were older (p = 0.03) and had a higher BMI (p = 0.01) than patients who were treated with ETI (Table 1). After propensity score matching, all baseline characteristics were adequately balanced between groups (Supplementary Materials, Supplementary Figure S1). No significant differences in the arterial blood gas parameters at the time of hospital admission were observed between groups after propensity score matching (Table 2). Missing entries amounted to 3.32% of the included data (Supplementary Materials, Supplementary Table S1).

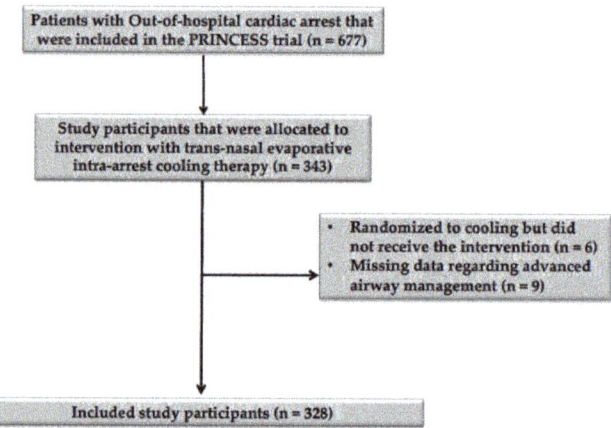

Figure 1. Flowchart describing patient inclusion and exclusion. A diagram describing the inclusion and exclusion of study participants, according to the inclusion and exclusion criteria mentioned in the methodology section of this article.

Table 1. Demographics before and after propensity score matching. Data after propensity score matching corresponded to that of one of the five imputed datasets that were generated following multiple imputation by chained equations (mice). Abbreviations: BMI = body mass index, CPR = cardiopulmonary resuscitation, EMS = emergency medical services, ETI = endotracheal intubation, SD = standard deviation, SGA = supraglottic airway, SMD = standardized mean difference, Q1 = first quartile, Q3 = third quartile.

	Unmatched			Matched		
	ETI (N = 259)	LMA (N = 69)	SMD	ETI (N = 126)	LMA (N = 67)	SMD
Sex						
Female	64 (24.7%)	18 (26.1%)	0.03	28 (22.2%)	18 (26.9%)	0.10
Male	195 (75.3%)	51 (73.9%)	−0.03	98 (77.8%)	49 (73.1%)	−0.10
Location						
At home	126 (55.5%)	46 (70.8%)	0.31	85 (67.5%)	47 (70.1%)	0.06
Other	16 (7.0%)	4 (6.2%)	−0.08	10 (7.9%)	4 (6.0%)	−0.06
Outside	54 (23.8%)	5 (7.7%)	−0.60	9 (7.1%)	5 (7.5%)	0.03
Public place	31 (13.7%)	10 (15.4%)	0.08	22 (17.5%)	11 (16.4%)	−0.06
Etiology						
Other	34 (14.3%)	13 (20.6%)	0.21	27 (21.4%)	15 (22.4%)	0.00
Suspected cardiac	204 (85.7%)	50 (79.4%)	−0.21	99 (78.6%)	52 (77.6%)	0.00
Bystander CPR						
No	89 (35.7%)	23 (35.9%)	0.07	48 (38.1%)	27 (40.3%)	0.03
Yes	160 (64.3%)	41 (64.1%)	−0.07	78 (61.9%)	40 (59.7%)	−0.03
EMS arrival time (minutes)						
Median (Q1–Q3)	7.0 (5.0, 10.0)	7.5 (4.0, 12.0)	0.04	8.0 (5.0, 11.0)	8.0 (4.5, 11.5)	−0.11
Time to ROSC (minutes)						
Median (Q1–Q3)	22.0 (15.0, 37.0)	23.5 (14.8, 29.5)	−0.28	24.0 (15.5, 40.5)	25.0 (17.0, 36.0)	0.11
Hospital admission time (minutes)						
Median (Q1–Q3)	48.0 (37.0, 59.0)	48.0 (39.0, 58.0)	−0.45	46.0 (35.0, 56.5)	51.0 (42.0, 58.8)	0.30
Initial rhythm						
Non-shockable	149 (57.8%)	47 (68.1%)	0.22	84 (66.7%)	45 (67.2%)	0.02
Shockable	109 (42.2%)	22 (31.9%)	−0.22	42 (33.3%)	22 (32.8%)	−0.02
Age (years)						
Mean (SD)	61.6 (12.1)	65.4 (12.3)	0.31	64.8 (10.7)	65.5 (12.2)	0.05
BMI						
Median (Q1–Q3)	26.2 (24.2, 29.3)	27.8 (25.4, 30.9)	0.31	27.8 (24.7, 30.1)	27.8 (25.0, 30.5)	0.02

Table 2. Patient characteristics at hospital admission. The presented results correspond to data obtained after propensity score matching for one of the five imputed datasets that were generated following multiple imputation by chained equations (mice). Abbreviations: $PaCO_2$ = partial pressure of carbon dioxide, PaO_2 = partial pressure of oxygen, SD = standard deviation, Q1 = first quartile, Q3 = third quartile.

	ETI	LMA	p Value
Lactate (mmol/L)	n = 24	n = 17	0.491
Mean (SD)	11.1 (4.9)	10.5 (5.3)	
Median (Q1–Q3)	11.2 (9.2, 13.2)	10.0 (7.0, 13.3)	
Range (Min–Max)	3.2–21.0	2.6–19.0	
$PaCO_2$ (mmHg)	n = 26	n = 19	0.491

Table 2. *Cont.*

	ETI	LMA	p Value
Mean (SD)	60.6 (25.5)	64.9 (32.2)	
Median (Q1–Q3)	54.0 (38.6, 84.0)	60.8 (46.9, 72.0)	
Range (Min–Max)	33.0–113.2	33.0–178.5	
PaO$_2$ (mmHg)	n = 26	n = 18	0.390
Mean (SD)	86.7 (48.1)	96.7 (46.6)	
Median (Q1–Q3)	74.8 (48.6, 106.3)	86.6 (65.7, 127.3)	
Range (Min–Max)	31.5–202.5	30.3–213.0	
pH	n = 24	n = 20	0.683
Mean (SD)	7.0 (0.2)	7.1 (0.2)	
Median (Q1–Q3)	7.0 (6.9, 7.2)	7.0 (6.9, 7.2)	
Range (Min–Max)	6.7–7.4	6.7–7.3	
Mean arterial pressure (mmHg)	n = 24	n = 17	0.233
Mean (SD)	82.9 (24.2)	90.3 (23.9)	
Median (Q1–Q3)	84.5 (63.0, 94.0)	92.0 (71.0, 107.0)	
Range (Min–Max)	43.0–140.0	55.0–132.0	

3.2. Outcome Measures

No significant differences between ETI and SGA were observed on the occurrence of survival with good neurologic outcome, CPC 1-2 at 90 days (OR 1.43, 95% CI 0.64–3.01), overall survival at 90 days (OR 1.26, 95% CI 0.57–2.55), survival with complete neurologic recovery at 90 days (OR 1.17, 95% CI 0.52–2.73) or hospital admission following sustained ROSC (OR 0.88, 95% CI 0.50–1.52), as can be seen in Figure 2.

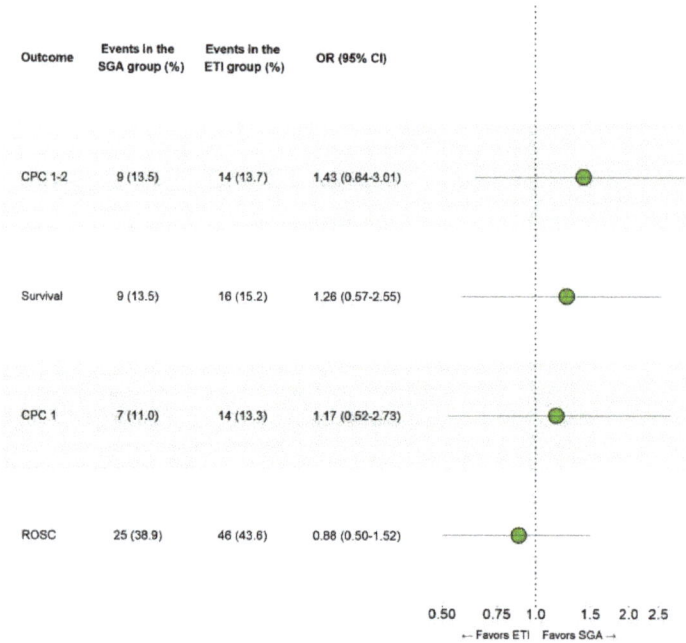

Figure 2. Comparison of endotracheal intubation and supraglottic airways. Results for the conditional logistic regression models that were fitted using propensity score matched data to examine the safety of ETI and SGA in patients with out-of-hospital cardiac arrest.

3.3. Time until Successful Airway Device Placement and the Initiation of Intra-Arrest Cooling

The time until airway management was available for 276 out of 328 study participants (84%). The median time from EMS arrival at the scene until successful airway management was 8 (interquartile range 4–12 min) minutes in the ETI group and 4 min in the SGA group (interquartile range 2–7 min), $p = 0.001$ (Figure 3A). However, we did not find any statistically significant difference between the SGA- and ETI groups regarding the time until the initiation of hypothermia treatment, which was on average 14 min in the ETI group (interquartile range 8–20) and 15 min in the SGA group (interquartile range 11–25), $p = 0.053$ (Figure 3B).

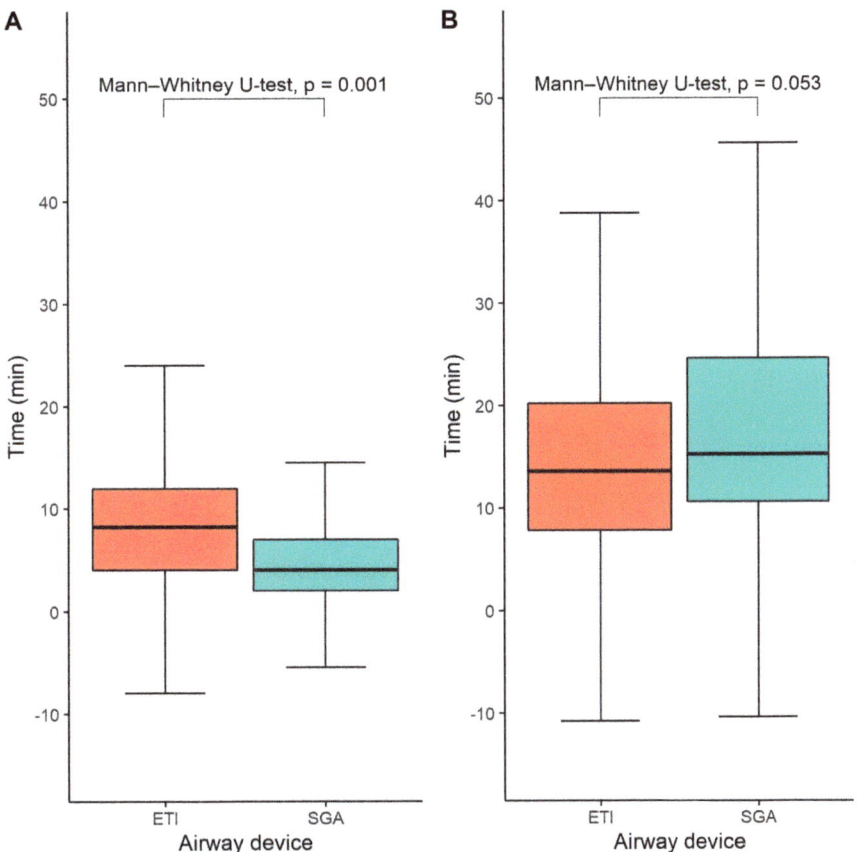

Figure 3. Time until successful advanced airway management (**A**) and time to start of intra-arrest cooling (**B**). Box-and-whisker plots depicting the time until successful airway management in the ETI and SGA groups, respectively. Medians and quartiles were estimated using quantile regression for each imputed dataset and subsequently averaged across all imputed datasets. Likewise, the Mann–Whitney U-test was performed in each imputed dataset and the results were pooled across all available imputed datasets.

The time until the initiation of intra-arrest cooling therapy was associated with survival with good neurological outcome (defined as CPC 1-2, OR 0.96 [0.92–1.00], $p = 0.045$), overall survival (OR 0.95 [0.91–0.99], $p = 0.017$), and survival with complete neurologic recovery at 90 days (defined as CPC 1, 0.95 [0.90–0.99], $p = 0.018$), as shown in the Supplementary Materials (Supplementary Table S2). In contrast, we did not observe any statistically significant association between the likelihood of achieving sustained ROSC and the time of intra-arrest cooling. Moreover, we found no statistically significant association between the endpoints of this study and the time until successful airway device placement. Thus, whereas the time until the initiation of intra-arrest cooling has a statistically significant association with both neurological outcomes and overall survival in OHCA patients, the time until successful airway device placement does not have any significant relationship to patient outcomes.

3.4. Infections

The incidence of infections prior to hospital discharge was reported in conjunction with the PRINCESS trial by all participating centers (Figure 4). Approximately 20% of patients suffered from some form of infection during their hospital stay, with pneumonia accounting for the majority of these cases. We found no statistically significant differences between the ETI- and SGA groups in the proportion of patients who suffered from pneumonia during their hospital stay ($p = 0.579$).

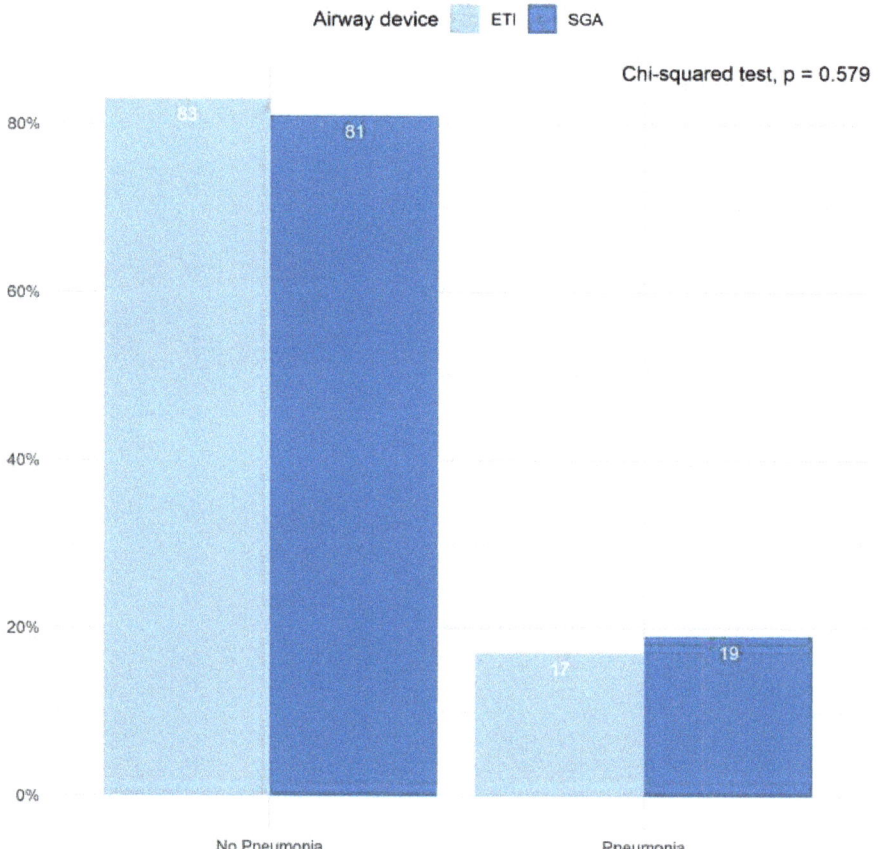

Figure 4. Pneumonia diagnosed during hospital stay. Bar plots depicting the proportion of patients in whom pneumonia was diagnosed prior to hospital discharge. Results are shown for the ETI group and the SGA group separately. The proportions were averaged across all imputed datasets. The Chi-squared test was performed in each imputed dataset and the results were pooled across all available imputed datasets.

4. Discussion

In this sub-analysis of the PRINCESS trial, we observed that SGA is feasible to use without any safety aspects reported prior to induction of trans-nasal evaporative cooling in OHCA and it significantly shortened the airway management time compared to ETI; SGA was not associated with any worsening in the gas exchange on arterial blood gas or with patient outcomes.

Trans-nasal evaporative intra-arrest cooling is an emerging therapeutic option in the management of OHCA patients which has, as the only cooling method, been shown to be safe and effective in inducing intra-arrest cooling at the scene of the arrest. Although not currently part of routine medical practice, trans-nasal evaporative intra-arrest cooling therapy has already been implemented in some clinical settings for the treatment of OHCA. Furthermore, trans-nasal evaporative intra-arrest cooling will continue to be investigated in clinical trials. Therefore, it is important to establish the safety of advanced airway management in the setting of trans-nasal evaporative intra-arrest cooling. In this study, we observed a shorter time period to successful airway management in the SGA group compared to intubation, but no differences in terms of sustained ROSC, overall survival, neurological recovery, the prevalence of pneumonia, or arterial blood gas parameters.

We observed that patients who were treated with SGA were on average older and had a higher BMI than patients who were treated with ETI. Although these imbalances were adjusted for in the subsequent analyses, we cannot dismiss the possibility of residual confounding due to one or several unmeasured parameters such as the lack of equipoise at the baseline including the expertise of centers. Therefore, we believe that there is a need for an external validation to confirm our results.

Despite concerns regarding an increased aspiration risk following trans-nasal evaporative cooling, we did not find any significant differences between the ETI and SGA groups concerning the proportion of patients suffering from pneumonia or arterial blood gas parameters on admission to hospital. Despite a limited sample size, these findings further support our other results, which suggest that ETI and SGA have similar safety profiles in the setting of trans-nasal evaporative intra-arrest cooling.

We observed a statistically significant difference between the ETI and SGA groups in the time elapsed until successful airway placement in the setting of trans-nasal evaporative intra-arrest cooling therapy. This result is in agreement with that of earlier studies on the topic of advanced airway management in OHCA [5,11]. However, we observed no statistically significant differences concerning the time until the initiation of trans-nasal evaporative intra-arrest cooling therapy. This result is most likely attributed to logistics, as the cooling device was carried by the second-tier vehicles and not by the paramedics in the first-tier ambulances. The pre-hospital physicians generally arrived at the site of the arrest later than the paramedics. Thus, although the patient's airway may have been secured using a SGA by the paramedic prior to the arrival of the pre-hospital emergency medicine physicians, intra-arrest cooling could only be initiated once the physician had arrived at the site of the arrest, making the time to hypothermia largely independent of the time until successful airway management.

This secondary analysis of the PRINCESS trial had several limitations. The study of two subgroups receiving different airway strategies within the intervention arm of the PRINCESS trial introduced a risk of selection bias. Although the treatment groups had similar baseline characteristics and propensity score matching was performed, the risk of residual confounding could not be eliminated. An additional limitation of this study is the fact that ETI and SGA could not be compared to bag-valve mask ventilation, as successful advanced airway management was specified as a requirement for inclusion in the PRINCESS trial [22]. In addition, the time elapsed from EMS arrival and successful ETI including the time interval between the arrival of the first- and second-tier vehicle and time interval for the ETI procedure, which may have enabled the SGA, could be undertaken by the first-tier team, to be placed faster. Furthermore, data on the quality of CPR such as information regarding chest compression interruption were unavailable and could thus not be included in this analysis. We also lacked information on the intubation attempts and where SGA was placed due to intubation failure.

5. Conclusions

In this sub-study of the PRINCESS trial, a shorter time period to successful airway management was observed in the SGA group when compared to ETI. No differences in clinically relevant outcomes such as survival with good neurologic outcome and overall survival were observed between groups. This study might help to design future trials using trans-nasal evaporative cooling to minimize the time to induce cooling.

Supplementary Materials: The following supporting information can be downloaded at: https://www.mdpi.com/article/10.3390/jcm11216370/s1. Figure S1: Covariate balance. Standardized mean differences before and after propensity score matching. Standardized Mean Differences (SMDs) at baseline (orange) and after propensity score matching (blue). The adjusted variables are displayed on the y-axis. SMD > 0.1 was considered to be indicative of a statistically significant group difference; Figure S2: Prehospital response times. Time from cardiac arrest to arrival of medical emergency services (EMS) and Acute life support (ALS) vehicle. The figure shows the arrival times (in minutes) of EMS and ALS for the ETI and SGA groups, respectively; Table S1: Missing data for the predictor variables (where present). Abbreviations: BMI = Body mass index in units of kg/m^2, CPR = Cardiopulmonary resuscitation, EMS = Emergency medical services; Table S2: The relationship between study endpoints and the time until the initiation of intra-arrest cooling and the time until successful airway device insertion, respectively. These results were obtained using univariate logistic regression in the unmatched dataset. Abbreviations: CPC = Cerebral Performance Category, OR = Odds ratio, CI = Confidence interval, Q1 = First quartile, Q3 = Third quartile.

Author Contributions: Conceptualization, J.T., E.D., F.S.T., A.T., S.F., J.H., M.J., L.S. and P.N.; Formal analysis, J.T. and M.J.; Funding acquisition, L.S. and P.N.; Investigation, T.H., E.D., F.S.T., A.T., S.F., J.H., M.R. and L.S.; Methodology, J.T., T.H., E.D., F.S.T., A.T., S.F., J.H., M.R., M.J., L.S. and P.N.; Resources, P.N.; Supervision, P.N.; Writing—original draft, J.T.; Writing—review & editing, T.H., E.D., F.S.T., A.T., S.F., J.H., M.R., M.J., L.S. and P.N. All authors have read and agreed to the published version of the manuscript.

Funding: Funding was provided by the Swedish Heart and Lung Foundation (Grant No. 20160637) and the Laerdal Foundation for Acute Medicine. The funders of the study had no role in the study design, data collection, analysis, or writing of the article.

Institutional Review Board Statement: Ethics and institutional committees in each participating country approved the study protocol and statistical analysis plan and the rationale and design of the trial have been published. An independent data and safety monitoring committee reviewed predefined end points at interim analyses after recruitment of 200 and 500 randomized patients.

Informed Consent Statement: The study was conducted according to the requirements of the Declaration of Helsinki. Written informed consent was obtained from the closest relative or a legal representative of each patient after hospital admission and, at a later stage, from each patient who regained mental capacity.

Data Availability Statement: The study present data from The PRINCESS randomized controlled Trial. The data are not publicly available in accordance with ethical approval and institutional regulations of patient data management.

Acknowledgments: We thank the study participants of the PRINCESS trial for making this study possible.

Conflicts of Interest: Nordberg reported grants from Swedish Heart-Lung Foundation and the Laerdal Foundation and nonfinancial support from BrainCool AB during the conduct of the study. Taccone reported personal fees from BARD outside the submitted work. Truhlar reported nonfinancial support from the Karolinska Institute during the conduct of the study. Svensson reported grants from the Swedish Heart and Lung foundation during the conduct of the study. No other disclosures were reported.

References

1. Atwood, C.; Eisenberg, M.S.; Herlitz, J.; Rea, T.D. Incidence of EMS-treated out-of-hospital cardiac arrest in Europe. *Resuscitation* **2005**, *67*, 75–80. [CrossRef] [PubMed]
2. Gräsner, J.T.; Wnent, J.; Herlitz, J.; Perkins, G.D.; Lefering, R.; Tjelmeland, I.; Koster, R.W.; Masterson, S.; Rossell-Ortiz, F.; Maurer, H.; et al. Survival after out-of-hospital cardiac arrest in Europe—Results of the EuReCa TWO study. *Resuscitation* **2020**, *148*, 218–226. [CrossRef] [PubMed]
3. Link, M.S.; Berkow, L.C.; Kudenchuk, P.J.; Halperin, H.R.; Hess, E.P.; Moitra, V.K.; Neumar, R.W.; O'Neil, B.J.; Paxton, J.H.; Silvers, S.M.; et al. Part 7: Adult advanced cardiovascular life support: 2015 American Heart Association guidelines update for cardiopulmonary resuscitation and emergency cardiovascular care. *Circulation* **2015**, *132*, S444–S464. [CrossRef] [PubMed]
4. McMullan, J.; Gerecht, R.; Bonomo, J.; Robb, R.; McNally, B.; Donnelly, J.; Wang, H.E. Airway management and out-of-hospital cardiac arrest outcome in the CARES registry. *Resuscitation* **2014**, *85*, 617–622. [CrossRef] [PubMed]
5. Stewart, R.D.; Paris, P.M.; Winter, P.M.; Pelton, G.H.; Cannon, G.M. Field endotracheal intubation by paramedical personnel. Success rates and complications. *Chest* **1984**, *85*, 341–345. [CrossRef] [PubMed]
6. Wang, H.E.; Yealy, D.M. Out-of-Hospital Endotracheal Intubation: Where Are We? *Ann. Emerg. Med.* **2006**, *47*, 532–541. [CrossRef]
7. Hasegawa, K.; Hiraide, A.; Chang, Y.; Brown, D.F.M. Association of prehospital advanced airway management with neurologic outcome and survival in patients with out-of-hospital cardiac arrest. *JAMA J. Am. Med. Assoc.* **2013**, *309*, 257–266. [CrossRef] [PubMed]
8. Wang, H.E.; Simeone, S.J.; Weaver, M.D.; Callaway, C.W. Interruptions in Cardiopulmonary Resuscitation From Paramedic Endotracheal Intubation. *Ann. Emerg. Med.* **2009**, *54*, 645–652.e1. [CrossRef] [PubMed]
9. Aufderheide, T.P.; Lurie, K.G. Death by hyperventilation: A common and life-threatening problem during cardiopulmonary resuscitation. *Crit. Care Med.* **2004**, *32*, S345–S351. [CrossRef]
10. Katz, S.H.; Falk, J.L. Misplaced endotracheal tubes by paramedics in an urban emergency medical services system. *Ann. Emerg. Med.* **2001**, *37*, 32–37. [CrossRef] [PubMed]
11. Kurola, J.; Harve, H.; Kettunen, T.; Laakso, J.P.; Gorski, J.; Paakkonen, H.; Silfvast, T. Airway management in cardiac arrest—Comparison of the laryngeal tube, tracheal intubation and bag-valve mask ventilation in emergency medical training. *Resuscitation* **2004**, *61*, 149–153. [CrossRef] [PubMed]
12. Kurz, M.C.; Prince, D.K.; Christenson, J.; Carlson, J.; Stub, D.; Cheskes, S.; Lin, S.; Aziz, M.; Austin, M.; Vaillancourt, C.; et al. Association of advanced airway device with chest compression fraction during out-of-hospital cardiopulmonary arrest. *Resuscitation* **2016**, *98*, 35–40. [CrossRef]
13. Benger, J.R.; Kirby, K.; Black, S.; Brett, S.J.; Clout, M.; Lazaroo, M.J.; Nolan, J.P.; Reeves, B.C.; Robinson, M.; Scott, L.J.; et al. Effect of a strategy of a supraglottic airway device vs tracheal intubation during out-of-hospital cardiac arrest on functional outcome the AIRWAYS-2 randomized clinical trial. *JAMA J. Am. Med. Assoc.* **2018**, *320*, 779–791. [CrossRef] [PubMed]
14. Wang, H.E.; Schmicker, R.H.; Daya, M.R.; Stephens, S.W.; Idris, A.H.; Carlson, J.N.; Riccardo Colella, M.; Herren, H.; Hansen, M.; Richmond, N.J.; et al. Effect of a strategy of initial laryngeal tube insertion vs endotracheal intubation on 72-hour survival in adults with out-of-hospital cardiac arrest a randomized clinical trial. *JAMA J. Am. Med. Assoc.* **2018**, *320*, 769–778. [CrossRef] [PubMed]
15. Benoit, J.L.; Gerecht, R.B.; Steuerwald, M.T.; McMullan, J.T. Endotracheal intubation versus supraglottic airway placement in out-of-hospital cardiac arrest: A meta-analysis. *Resuscitation* **2015**, *93*, 20–26. [CrossRef]
16. Mild Therapeutic Hypothermia to Improve the Neurologic Outcome after Cardiac Arrest. *N. Engl. J. Med.* **2002**, *346*, 549–556. [CrossRef]
17. Abella, B.S.; Zhao, D.; Alvarado, J.; Hamann, K.; Vanden Hoek, T.L.; Becker, L.B. Intra-arrest cooling improves outcomes in a murine cardiac arrest model. *Circulation* **2004**, *109*, 2786–2791. [CrossRef] [PubMed]
18. Awad, A.; Taccone, F.S.; Jonsson, M.; Forsberg, S.; Hollenberg, J.; Truhlar, A.; Ringh, M.; Abella, B.S.; Becker, L.B.; Vincent, J.-L.; et al. Time to intra-arrest therapeutic hypothermia in out-of-hospital cardiac arrest patients and its association with neurologic outcome: A propensity matched sub-analysis of the PRINCESS trial. *Intensive Care Med.* **2020**, *46*, 1361–1370. [CrossRef] [PubMed]
19. Taccone, F.S.; Hollenberg, J.; Forsberg, S.; Truhlar, A.; Jonsson, M.; Annoni, F.; Gryth, D.; Ringh, M.; Cuny, J.; Busch, H.J.; et al. Effect of intra-arrest trans-nasal evaporative cooling in out-of-hospital cardiac arrest: A pooled individual participant data analysis. *Crit. Care* **2021**, *25*, 198. [CrossRef]
20. Nordberg, P.; Taccone, F.S.; Truhlar, A.; Forsberg, S.; Hollenberg, J.; Jonsson, M.; Cuny, J.; Goldstein, P.; Vermeersch, N.; Higuet, A.; et al. Effect of Trans-Nasal Evaporative Intra-arrest Cooling on Functional Neurologic Outcome in Out-of-Hospital Cardiac Arrest: The PRINCESS Randomized Clinical Trial. *JAMA* **2019**, *321*, 1677–1685. [CrossRef]
21. Castrén, M.; Nordberg, P.; Svensson, L.; Taccone, F.; Vincent, J.L.; Desruelles, D.; Eichwede, F.; Mols, P.; Schwab, T.; Vergnion, M.; et al. Intra-arrest transnasal evaporative cooling: A randomized, prehospital, multicenter study (PRINCE: Pre-ROSC IntraNasal cooling effectiveness). *Circulation* **2010**, *122*, 729–736. [CrossRef] [PubMed]
22. Nordberg, P.; Taccone, F.S.; Castren, M.; Truhlár, A.; Desruelles, D.; Forsberg, S.; Hollenberg, J.; Vincent, J.L.; Svensoon, L. Design of the PRINCESS trial: Pre-hospital resuscitation intra-nasal cooling effectiveness survival study (PRINCESS). *BMC Emerg. Med.* **2013**, *13*, 21. [CrossRef] [PubMed]
23. Abou-Chebl, A.; Sung, G.; Barbut, D.; Torbey, M. Local brain temperature reduction through intranasal cooling with the rhinochill device: Preliminary safety data in brain-injured patients. *Stroke* **2011**, *42*, 2164–2169. [CrossRef] [PubMed]

24. Jennett, B.; Bond, M. Assessment of outcome after severe brain damage. *Lancet* **1975**, *1*, 480–484. [CrossRef]
25. van Buuren, S.; Groothuis-Oudshoorn, K. Mice: Multivariate imputation by chained equations in R. *J. Stat. Softw.* **2011**, *45*, 1–67. [CrossRef]
26. Ling, A.Y.; Montez-Rath, M.E.; Mathur, M.B.; Kapphahn, K.; Desai, M. How to apply multiple imputation in propensity score matching with partially observed confounders: A simulation study and practical recommendations. *J. Mod. Appl. Stat. Methods* **2019**, *19*, eP3439. [CrossRef]

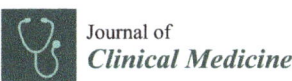

Article

Risk Factors of Sudden Cardiac Arrest during the Postoperative Period in Patient Undergoing Heart Valve Surgery

Piotr Duchnowski

Cardinal Wyszynski National Institute of Cardiology, Alpejska 42, 04-628 Warsaw, Poland; pduchnowski@ikard.pl

Abstract: Background: Sudden cardiac arrest (SCA) is the sudden cessation of normal cardiac activity with hemodynamic collapse. This usually leads to sudden cardiac death (SCD) when cardiopulmonary resuscitation is not undertaken. In patients undergoing heart valve surgery, postoperative SCA is a complication with a high risk of death, cerebral hypoxia and multiple organ dysfunction syndrome (MODS). Therefore, knowledge of the predictors of postoperative SCA is extremely important as it enables the identification of patients at risk of this complication and the application of the special surveillance and therapeutic management in this group of patients. The aim of the study was to evaluate the usefulness of selected biomarkers in predicting postoperative SCA in patients undergoing heart valve surgery. Methods: This prospective study was conducted on a group of 616 consecutive patients with significant valvular heart disease that underwent elective valve surgery with or without coronary artery bypass surgery. The primary end-point at the intra-hospital follow-up was postoperative SCA. The secondary end-point was death from all causes in patients with postoperative SCA. Patients were observed until discharge from the hospital or until death. Logistic regression was used to assess the relationships between variables. Results: The postoperative SCA occurred in 14 patients. At multivariate analysis, only NT-proBNP (odds ratio (OR) 1.022, 95% confidence interval (CI) 1.012–1.044; $p = 0.03$) remained independent predictors of the primary end-point. Age and NT-proBNP were associated with an increased risk of death in patients with postoperative SCA. Conclusions: The results of the presented study indicate that SCA in the early postoperative period in patients undergoing heart valve surgery is an unpredictable event with high mortality. The potential predictive ability of the preoperative NT-proBNP level for the occurrence of postoperative SCA and death in patients after SCA demonstrated in the study may indicate that the overloaded and damaged myocardium in patients undergoing heart valve surgery is particularly sensitive to non-physiological conditions prevailing in the perioperative period, which may cause serious hemodynamic disturbances in the postoperative period and lead to death.

Keywords: sudden cardiac arrest; N-terminal of the prohormone brain natriuretic peptide predicts postoperative (NT-proBNP); valve surgery

Citation: Duchnowski, P. Risk Factors of Sudden Cardiac Arrest during the Postoperative Period in Patient Undergoing Heart Valve Surgery. *J. Clin. Med.* **2022**, *11*, 7098. https://doi.org/10.3390/jcm11237098

Academic Editors: Nicola Cosentino, Michael Behnes, Tobias Schupp and Chirag Bavishi

Received: 20 October 2022
Accepted: 28 November 2022
Published: 30 November 2022

Publisher's Note: MDPI stays neutral with regard to jurisdictional claims in published maps and institutional affiliations.

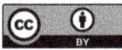

Copyright: © 2022 by the author. Licensee MDPI, Basel, Switzerland. This article is an open access article distributed under the terms and conditions of the Creative Commons Attribution (CC BY) license (https://creativecommons.org/licenses/by/4.0/).

1. Introduction

Sudden cardiac arrest (SCA) is by definition the cessation of mechanical heart function, which occurs within 1 h of the onset of new or worsening symptoms. It usually leads to sudden cardiac death (SCD) when cardiopulmonary resuscitation is not undertaken. The main recognized reasons for the occurrence of SCA are: a canalopathies and cardiomyopathies as well as myocarditis and coronary anomalies that predominate among the young. Over the age of 40, SCD is largely associated with the presence of structural diseases of the heart muscle, among which coronary heart disease predominates, in addition to valvular heart disease and heart failure [1–5]. The prediction of SCA is the philosopher's stone of arithmology. It is now known that the propensity to develop sudden cardiac arrhythmias that may lead to SCA (such as asystole, pulseless electrical activity, ventricular fibrillation or ventricular tachycardia) is associated with an unfavorable coincidence of interaction of a susceptibility substrate (e.g., genetic or acquired changes in the electrical or mechanical properties of the heart) with many temporary factors [1,2,6]. To date, the only indicator that shows a consistent relationship with an increased risk of SCA and left ventricular (LV) dysfunction is left ventricular ejection fraction (LVEF). Other new parameters of promise for SCD prediction include biochemical indices such as high-sensitivity Troponin T (hs-TnT) and the concentration of BNP, for which encouraging results were obtained in preliminary studies. The postoperative SCA in patients undergoing heart valve surgery is a complication which significantly increases the risk of hospital death as well as cerebral hypoxia and multiple organ dysfunction syndrome (MODS) [7–11]. Knowledge of the predictive factors of postoperative SCA is very important because it enables the preoperative selection of patients at risk of this complication, particular attention during the process of qualifying for interventional treatment, vigilant supervision of the patient in the perioperative period and taking an immediate response in the event of any warning symptoms. Therefore, we made an attempt to check the usefulness of selected biomarkers in predicting the occurrence of SCA in the early postoperative period in patients with heart valve disease undergoing cardiac surgery.

2. Methods

The current prospective study was performed on consecutive patients with hemodynamically significant valve defects who underwent elective replacement or repair of the valve with or without additional procedures at the Cardinal Wyszynski National Institute of Cardiology in Warsaw, Poland. Patients under 18 years of age, unwilling to participate, or diagnosed with active malignancy, autoimmune diseases, chronic inflammatory bowel disease and significant atherosclerotic lesions in the carotid arteries were excluded from the study. The day before surgery a blood sample for biomarkers was collected from each patient. Full blood counts were measured from K2EDTA samples using a Sysmex K-4500 (Sysmex, Kobe, Japan) electronic counter. The plasma levels of NT-proBNP concentrations were measured by electrochemiluminescent immunoassays Elecsys 2010 (Roche, Munich, Germany). All treatments were performed through median sternotomy under general anesthesia and normothermic conditions. Cold cardioplegia was used in each case. The primary endpoint in in-hospital follow-up is SCA during the early postoperative period, defined as cardiac arrest within one hour of the onset of acute symptoms, regardless of whether it was reversed by resuscitation. The secondary end-point was death from all causes in patients with postoperative SCA. The observation period was until discharge from hospital or death. The Institutional Ethics Committee approved the study protocol, number 1705.

3. Statistical Analysis

All analyses were performed using IBM SPSS software. The collected data are presented as mean ± SD and frequency (%). Comparisons between individual groups of variables were performed using the Mann–Whitney U test, the Pearson χ^2 test or the Student's t test. The Shapiro–Wilk normality test was used to test the sample distribution. Logistic regression was used to assess relationships between variables. The following covariates were investigated for association with the primary and secondary end-points in univariate analysis: age, aortic cross-clamp time, cardiopulmonary bypass time, atrial fibrillation, body mass index, chronic obstructive airway disease, coronary artery disease, coronary artery bypass grafting (CABG) procedure, GFR, high-sensitivity troponin T (hs-TnT), hemoglobin, left ventricular ejection fraction (LVEF), the functional class of heart failure according the New York Heart Association (NYHA classes), N-terminal of the prohormone brain natriuretic peptide (NT-proBNP), peripheral atherosclerosis, pulmonary blood pressure, tricuspid annulus plane systolic excursion (TAPSE), aortic valve replacement (AVR), mitral valve plasty (MVP), mitral valve replacement (MVR), AVR plus MVR, and postoperative major blending. Significant determinants ($p < 0.05$) identified on the basis of univariate analysis were subsequently introduced into multivariate models.

The Spearman rank correlation analysis was used to search for associations between the preoperative value of NT-proBNP level and LVEF, NYHA classes and hs-TnT.

4. Results

This study included 616 patients undergoing heart valve surgery with or without coronary artery bypass surgery. The mean (SD) age in the study population was 63 [12] years. Significantly impaired left ventricular systolic function (ejection fraction $\leq 35\%$) in the preoperative period was reported in forty-eight (8%) patients. The mean preoperative NT-proBNP level was 1993 pg/mL (standard deviation (SD) ± 1498). Table 1 shows the characteristics of the patients studied. Postoperative SCA occurred in 14 patients (during the monitoring, the ecg was found: ventricular fibrillation in six patients, ventricular tachycardia in four patients, pulseless electrical activity in one patient, and asystole in three patients). The average period from the end of surgery to the occurrence of SCA was 2 days ((SD) ± 1.5). In each case of SCA, cardiopulmonary resuscitation was used, which resulted in the restoration of a hemodynamically stable heart rhythm in 10 patients (among which two patients required permanent pacemaker implantation). In four cases, death occurred despite resuscitation. In a further follow-up with 10 patients who survived SCA, five patients died due to progressive MODS. The statistically significant predictors of postoperative sudden cardiac arrest at univariate and multivariate analyses are presented in Table 2. At multivariate analysis, only NT-proBNP (odds ratio (OR) 1.022; 95% confidence interval (CI) 1.012–1.044; $p = 0.03$) remained an independent predictor of the primary endpoint. In the group of patients with SCA, the mean LVEF value was 52% (±14%) and was significantly lower compared to patients with no SCA 58% (±12%) ($p < 0.05$). Moreover, the mean preoperative value of NT-proBNP in patients with SCA was 5346 pg/mL (±3582) and was significantly higher compared to patients with no SCA 1910 pg/mL (±1398) ($p < 0.05$). A significant correlation was found between the level of preoperative NT-proBNP and pre-operative LVEF ($r = -0.39$; $p < 0.001$), level of hs-TnT ($r = 0.38$; $p < 0.001$) and NYHA classes ($r = 0.41$, $p < 0.001$). A secondary end-point occurred in nine patients (1.5% of total patients). Statistically significant predictors of death from all causes in patients with postoperative SCA at univariate analysis were NT-proBNP (OR 1.021; 95% CI: 1.011–1.022; $p = 0.001$) and age (OR 1.086; 95% CI 1.002–1.176; $p = 0.04$) (multivariate analysis was not performed due to an insufficient number of events) (Table 3). The mean NT-proBNP value in the group with postoperative SCA who died was 6978 pg/mL (±3582) and was significantly higher compared to patients with SCA who survived 2410 pg/mL (±943) ($p < 0.05$). The total in-hospital mortality was 3.7%.

Ninety-eight patients (16% of the total group with severe valvular disease) had concomitant coronary artery disease. Of these, 95 patients (15% of the entire group) underwent an additional coronary artery bypass procedure. Importantly, however, no significantly higher NT-proBNP concentration was found in patients with concomitant coronary artery disease ($p = 0.30$) and in patients who underwent additional coronary artery bypass grafting ($p = 0.33$) compared to the remaining group of 518 patients with severe valvular heart without coexisting coronary artery disease. Among the 98 patients with severe valvular heart disease and concomitant coronary artery disease undergoing cardiac surgery, 3 patients experienced sudden cardiac arrest in the early postoperative period. In the univariate logistic regression analysis, both the coexistence of coronary artery disease ($p = 0.29$) and the additional coronary artery bypass procedure ($p = 0.12$) in patients undergoing heart valve surgery were not predictors of sudden cardiac arrest in the early postoperative period.

Table 1. Baseline characteristics of the study population.

Preoperative Characteristics of Patients (n = 616)	Values
Age, years *	63 ± 12
Atrial fibrillation, n (%)	268 (43%)
Coronary artery disease, n (%)	98 (15%)
Chronic kidney disease (GFR < 60 mL/min/1.73 m^2), n (%)	196 (31%)
Creatinine, mg/dL *	0.8 ± 0.5
Hemoglobin, g/dL *	13.7 ± 1.4
LV ejection fraction, (%) *	57 ± 12
Male: men, n (%)	355 (58%)
NYHA, (classes) *	2.6 ± 0.6
Hs-TnT, ng/L *	26 ± 21
Nt-proBNP, pg/mL *	1993 ± 1498
Intraoperative and postoperative characteristics of patients	Values
Aortic cross-clamp time, min *	101 ± 41
Cardiopulmonary bypass time, min *	132 ± 53
The day of sudden cardiac arrest, days *	2 ± 1.5
Postoperative major blending, n (%)	45 (7%)
Main procedures:	
AVR, n (%)	319 (52%)
AVR + MVR, n (%)	54 (9%)
AVP, n (%)	17 (3%)
MVR, n (%)	111 (18%)
MVP, n (%)	115 (18%)
Concomitant procedures:	
CABG, n (%)	95 (15%)
TVP, n (%)	115 (18%)

Values are represented by the mean * and a measure of the variation of the internal standard deviation. Abbreviations: AVP = aortic valve plasty; AVR = aortic valve replacement; CABG = coronary artery bypass grafting; MVP = mitral valve plasty; MVR = mitral valve replacement; GFR = glomerular filtration rate; LV = left ventricle; NYHA = New York Heart Association; TVP = tricuspid valve plasty.

Table 2. Analysis of predictive factors for the occurrence of postoperative sudden cardiac arrest.

	Univariable			Multivariable		
Variable	Odds Ratio	95% Cl	p-Value	Odds Ratio	95% Cl	p-Value
Nt-proBNP, pg/mL	1.026	1.009–1.046	0.003	1.022	1.012–1.044	0.03
NYHA, classes	3.255	1.254–8.454	0.01			

Abbreviations: Nt-proBNP = N-terminal of the prohormone brain natriuretic peptide, NYHA = New York Heart Association. Univariate analysis followed by multivariate regression analysis was performed.

Table 3. Univariate analysis of predictive factors for the occurrence of death in patients with SCA.

Variable	Odds Ratio	95% Cl	p-Value
Nt-proBNP, pg/mL	1.021	1.011–1.022	0.003
Age, years	1.086	1.002–1.176	0.04

Abbreviation: Nt-proBNP = N-terminal of the prohormone brain natriuretic peptide. Multivariate analysis was not performed due to insufficient number of events.

5. Discussion

The occurrence of SCA in the early postoperative period in patients undergoing heart valve surgery is a critical event. The alertness of the medical staff and the reaction time can be decisive in reversing the further fate of the patient. Additionally, the presence of a postoperative wound poses a major challenge for the team undertaking resuscitation in saving the patient's life. Therefore, the knowledge of predictive factors for SCA in the early postoperative period in this group of patients gives the patient a chance to survive through the special surveillance of patients in the critical postoperative period and early response in the event of predictive symptoms [12,13].

Arrhythmias are a fairly common complication occurring in the early postoperative period in patients undergoing cardiac surgery. The most common arrhythmia in this group of patients is postoperative atrial fibrillation. In turn, sustained ventricular tachycardia and ventricular fibrillation (main direct mechanism of occurrence of postoperative SCA) are quite rare and, ranging from 0.7% to 3.1% according to various investigators, and are associated with a high risk of death [3,14–19]. In the present study, SCA occurred in 14 patients, which is approximately 2% of patients undergoing heart valve surgery. Of the 14 patients who experienced SCA, in-hospital death was observed in nine patients.

The present study showed that the preoperative NT-proBNP level may be a potential predictor of SCA and death in the early postoperative period in patients undergoing heart valve surgery. Due to the fact that the active form of BNP is involved in maintaining the homeostasis of the cardiovascular system, NT-proBNP is currently widely used in the diagnosis, assessment of progression, and the degree of myocardial damage. NT-proBNP is mainly released by left ventricular cardiomyocytes in response to myocardial tone and increased intravascular volume. In severe valvular heart disease, there is a significant pressure and/or volume overload of the left ventricular muscle, which leads to an increase in NT-proBNP release from cardiomyocytes. However, long-lasting overload of the heart muscle, may be the cause of a progressive degenerative process associated with slow cardiomyocyte necrosis and the occurrence of fibrosis [20–31]. Very high NT-proBNP values present in the blood serum of patients with severe valvular heart disease may indicate significant damage to the overloaded left ventricular muscle, which may be confirmed by the significant correlation shown in the study between the preoperative NT-proBNP concentration and the NYHA class, preoperative hs-TnT level and left ventricular systolic function assessed using LVEF. The potential predictive ability of NT-proBNP levels for the primary and secondary endpoints demonstrated in the study may indicate that the overloaded and damaged myocardium in a patient undergoing heart valve surgery is particularly sensitive to non-physiological conditions during cardiac surgery on cardiac arrest. It seems that the conditions prevailing during extracorporeal circulation may favor further myocardial damage and contribute to the occurrence of electrical disturbances underlying mechanical cardiac arrest. The above thesis may be confirmed by the results of previously published studies, which showed a significant correlation between aortic cross-clamp time and cardiopulmonary bypass time with the postoperative high-sensitivity Troponin T level [3,32–34]. In addition, the presence of electrolyte disturbances, such as hypokalemia and hypomagnesaemia, metabolic acidosis, decrease in hemoglobin level, or increased supply of sympathomimetics in the early postoperative period may be a direct factor causing dangerous ventricular arrhythmia in the myocardium damaged by long-term valvular heart disease [15].

It is worth mentioning that out of 616 patients who underwent surgical treatment of valvular heart disease, 98 patients had significant atherosclerotic changes in the coronary arteries and 95 underwent coronary artery bypass grafting at the same time. However, the statistical analysis performed showed that the coexistence of significant stenosis in the coronary arteries does not increase the risk of sudden cardiac arrest in the early postoperative period.

Additionally, although the results of the presented study indicate that the preoperative level of NT-proBNP may be a potential predictor of SCA and death in patients with previous SCA in the early postoperative period, the essence of the above study is the fact that SCA is an unpredictable event with a high risk of death. Both the previously presented studies and the above results indicate a significant problem of preoperative myocardial damage resulting from the long-term impact of severe valvular defects/defects on the heart muscle and thus the possibility of serious events in the postoperative period, including hemodynamic instability, shock, and the possibility of SCA and death in the early postoperative period [3,22,35]. Therefore, the group of patients with severe heart valve disease and very high NT-proBNP values requires special attention and professionalism during surgery and in the postoperative period, including intensive medical supervision and ECG monitoring. In addition, the study results may also suggest that earlier qualification for surgery with less advanced myocardial damage and lower NT-proBNP, or qualification for less burdensome procedures such as TAVI or percutaneous valve repair, may be associated with a reduction in the incidence of severe postoperative complications and death.

6. Conclusions

The results of the presented study indicate that SCA in the early postoperative period in patients undergoing heart valve surgery is an unpredictable event with high mortality. The potential predictive ability of the preoperative NT-proBNP level for the occurrence of postoperative SCA and death in patients after SCA demonstrated in the study may indicate that the overloaded and damaged myocardium in a patient undergoing heart valve surgery is particularly sensitive to the non-physiological conditions prevailing in the perioperative period, which may cause serious hemodynamic disturbances in the postoperative period, and consequently, may be the cause of death. In future studies, enlarging the group may enable confirming the obtained results. In addition, the extension of the study will also enable confirming whether the coexistence of ischemic heart disease is conducive to sudden cardiac arrest in the early postoperative period. Knowledge of the predictors of postoperative complications is extremely important because it allows the implementation of an appropriate perioperative strategy, which in turn can improve treatment outcomes in patients with valvular heart disease.

Funding: This research received no external funding.

Institutional Review Board Statement: The study was conducted in accordance with the Declaration of Helsinki, and approved by Institutional Ethics Committee of the Institute of Cardiology, Warsaw, Poland (number 1705).

Informed Consent Statement: Informed consent was obtained from all subjects involved in the study.

Data Availability Statement: Research data available from the author of the publication.

Conflicts of Interest: The author declares no conflict of interest.

References

1. Zeppenfeld, K.; Tfelt-Hansen, J.; de Riva, M.; Gregers Winkel, B.; Behr, E.R.; Blom, N.A.; Charron, P.; Corrado, D.; Dagres, N.; de Chilou, C.; et al. ESC Guidelines for the management of patients with ventricular arrhythmias and the prevention of sudden cardiac death: Developed by the task force for the management of patients with ventricular arrhythmias and the prevention of sudden cardiac death of the European Society of Cardiology (ESC) Endorsed by the Association for European Paediatric and Congenital Cardiology (AEPC). *Eur. Heart J.* **2022**, *43*, 3997–4126. [PubMed]
2. Priori, S.; Blomström-Lundqvist, C.; Mazzanti, A.; Blom, N.; Borggrefe, M.; Camm, J.; Elliot, P.M.; Fitzsimons, D.; Hatala, R.; Hindricks, G.; et al. The Task Force for the Management of Patients with Ventricular Arrhythmias and the Prevention of Sudden Cardiac Death of the European Society of Cardiology (ESC) Endorsed by: Association for European Paediatric and Congenital Cardiology (AEPC). *Eur. Heart J.* **2015**, *36*, 2793–2867. [CrossRef] [PubMed]
3. Duchnowski, P.; Hryniewiecki, T.; Kuśmierczyk, M.; Szymański, P. Postoperative high-sensitivity troponin T as a predictor of sudden cardiac arrest in patients undergoing cardiac surgery. *Cardiol. J.* **2019**, *26*, 777–781. [CrossRef]
4. Eckart, R.E.; Shry, E.A.; Burke, A.P.; McNear, J.A.; Appel, D.A.; Castillo-Rojas, L.M.; Avedissian, L.; Pearse, L.A.; Potter, R.N.; Tremaine, L.; et al. Sudden death in young adults: An autopsy-based series of a population undergoing active surveillance. *J. Am. Coll. Cardiol.* **2011**, *58*, 1254–1261. [CrossRef]
5. Van Camp, S.P.; Bloor, C.M.; Mueller, F.O.; Cantu, R.C.; Olson, H.G. Nontraumatic sports death in high school and college athletes. *Med. Sci. Sport. Exerc.* **1995**, *27*, 641–647. [CrossRef]
6. Myerburg, R.J.; Kessler, K.M.; Castellanos, A. Sudden cardiac death. Structure, function, and time-dependence of risk. *Circulation* **1992**, *85*, 2–10.
7. Scott, P.A.; Barry, J.; Roberts, P.R.; Morgan, J.M. Brain natriuretic peptide for the prediction of sudden cardiac death and ventricular arrhythmias: A meta-analysis. *Eur. J. Heart Fail.* **2009**, *11*, 958–966. [CrossRef] [PubMed]
8. Levine, Y.C.; Rosenberg, M.A.; Mittleman, M.; Samuel, M.; Methachittiphan, N.; Link, M.; Josephon, M.E.; Buxton, A.E. B-type natriuretic peptide is a major predictor of ventricular tachyarrhythmias. *Heart Rhythm.* **2014**, *11*, 1109–1116. [CrossRef] [PubMed]
9. Zipes, D.P.; Wellens, H.J. Sudden cardiac death. *Circulation* **1998**, *98*, 2334–2351. [CrossRef] [PubMed]
10. Drory, Y.; Turetz, Y.; Hiss, Y.; Lev, B.; Fisman, E.Z.; Pines, A.; Kramer, M.R. Sudden unexpected death in persons less than 40 years of age. *Am. J. Cardiol.* **1991**, *68*, 1388–1392. [CrossRef] [PubMed]

11. Maisel, A.; Mueller, C.; Adams, K., Jr.; Anker, S.D.; Aspromonte, N.; Cleland, J.G.F.; Cohen-Solal, A.; Dahlstrom, U.; DeMaria, A.; Di Somma, S.; et al. State of the art: Using natriuretic peptide levels in clinical practice. *Eur. J. Heart Fail.* **2008**, *10*, 824–839. [CrossRef] [PubMed]
12. Carvajal-Zarrabal, O.; Hayward-Jones, P.M.; Nolasco-Hipolito, C.; Barradas-Dermitz, D.M.; Calderón-Garcidueñas, A.L.; López-Amador, N. Use of cardiac injury markers in the postmortem diagnosis of sudden cardiac death. *J. Forensic Sci.* **2017**, *62*, 1332–1335. [CrossRef] [PubMed]
13. Rahimi, R.; Dahili, N.D.; Anuar Zainun, K.; Mohd Kasim, N.A.; Md Noor, S. Post mortem troponin T analysis in sudden death: Is it useful? *Malays. J. Pathol.* **2018**, *40*, 143–148. [PubMed]
14. Urena, M.; Webb, J.G.; Eltchaninoff, H.; Muñoz-García, A.J.; Bouleti, C.; Tamburino, C.; Nombela-Franco, L.; Nietlispach, F.; Moris, C.; Ruel, M.; et al. Late cardiac death in patients undergoing transcatheter aortic valve replacement: Incidence and predictors of advanced heart failure and sudden cardiac death. *J. Am. Coll. Cardiol.* **2015**, *65*, 437–448. [CrossRef]
15. Rho, R.W.; Bridges, C.R.; Kocovic, D. Management of postoperative arrhythmias. *Semin. Thorac. Cardiovasc. Surg.* **2000**, *12*, 349–361. [CrossRef] [PubMed]
16. Gottipatty, V.; Kocovic, D.; Kinchla, N.; Couper, G.; Friedman, P.L. Timing and impact of survival of in-hospital cardiac arrest after coronary artery bypass graft surgery (abstr.) *Circulation* **1993**, *88*, 1–166.
17. Topol, E.J.; Lerman, B.B.; Baughman, K.L.; Platia, E.V.; Griffith, L.S. De novo refrectory ventricular tachyarrhythmias after coronary revascularization. *Am. J. Cardiol.* **1986**, *57*, 57–59. [CrossRef] [PubMed]
18. Kron, I.L.; DiMarco, P.J.; Harman, P.K.; Crosby, I.K.; Mentzer, R.M., Jr.; Nolan, S.P.; Wellons, H.A., Jr. Unanticipated postoperative ventricular tachyarrhythmias. *Ann. Thorac. Surg.* **1984**, *38*, 317–322. [CrossRef] [PubMed]
19. Steinberg, J.S.; Gaur, A.; Sciacca, R.; Tan, E. New-onset Sustained ventricular tachycardia after cardiac surgery. *Circulation* **1999**, *99*, 903–908. [CrossRef] [PubMed]
20. Roberts, E.; Ludman, A.J.; Dworzynski, K.; Al-Mohammad, A.; Cowie, M.R.; McMurray, J.J.V.; Mant, J.; NICE Guideline Development Group for Acute Heart Failure. The diagnostic accuracy of the natriuretic peptides in heart failure: Systematic review and diagnostic meta-analysis in the acute care setting. *BMJ* **2015**, *350*, h910. [CrossRef] [PubMed]
21. Sezai, A.; Shiono, M. Natriuretic peptides for perioperative management of cardiac surgery. *J. Cardiol.* **2016**, *67*, 15–21. [CrossRef] [PubMed]
22. Duchnowski, P. N-Terminal of the Prohormone Brain Natriuretic Peptide Predicts Postoperative Cardiogenic Shock Requiring Extracorporeal Membrane Oxygenation. *J. Clin. Med.* **2022**, *11*, 5493. [CrossRef] [PubMed]
23. Jiang, H.; Vánky, F.; Hultkvist, H.; Holm, J.; Yang, Y.; Svedjeholm, R. NT-proBNP and postoperative heart failure in surgery for aortic stenosis. *Open Heart* **2019**, *6*, e001063. [CrossRef] [PubMed]
24. Zaphiriou, A.; Robb, S.; Murray-Thomas, T.; Mendez, G.; Fox, K.; McDonagh, T.; Hardman, S.M.C.; Dargie, H.J.; Cowie, M.R. The diagnostic accuracy of plasma BNP and NTproBNP in patients referred from primary care with suspected heart failure: Results of the UK natriuretic peptide study. *Eur. J. Heart Fail.* **2005**, *7*, 537–541. [CrossRef] [PubMed]
25. Chin, C.; Shah, A.S.; McAllister, D.; Cowell, S.J.; Alam, S.; Langrish, J.P.; Strachan, F.E.; Hunter, A.L.; Choy, A.M.; Lang, C.C.; et al. High-sensitivity troponin I concentrations are a marker of an advanced hypertrophic response and adverse outcomes in patients with aortic stenosis. *Eur. Heart J.* **2014**, *35*, 2312–2321. [CrossRef] [PubMed]
26. Weidemann, F.; Hermann, S.; Störk, S.; Niemann, M.; Frantz, S.; Lange, V.; Beer, M.; Gattenlöhner, S.; Voelker, W.; Ertl, G.; et al. Impact of myocardial fibrosis in patients with symptomatic severe aortic stenosis. *Circulation* **2009**, *120*, 577–584. [CrossRef] [PubMed]
27. Ponikowski, P.; Voors, A.; Anker, S.; Bueno, H.; Cleland, J.G.F.; Coats, A.J.S.; González-Juanatey, J.R.; Harjola, V.-P.; Jankowska, E.A.; Jessup, M.; et al. 2016 ESC guidelines for the diagnosis and treatment of acute and chronic heart failure: The taskforce for the diagnosis and treatment of acute and chronic heart failure of the European Society of Cardiology (ESC) Developed with thespecial contribution of the Heart Failure Association (HFA) of the ESC. *Eur. Heart J.* **2016**, *37*, 2129–2200. [PubMed]
28. van Peet, P.G.; de Craen, A.J.; Gussekloo, J.; de Ruijter, W. Plasma NT-proBNP as predictor of change in functional status, cardiovascular morbidity and mortality in the oldest old. Leiden 85-plus study. *Age* **2014**, *36*, 9660. [CrossRef]
29. Filsoufi, F.; Rahmanian, P.B.; Salzberg, S.; von Harbou, K.; Bodian, C.A.; Adams, D.H. B-type natriuretic peptide (BNP) in patients undergoingmitral valve surgery. *J. Card. Surg.* **2008**, *23*, 600–605. [CrossRef] [PubMed]
30. Georges, A.; Forestier, F.; Valli, N.; Plogin, A.; Janvier, G.; Bordenave, L. Changes in type B natriuretic peptide (BNP) concentrations during cardiac valve replacement. *Eur. J. Cardio-Thorac. Surg.* **2004**, *25*, 941–945. [CrossRef] [PubMed]
31. Perreas, K.; Samanidis, G.; Dimitriou, S.; Athanasiou, A.; Balanika, M.; Smirli, A.; Antzaka, C.; Politis, K.; Khoury, M.; Michalis, A. NT-proBNP in the mitral valve surgery. *Crit. Pathw. Cardiol.* **2014**, *13*, 55–61. [CrossRef] [PubMed]
32. Reichlin, T.; Schindler, C.; Drexler, B.; Twerenbold, R.; Reiter, M.; Zellweger, C.; Moehring, B.; Ziller, R.; Hoeller, R.; Gimenez, M.R.; et al. One-hour rule-out and rule-in of acute myocardial infarction using high-sensitivity cardiac troponin T. *Arch. Intern. Med.* **2012**, *172*, 1211–1218. [CrossRef] [PubMed]
33. Abramov, D.; Abu-Tailakh, M.; Frieger, M.; Ganiel, A.; Tuvbin, D.; Wolak, A. Plasma troponin levels after cardiac surgery vs. after myocardial infarction. *Asian Cardiovasc. Thorac. Ann.* **2006**, *14*, 530–535. [CrossRef] [PubMed]

34. Opfermann, U.T.; Peivandi, A.A.; Dahm, M.; Hilgenstock, H.; Hafner, G.; Loos, A.; Oelert, H. Postoperative patterns and kinetics of cTnI, cTnT, CK-MB-activity and CK-activity after elective aortic valve replacement. *Swiss Med. Wkly.* **2001**, *131*, 550–555.
35. Duchnowski, P.; Hryniewiecki, T.; Kuśmierczyk, M.; Szymanski, P. N-terminal of the prohormone brain natriuretic peptide is a predictor of hemodynamic instability in valve disease. *Biomark. Med.* **2019**, *13*, 353–358. [CrossRef]

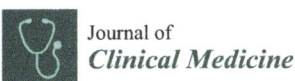

Review

Advanced and Invasive Cardiopulmonary Resuscitation (CPR) Techniques as an Adjunct to Advanced Cardiac Life Support

Manuel Obermaier *, Stephan Katzenschlager, Othmar Kofler, Frank Weilbacher and Erik Popp

Department of Anaesthesiology, Heidelberg University Hospital, 69120 Heidelberg, Germany
* Correspondence: manuel.obermaier@med.uni-heidelberg.de; Tel.: +49-6221-56-36529

Abstract: Background: Despite numerous promising innovations, the chance of survival from sudden cardiac arrest has remained virtually unchanged for decades. Recently, technological advances have been made, user-friendly portable devices have been developed, and advanced invasive procedures have been described that could improve this unsatisfactory situation. Methods: A selective literature search in the core databases with a focus on randomized controlled trials and guidelines. Results: Technical aids, such as feedback systems or automated mechanical cardiopulmonary resuscitation (CPR) devices, can improve chest compression quality. The latter, as well as extracorporeal CPR, might serve as a bridge to treatment (with extracorporeal CPR even as a bridge to recovery). Sonography may be used to improve thoracic compressions on the one hand and to rule out potentially reversible causes of cardiac arrest on the other. Resuscitative endovascular balloon occlusion of the aorta might enhance myocardial and cerebral perfusion. Minithoracostomy, pericardiocentesis, or clamshell thoracotomy might resolve reversible causes of cardiac arrest. Conclusions: It is crucial to identify those patients who may benefit from an advanced or invasive procedure and make the decision to implement the intervention in a timely manner. As with all infrequently performed procedures, sound education and regular training are paramount.

Keywords: cardiac arrest; sudden cardiac death; emergency treatment; invasive procedures; heart massage; circulation; clamshell thoracotomy; extra-corporeal membrane oxygenation; echocardiography; resuscitative endovascular balloon occlusion of the aorta

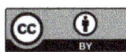

1. Introduction

The cornerstones of cardiopulmonary resuscitation (CPR) as we know it today have been laid in 1960 through the revolutionary principle of closed-chest cardiac massage introduced by Kouwenhoven, Jude, and Knickerbocker [1], and the pioneering works on artificial respiration by Safar [2]. Six decades later, and despite major efforts in research and all advancements in technology, little has changed in the poor prognosis of patients suffering sudden cardiac arrest [3].

In order to remedy this highly unsatisfactory situation, clinician scientists worldwide strive to enhance treatment and markedly improve survival. Some of these supposedly revolutionary treatment approaches had to be abandoned again due to lack of efficacy [4], while others are now an integral part of the international guidelines concerning CPR [5]. In addition to various educational concepts and abundant awareness campaigns which address the broad public [6], some most recent developments concerning advanced therapeutic options focus on hyperinvasive strategies and approaches [7]. It is recognized that maintaining blood pressure targets during cardiac arrest and, after the return of spontaneous circulation (ROSC), affects survival rates [8,9]. As Brede concisely determines in a current editorial, each "long term survival" is preceded by a ROSC and, therefore, "all potential adjunct treatments to increase the rate of ROSC should be assessed" [10].

In cases where ROSC cannot be achieved immediately, chest compression continuity and its quality are key determinants for survival in cardiac arrest [11,12]. Conventional manual chest compressions are demanding, leading to increased interruptions [13], and are insufficiently performed [14] due to rescuers' exhaustion. Subsequently, no- and low-flow times are increasing which affects the hemodynamic situation [15]. This is considered a main determinant that prevents ROSC and, subsequently, survival due to impaired myocardial and brain perfusion [16,17].

There are several advanced and invasive techniques readily available in hospital emergency departments, which seem to stay unused in the out-of-hospital emergency setting. Consequently, in a new approach, the attempt is made to bring these techniques, devices, and qualified personnel who routinely apply these techniques in an in-hospital cardiac arrest (IHCA) setting to patients suffering an out-of-hospital cardiac arrest (OHCA) [18,19].

We aim to provide a narrative overview of currently discussed advanced principles and invasive techniques as adjuncts to advanced life support (ALS).

2. Methods

We conduct a selective literature search in established scientific databases as well as preprint servers, clinical trials registry platforms (Tables S1 and S2), and internet search engines for publications with a focus on randomized controlled trials (RCT), recommendations from scientific societies and official guidelines concerning advanced and invasive technical therapeutic options in the treatment of cardiac arrest.

We define those resuscitation techniques as "advanced and invasive" that go beyond routine application under the "standard" ALS algorithm.

3. Results and Discussion of Advanced and Invasive Techniques

As with any complex and seldomly utilized technique, situation awareness, sound education, and continuous training in technical and non-technical skills are paramount. The basis for all advanced resuscitation measures is the uninterrupted and effective basic resuscitation that has been started as quickly as possible [6,11]. This is crucial for patient survival and often advanced and invasive techniques are not useful unless lay resuscitation has taken place [5,20]. Consequently, every person working in the medical field should regularly participate in CPR training courses according to his or her qualifications.

There is a broad array of courses offered for learning and training in advanced invasive procedures that go beyond the "standard" ALS, as well as sonography and non-technical skills, such as crisis resource management [21–23]. In addition, cognitive aids can help to work through complex situations in a structured way [24]. It must be emphasized that all trials discussed in this work refer to well-trained and experienced experts in specialized centers. This level cannot usually be achieved by attending courses alone, but also requires regular work in a center with a correspondingly high number of cases.

3.1. Real-Time Audio or Audiovisual CPR Feedback Devices

Considerations that poor CPR quality with frequent interruptions may entail low survival rates [25,26], as previously stated, led to the development of feedback devices that are designed to measure important CPR quality parameters (i.e., compression depth, relief, frequency, and hands-off time) and give real-time audio (clickers for tactile feedback) or audiovisual feedback. This enables life support providers to continuously monitor and, when appropriate, to self-adjust their external chest compressions in real-time. Furthermore, most systems allow the users to retrospectively analyze the performance for educational purposes. Therefore, real-time feedback devices are expected to improve CPR quality and possibly patient survival [27].

This review focuses on audio or audiovisual feedback devices but does neither address functions such as metronome sound, which occasionally are referred to as feedback devices [11], nor software applications for mobile communication devices.

Several trials report partially contradictory or ambivalent results concerning the effect of real-time feedback systems on CPR quality and patient outcome (Table 1) [27,28]. In addition to several observational studies, mainly from simulated training scenarios, only two RCTs could be identified. An individualized RCT and its secondary analysis evaluating an audio-only feedback device in a hospital setting found better adherence to resuscitation guidelines, as well as significantly higher rates of ROSC and survival until intensive care unit (ICU) and hospital discharge [29,30]. A large cluster RCT evaluating an audiovisual device in an out-of-hospital setting confirms the findings regarding improved CPR quality, but this was not associated with improved survival rates [31]. This result calls into question the previously assumed clinical relevance of improved chest compressions.

Table 1. Overview of RCTs on real-time audio or audiovisual CPR feedback systems vs. conventional manual chest compression.

Trial Abbreviation and Quotation	Design and Inclusion Criteria	Main Findings and Limitations
Compression Feedback for Patients with In-hospital Cardiac Arrest [29]	Cardio First Angel® vs. conventional manual CPR; prospective individualized RCT, multi-center (Iran); in-hospital; 2015; 450 vs. 450 cases out of 1454 Inclusion criteria: age $\geq$ 18 years, admitted to ICU, resuscitation status (full code), and informed consent	↑ ROSC, ↑ ICU discharge, ↑ hospital discharge Limitations: selection bias (no primary cardiac entity), performance bias (quality monitoring), and training effect
Automated Real-time Feedback on CPR Study [31]	HeartStart-MRx® vs. conventional manual CPR; prospective cluster RCT, multi-center (USA, Canada); out-of-hospital; 2007–2009; 815 vs. 771 cases out of 1819 Inclusion criteria: age $\geq$ 20, defibrillation or chest compressions by study vehicle team and non-TCA	↑ hands-on time, ↑ compression depth, ↑ complete release, ± ROSC, ± admission, ± discharge, ± CPC Limitations: design (allocation concealment and no regression analysis), selection bias (trial vehicle), and training effect

Legend: ± = equal, comparable, and no statistically significant difference; ↑ = more, higher, better, and superior; ↓ = less, lower, worse, and inferior. Abbreviations: RCT = randomized controlled trial, CPR = cardiopulmonary resuscitation, ICU = intensive care unit, ROSC = return of spontaneous circulation, CPC = Glasgow–Pittsburgh cerebral performance category, and TCA = traumatic cardiac arrest.

There seems to be sufficient objective evidence that the application of real-time audio or audiovisual feedback devices contributes to an improvement of chest compression quality and continuity, as laid down in resuscitation guidelines. In order to either confirm or refute the hypothesis that improved chest compressions actually lead to higher survival rates with favorable neurological outcomes, further well-designed, sufficiently powered, and properly conducted studies are necessary.

Nevertheless, currently, valid guidelines recommend the use of real-time audiovisual feedback devices in order to improve CPR quality as a part of a comprehensive quality improvement program [11,32].

3.2. Automated Mechanical CPR (mCPR)

Whilst feedback devices might contribute to improving chest compression quality, they cannot resolve the problem of increasing exhaustion of staff members during prolonged CPR attempts or the impaired quality of chest compression in certain situations (i.e., on transport). Automated mCPR devices have been developed for this purpose and perform consistent chest compressions, either by a semi-circumferential load-distributing band or a vertical piston. It is a matter of in-depth discussion on whether their application might improve patient survival rates (Table 2).

3.2.1. Rationale

A large RCT, the ASPIRE trial was terminated prematurely by the data and safety monitoring board, after there was—despite similar survival rates at 4 h after the incident—a trend to impaired survival until hospital discharge and neurologic state [33]. Despite slightly distinctive definitions of ROSC, none of the other studies revealed any statistically significant different rates of ROSC at any time or sustaining ROSC until hospital admission, respectively. The CIRC trial, an RCT that compares an automated mCPR device utilizing a load-distributing band to conventional manual CPR, found a slightly diminished rate of sustaining ROSC (odds ratio (OR) 0.84, 95% confidence interval (CI) 0.73–0.96) and survival after 24 h (OR 0.86, 95% CI 0.74–0.998) in the mCPR group. This observation is recouped during the stay in the hospital, as the rate of survival until hospital discharge (OR 0.89, 95% CI 0.72–1.10) and neurologic state at discharge according to the modified Rankin Scale (mRS) (OR 0.80, 95% CI 0.47–1.37) do not show any statistically significant differences [34]. Two other well-conducted multi-center RCTs, the LINC trial [35] and the PARAMEDIC trial [36], found equal survival rates until hospital discharge. In the latter, this was associated with a slightly but significantly worse neurologic outcome in the intervention group receiving automated mechanical chest compressions through a vertical piston device. Adjusted OR for the risk of favorable neurologic outcome (defined as CPC 1–2) was 0.72 (95% CI 0.52–0.99) [36]. Apart from these exceptions, no statistically significant differences in survival rates and neurological outcomes were observed in any of the large RCTs [34–37]. In the as-treated analysis, the MECCA investigators found improved survival rates compared to conventional manual CPR, if the automated mCPR device utilizing a vertical piston was attached "early" during the course, viz., before moving the patient to the ambulance [37]. In all these studies, it is of key importance to consider that the results and, thereby, the conclusions of superiority or inferiority of any technique mainly depend on the quality of conventional manual CPR delivered in the respective control groups [38,39].

3.2.2. Significance of the Time Aspect

The observations regarding the importance of time correspond with observations from a retrospective registry analysis, where a higher rate of ROSC was found in the mechanical CPR groups, which is mainly attributable to lower risk factors among the population within this group. Compared with the predicted rate of ROSC (the ROSC after cardiac arrest (RACA) score), patients in the load-distributing band group achieved ROSC significantly more frequently (predicted 46.6%; achieved 57.1%, 95% CI 49.5–64.5%), while patients in the mechanical piston group (predicted 43.4%; achieved 46.5%, 95% CI 38.4–54.7%) and manual CPR group (predicted 39.9%; achieved 40.1%; 95% CI 39.2–41.1) only fulfilled the predicted outcome. Adjusted for epidemiologic and therapeutic factors, OR for ROSC was 1.70 (95% CI 1.12–2.57) for the load-distributing band system and 1.66 (95% CI 1.09–2.51) for the mechanical piston system [40]. On the contrary, in a pilot study, which neither excluded resuscitations shorter than 5 min nor considered CPR duration in its regression analysis, we found an OR for ROSC of 0.82 (95% CI 0.64–1.07) for the load-distributing band system and 0.48 (95% CI 0.36–0.64) for the mechanical piston system [41]. This is consistent with a secondary analysis of the CIRC trial utilizing a logistic regression analysis that identified an increased probability for survival until hospital discharge after automated mCPR (OR 1.46; 95% CI 1.03–2.07) if adjusted for emergency medical service (EMS) response time [42]. In the original publication of the CIRC trial, response times > 16 min have been excluded [34]. A longitudinal, phased cohort study from Singapore shows a higher rate of survival until hospital discharge in the load-distributing band mCPR group (8.1% vs. 1.9% in the manual CPR group) if the EMS response time was < 8 min. If response times were > 8 min, only a few patients survived in both groups [43].

The installation of automated mCPR devices may delay the time until the first defibrillation, depending on which source is consulted, for a period of up to 2.1 min [33–35,38]. A Cochrane review suggests that these negative impacts on CPR quality, namely lag-times until the application of the device with increased hands-off time and delay of the first defibrillation in shockable rhythms, may negate "any physiologic benefit observed in preclinical studies" [39]. Nevertheless, defibrillation is feasible and safe during ongoing automated mechanical chest compressions and, thereby, reduces the hands-off time during the later course [5,35].

Table 2. Overview of selected studies on automated mechanical vs. conventional manual chest compression.

Trial Abbreviation and Quotation	Design and Inclusion Criteria	Main Findings and Limitations
(a) RCTs on automated mCPR vs. conventional manual chest compression		
ASPIRE [33]	mCPR (AutoPulse®) vs. conventional manual CPR; prospective cluster RCT, multi-center (Canada, USA); out-of-hospital; 2004–2005; 394 vs. 373 cases out of 1377 Inclusion criteria: age ≥ 18 and non-TCA	Stopped by DSMB, ±survival (after 4 h), ↓ discharge, ↓ CPC Limitations: design (allocation concealment and not powered for secondary analyses), selection bias (trial vehicles), performance bias (device implementation, noncompliance, quality monitoring), training effect, and COI (funding by manufacturer)
CIRC [34]	mCPR (AutoPulse®) vs. conventional manual CPR; prospective individually RCT, multi-center (USA, Austria, Netherlands); out-of-hospital; 2009–2011; 2099 vs. 2132 cases out of 4753 Inclusion criteria: age ≥ 18, presumed cardiac origin (non-TCA), and response time ≤ 16 min	↓ "sustained" ROSC, ↓ survival (after 24 h), ±discharge, ±CPC Limitations: selection bias (response time), performance bias (guideline revision, quality monitoring), reporting bias (post-randomization exclusions), training effect, and COI (co-author is an employee of the manufacturer)
LINC [35]	mCPR (LUCAS®) with simultaneous defibrillation vs. conventional manual CPR with sequential defibrillation; prospective individually RCT, multi-center (Sweden, UK, Netherlands); out-of-hospital; 2008–2013; 1300 vs. 1289 cases out of 4998 Inclusion criteria: age ≥ 18, non-TCA, and no defibrillation before the device arrived on scene	±ROSC, ±admission, ± survival (after 4 h and 1 and 6 months), ±discharge, ±CPC Limitations: performance bias (defibrillation simultaneous vs. sequential, guideline revision, quality monitoring, noncompliance), training effect, and COI (device developed by investigating university)
PARAMEDIC [36]	mCPR (LUCAS®) vs. conventional manual CPR; prospective cluster RCT, multi-center (UK); out-of-hospital; 2010–2013; 1652 vs. 2818 cases out of 4689 Inclusion criteria: trial vehicle first on the scene, age ≥ 18, and non-TCA	±ROSC, ±admission, ±survival (after 1, 3 & 12 months), ↓ CPC Limitations: design (allocation concealment and the sample size was increased), selection bias (trial vehicles), performance bias (guideline revision, quality monitoring), and training effect
MECCA [37]	mCPR (LUCAS®) vs. conventional manual CPR; prospective cluster RCT, multi-center (Singapore); out-of-hospital; 2011–2012; 302 vs. 889 cases out of 1274 Inclusion criteria: age ≥ 21, presumed cardiac entity (non-TCA), and attended to by ambulance crew	±ROSC, ±survival (after 24 h and 30 days), ±discharge; as-treated analysis: any outcome ↑ if mCPR device attached early Limitations: design (not powered for secondary analyses and allocation concealment), performance bias (quality monitoring and noncompliance), training effect, and COI not reported
(b) Non-RCTs on automated mCPR vs. conventional manual chest compression		
German Resuscitation Registry [38,40]	mCPR (LUCAS®, AutoPulse®) vs. conventional manual CPR; retrospective registry analysis, multi-center (Germany); out-of-hospital; 2007–2014; 912 vs. 18,697 cases out of 35,593 Inclusion criteria: cases documented in the registry, age ≥ 18, and non-TCA	↑ (AutoPulse®) or ± (LUCAS®) ROSC (if CPR duration considered, ±(AutoPulse®) or ↓ (LUCAS®) with general application) Limitations: design (retrospective), selection bias (voluntary participation in the registry), performance bias (registry data, quality of documentation, and voluntary), and loss of follow-up
LDB device for OHCA resuscitation [43]	mCPR (AutoPulse®) vs. conventional manual CPR; prospective phased longitudinal observational cohort study, single-center (USA); out-of-hospital; 2001–2005; 284 vs. 499 cases out of 2294 Inclusion criteria: age ≥ 18 and non-TCA	↑ ROSC, ↑ admission, ↑ discharge, ±CPC, few survivors if response time > 8 min Limitations: design (observational), performance bias (hypothermia and device implementation), training effect, and COI (funding by manufacturer, co-author is an advisor for the manufacturer)

Legend: ± = equal, comparable, and no statistically significant difference; ↑ = more, higher, better, and superior; ↓ = less, lower, worse, and inferior. Abbreviations: RCT = randomized controlled trial, CPR = cardiopulmonary resuscitation, mCPR = (automated) mechanical CPR, DSMB = data and safety monitoring board, CPC = Glasgow–Pittsburgh cerebral performance category, ROSC = return of spontaneous circulation, COI = conflict of interest, TCA = traumatic cardiac arrest, and OHCA = out-of-hospital cardiac arrest.

3.2.3. Decision Criteria

Further data regarding secondary outcomes, such as long-term survival (e.g., after 1, 3, 6, or 12 months) or CPR quality surrogates (e.g., compression depth and frequency, hands-off time, injuries, blood pressure, coronary or cerebral perfusion pressures, respiratory, metabolic, and other laboratory parameters) show heterogeneous and, in parts, contradictory results. The later the endpoints, the slighter the difference between mechanical and manual CPR outcomes—a frequent observation within longitudinal resuscitation studies [38,39,44,45]. Trauma due to chest compression may occur both after conventional manual and automated mCPR in the same frequency, but the injury patterns seem to differ. Patients who received conventional manual chest compressions typically show anterior rib fractures, sternum fractures, unshaped midline chest abrasions along the sternum, visceral bleeding, and retrosternal hematoma. In contrast, patients who received automated mechanical chest compressions show posterior rib fractures, vertebral fractures, shaped skin abrasions along the anterolateral chest and shoulder, visceral bleeding including liver and splenic lacerations, and retroperitoneal hematoma [46–49].

Automated mCPR cannot reverse any cause of cardiac arrest, nor does it lead to higher survival rates compared to manual CPR. Hence, manual chest compression should be the standard technique, but under special circumstances and in particular fields of application, the devices may provide effective and safe chest compressions until an adequate health care facility is reached, where the definitive treatment can be performed. Thus, these systems may be beneficial as a bridge to treatment tool or as a bridge to decision on further treatment, and may be considered especially during prolonged resuscitation attempts. This might arise under specific conditions, such as, for example, sustaining ventricular fibrillation (VF) [50] or hypothermic cardiac arrest [50–54], patient transportation [5,55–57], diagnostics, such as computed tomography (CT) [5,58–60] (not chest X-rays [61]), and interventions, such as percutaneous coronary intervention (PCI) [5,58,62], fibrinolysis [60,63], dialysis [54], extra-corporeal membrane oxygenation (ECMO) [5], transcatheter aortic valve implantation (TAVI) [64], surgery [65,66], or organ preservation until retrieval [5,67]. On the other hand, after the implementation of mechanical CPR devices in a German EMS system, a dramatic increase in transportation with ongoing CPR, even for patients with unfavorable prognoses, has been observed [68].

3.2.4. Therapeutic Strategy

Thus, appropriate patients with potentially reversible and, therefore, treatable causes of cardiac arrest should be carefully identified and selected, as they might profit from transportation to a suitable hospital under ongoing automated mCPR with clear therapeutic approaches [54]. This interpretation is consistent with the manufacturers' original intention, as laid down in the 1979 US Food and Drug Administration (FDA) classification report: "(. . .) the device is not designed to replace manual CPR. The literature seems to recommend it for certain situations (. . .)" [69]. Currently, valid guidelines recommend trained teams that are familiar with the device to consider automated mCPR "only if high-quality manual chest compression is not practical or compromises provider safety" [5], and under special circumstances, such as hypothermia, metabolic disorders, low cardiac output state, obesity, the need of prolonged transportation, difficult terrain, and restricted space conditions, for example, helicopter flights due to a limited cabin size [54].

3.3. Extra-Corporeal Cardiopulmonary Resuscitation (eCPR)

As previously stated, it is necessary to keep the low-flow time during CPR as short as possible. In the setting of an OHCA, it is essential to identify patients early who could benefit from an advanced or invasive procedure, such as extra-corporeal life support (ECLS), often synonymously referred to as extra-corporeal CPR (eCPR). As this approach involves a specialized multidisciplinary team, the decision should be made involving all parties.

3.3.1. Rationale

eCPR has proven to increase the chances of survival with good neurological outcomes in patients with refractory cardiac arrest treated in experienced centers by expert teams. Two randomized controlled trials demonstrated the effect of eCPR and a subsequent invasive diagnostic and treatment strategy, such as PCI. Early invasive treatment is the cornerstone of increased survival in these patients (Table 3). Bělohlávek et al. demonstrated in a secondary analysis a favorable neurological outcome in 22% of patients who received eCPR, which is the same proportion as patients in the standard-of-care group. Compared with 31.5% in their intervention group, this demonstrates the effect of an early invasive treatment strategy even without eCPR [7]. A smaller phase 2 RCT, the ARREST trial, was stopped early by the DSMB, as superiority exceeded the prespecified monitoring boundary in a planned interim analysis. The survival rate in the eCPR group was significantly higher than in the control group, but the case number was too small to demonstrate benefits in neurological outcomes [70]. In a secondary analysis from the original Prague OHCA trial, Rob et al. found a significantly higher rate of survivors in patients without prehospital ROSC and eCPR compared to standard ACLS. Furthermore, a good neurological outcome (CPC 1 or 2) was only achieved by 1.2% of patients treated with standard ACLS without prehospital ROSC. This compares to 21.7% in the eCPR group and 56.6% when prehospital ROSC was achieved [71]. All studies that are assessing the effect of eCPR in patients with OHCA have a high rate of bystander CPR. Although it should not be limited to this factor, bystander CPR has been shown to be crucial in all OHCA cases [72].

Currently, there is no consensus on when eCPR should be performed. Some studies suggest that the latest decision point should be around 30 min after cardiac arrest [73]. Recent studies in Prague [7] and Denmark [74] showed a beneficial effect in patients with >30 min of low-flow time. Furthermore, the study by Mørk et al. showed a neurologic intact survival in 20% of the patients receiving eCPR with a low-flow time of >75 min [74]. In contrast, earlier studies have shown no benefit when eCPR was initiated after 60 min of cardiac arrest [73].

Table 3. Overview of selected studies on eCPR alone or as a part of a combined hyperinvasive approach vs. conventional manual chest compression.

Trial Abbreviation and Quotation	Design and Inclusion Criteria	Main Findings and Limitations
(a) RCTs on eCPR vs. conventional manual chest compression or automated mCPR		
ARREST [70]	eCPR vs. conventional manual CPR or automated mCPR in patients with VF; prospective individualized RCT, single-center (USA); emergency department; 2019–2020; 15 vs. 15 patients out of 36 inclusion criteria: age 18–75, initially documented OHCA rhythm VF or pulseless ventricular tachycardia, no ROSC following three defibrillations, body morphology allows mCPR, and estimated transfer time < 30 min	Stopped by DSMB, superiority exceeded prespecified monitoring boundary; ↑ discharge, ↑ survival (after 3 and 6 months), ±CPC Limitations: design (single-center), performance bias (high eCPR expertise), low number of participants since stopped early, and training effect
(b) RCTs on a combined hyperinvasive approach vs. conventional manual chest compression		
Prague OHCA study [7]	mCPR (LUCAS®), early intra-arrest transport, eCPR, invasive assessment and treatment vs. conventional manual CPR; prospective individually RCT, single-center (Czech Republic); out-of-hospital; 2013–2020; 124 vs. 132 cases out of 256 Inclusion criteria: age 18–65, witnessed collapse, presumed cardiac cause, ≥ 5 min ALS without sustained ROSC, unconsciousness (Glasgow Coma Score < 8), eCPR team, and ICU bed capacity available	Stopped by DSMB, possibly underpowered; ± "sustained" ROSC, ± "neurologic recovery" [survival with CPC 1–2] (↑ after 30 days, ± after 180 days), ± "cardiac recovery" Limitations: design (single-center, limited enrollment, power, and crossover), performance bias (high eCPR expertise and noncompliance), selection bias (high bystander CPR rates), and training effect
(c) retrospective cohort studies on mechanical circulatory support vs. mCPR		

Table 3. Cont.

Trial Abbreviation and Quotation	Design and Inclusion Criteria	Main Findings and Limitations
Survival and neurological outcome after OHCA treated with and without mechanical circulatory support [74]	eCPR (with or without Impella) vs. mCPR; retrospective cohort study, single-center (Denmark); emergency department; 2015–2019; 101 vs. 216 cases out of 1015 Inclusion criteria: age $\geq$ 18 and transport to the hospital with refractory OHCA	↑ ICU admission, ↑ discharge, ↑ survival (after 30 days and 1 year), ↑ CPC Design (retrospective), selection bias (voluntary participation in the registry), performance bias (registry data, quality of documentation, and voluntarily), and loss of follow-up

Legend: $\pm$ = equal, comparable, and no statistically significant difference; ↑ = more, higher, better, and superior; ↓ = less, lower, worse, and inferior. Abbreviations: RCT = randomized controlled trial, CPR = cardiopulmonary resuscitation, eCPR = extracorporeal CPR, mCPR = (automated) mechanical CPR, VF = ventricular fibrillation, DSMB = data and safety monitoring board, CPC = Glasgow–Pittsburgh cerebral performance category, OHCA = out-of-hospital cardiac arrest, ALS = advanced life support, ROSC = return of spontaneous circulation, and ICU = intensive care unit.

3.3.2. Decision Criteria

As important as the optimal timing of eCPR cannulation are the decision criteria for eCPR initiation. National [75] and international [5,20] guidelines are available to answer this question. Overlapping inclusion criteria are younger age, witnessed arrest, duration of no-flow time <5 min, and time until eCPR initiation <60 min. Further criteria to consider are signs of life under CPR [76], intermittent ROSC or recurrent VF, neuroprotective circumstances, availability of cardiac arrest center with PCI capability, blood gas analysis, known diseases and, if known, the patient's request. Signs of life under CPR were independently associated with a favorable neurological outcome. In a study analyzing 434 individuals undergoing eCPR, any sign of life before or throughout CPR was associated with an OR for a favorable neurological outcome of 7.35 (95% CI 2.71–19.97). This was further assessed for different types of signs of life, such as gasping, pupillary light reaction, and increased level of consciousness. Those signs had an OR of 1.75 (95% CI 0.95–3.21), 5.86 (95% CI 2.28–15.06), and 4.79 (95% CI 2.16–10.63), respectively. Patients with pulseless electrical activity (PEA) or asystole had a 12% (95% CI 5–25) chance of 30-day survival with CPC 1–2 when any sign of life was present. In contrast, patients without signs of life in PEA or asystole had a 0% (95% CI 0–7%) 30-day survival with CPC 1–2. This effect is also seen in patients with a shockable rhythm, where 23% (95% CI 17–30%) with any sign of life and only 4% (95% CI 1–11%) without any sign of life had a good neurological outcome, respectively [76].

3.3.3. Cannulation

It remains unclear which cannulation strategy is the best for eCPR in OHCA patients. Kashiura et al. demonstrated that patients who underwent eCPR cannulation with both ultrasound guidance and fluoroscopy had an independently associated lower complication rate compared to ultrasound guidance alone (adjusted OR 0.14, p = 0.024). Furthermore, the time until eCPR started was the same in both groups, with a median of 17 min [77].

This compares to a mean cannula insertion time of 22.5 $\pm$ 9.9 min when a hybrid cutdown technique is performed by non-surgeons [78]. For all three approaches, failure rates were low with a change to surgical approach in four cases (8%) if ultrasound was the only method used. The overall failure rate for the hybrid approach was as low as 7.4%.

Danial et al. assessed the impact of cannulation techniques in 814 patients. Until November 2016, all patients were cannulated using a surgical approach, while hospital policy changed in November 2016 and a percutaneous approach was used from there on. Using this retrospective data, a propensity score-matched cohort study for cannulation techniques in 532 veno-arterial ECMO patients was performed. Patients were divided into a surgical and percutaneous group, with 266 patients each. Compared to a surgical approach, percutaneous access, performed via doppler ultrasound, had a higher 30-day overall survival rate (63.8% vs. 56.3%, p = 0.034) and more vascular complications after cannula removal (14.7% vs. 3.4%, p < 0.001), which mainly resulted in surgical revision for persistent bleeding. Furthermore, a lower infection rate at the cannulation site was recorded (16.5% vs. 27.8%, $p = 0.001$) [79].

Especially if a contralateral approach is used, the risk of arterio-arterial or veno-venous cannulation is given; this can be limited with ultrasound guidance.

3.3.4. Therapeutic Strategy

Similar to automated mCPR, eCPR should not be considered a definitive treatment in cardiac arrest, but as a bridge to decision or bridge to treatment while organ perfusion (particularly cerebral and coronary) is maintained. Moreover, eCPR might have the potential to serve as a bridge to recovery. Again, it is crucial to identify patients with potentially reversible entities of cardiac arrest who might profit from this invasive treatment; for example, therapy-refractory ventricular fibrillation or severe hypothermia. In-depth expertise is essential for the implementation of this measure, which requires comprehensive technical and non-technical skills and correspondingly high case numbers at the institutions providing the training. In addition to human resources, the receiving hospital must also have the equipment and capacity for this highly critical patient population. Moreover, it requires a system with highly skilled care providers, as well as the equipment and capacity necessary to provide adequate continuing care for patients.

In addition, eCPR might also serve as a bridge to donation. Although this should never be the main purpose of initiation, it can be a secondary benefit to others when, despite the best effort, ECMO weaning is not possible or severe brain damage has already occurred.

3.4. Sonography

Sonography (point-of-care ultrasound, POCUS) is increasingly becoming a key skill for the evaluation of CPR quality, reversible causes of cardiac arrest, and hemodynamic situations after sustained ROSC. Despite all the versatility of its applications, to date, no RCT has demonstrated an improvement in patient outcomes due to the performance of sonography and the resulting therapeutic consequences.

There are an increasing number of courses to learn emergency ultrasonography, although its performance under emergency conditions and, especially, during ongoing CPR, requires appropriate experience to obtain reliable images and draw clinical conclusions from it.

The extended Focused Assessment with Sonography for Trauma (eFAST) protocol has been established for the rapid assessment of critically injured patients [80]. This protocol specifies defined ultrasound positions with a focus on the detection of pericardial effusion, pneumothorax, and free abdominal and thoracic fluid, which are considered potentially reversible causes of cardiac arrest [5]. In addition, the Focused Echocardiographic Evaluation in Life Support (FEEL) protocol has been established to address cardiac causes of hypotension and cardiac arrest by basic trans-thoracic echocardiography (TTE) [81]. Using these protocols has the potential to detect reversible causes of cardiac arrest and improve hemodynamic therapies in patients during shock. Although the importance of early detection of reversible causes of circulatory arrest seems obvious, evidence of improved survival rates based on ultrasonography and the resulting therapeutic consequences is still lacking.

Accordingly, current guidelines do not state at which time in a cardiac arrest case ultrasound should be used. Guidelines from the European resuscitation council explicitly say that only experienced providers should use ultrasound in emergency situations [32]. This increases image quality and the ability to draw therapeutic conclusions from it. In order to minimize hands-off time, the ultrasound probe should be placed at the subxiphoidal position during ongoing chest compressions. One team member, who is not responsible for the conduction of the ultrasound exam, should count from five backward and chest compressions should be resumed automatically. Image storage can be used if reassessment is necessary.

There are cases where TTE is not possible or visualization is severely limited. In such cases, trans-oesophageal echocardiography (TOE) can be used to identify reversible causes of cardiac arrest with ongoing chest compressions.

3.4.1. Optimisation of Chest Compressions

High-quality chest compression is the cornerstone in the treatment of each cardiac arrest case. The "middle of the chest" has been proven to be an unreliable place when the left ventricle (LV) should be compressed [82–84]. One approach would be to continuously assess the capnography waveform and change hand positions based on three pre-defined positions (Figure 1).

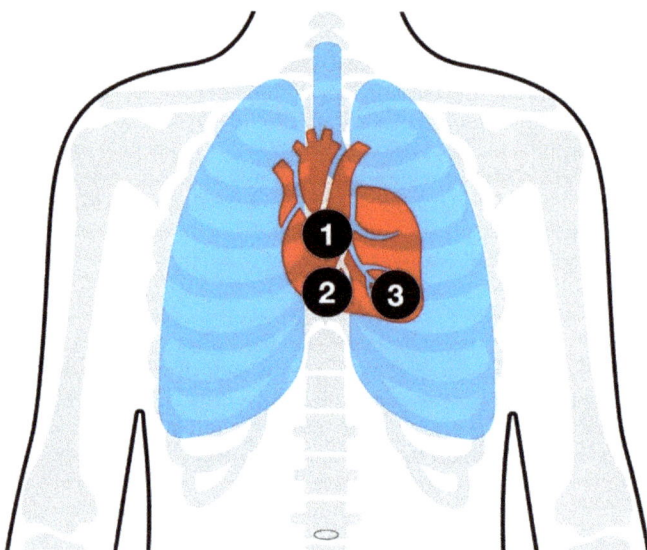

Figure 1. Schematic diagram of chest compression points. (**1**) "classic" hand position according to current guidelines [11,32]; (**2**) a more caudal approach with the hand still on the sternum; (**3**) a more caudal and left lateral approach in order to provide the maximum compression upon the left ventricle (LV).

As this "blind" approach can be time-consuming and waveform capnography can be impaired due to various circumstances, such as the underlying pathology, echocardiography during CPR is a powerful tool for the detection of the area of maximal compression (AMC), and following the optimization of chest compression.

Although availability can be limited, the TOE probe can be inserted during ongoing chest compressions. Assessment of the AMC is performed in the midoesophageal 4-chamber view (ME4CH) and the midoesophageal long axis (MELAX). As soon as the AMC is identified over the left ventricular outflow tract (LVOT) or the right ventricle (RV) (Video S1), hand positioning should be optimized. Continuous assessment of the AMC is now possible while maintaining high-quality chest compressions.

Blaivas described the performance of TOE under CPR in 2008 with a case series from an emergency department highlighting the benefits of continuous chest compressions while seeking reversible causes that led to cardiac arrest [85].

A 4-view approach was used in an emergency department in a prospective observational study. Teran et al. performed four standardized TOE views: the ME4CH, MELAX, midoesophageal bicaval (ME Bicaval), and transgastric short axis (TGSAX). Out of 33 total cases with OHCA, they were able to assess the AMC in 17 patients during ongoing CPR, while the other 16 patients achieved ROSC before resuscitative TOE was conducted. TOE was performed within 12 min (SD 8.16) after the patient's arrival. This revealed nine cases (53%) with an AMC over the LVOT or aortic root. Changes in the compression position resulted in an observable improvement of the end-tidal carbon dioxide partial pressure (etCO$_2$) and perfusion. Although TOE identified RV dilation in thirteen patients (39%), pulmonary embolism (PE) was only suspected in two cases. This is in line with the negative association of ROSC and intra-arrest RV dilation with an OR of 0.7 (95% CI 0.01–0.82). Although no benefit regarding favorable neurological survival was found when AMC was adjusted, TOE influenced clinical management with regard to diagnostic, therapeutic, and prognostic consequences in 97% (32/33) of the cases [86]. Further studies should focus on the change in etCO$_2$ and hemodynamic parameters when AMC is adjusted.

3.4.2. Detecting and Addressing Reversible Causes of Cardiac Arrest

Hypovolaemia: In traumatic cardiac arrest, hypovolaemia due to exsanguination is one of the most common reversible causes, and invasive therapeutic options are available. In order to enhance certainty before performing invasive interventions, the eFAST protocol can be applied to detect free abdominal or thoracic fluid. Venous congestion during CPR can limit the significance of inferior vena cava (IVC) assessment. Current guidelines state limited knowledge about the use of ultrasound for the detection of hypovolemia in cardiac arrest [5,32].

Thromboembolism: Thrombosis, either cardiac or pulmonary, is one of the most frequent causes of sudden cardiac death. As PE has non-specific clinical signs and symptoms that may lead to PEA, it is crucial to look for specific echocardiographic signs before the patient further deteriorates [87,88]. Therefore, visual assessment should be the main priority, as this can be performed in every setting with a handheld ultrasound device.

In patients with cardiac arrest, RV dilation is a common finding, especially if resuscitation has been ongoing for a prolonged period [89]. This weak association between RV dilation and PE brings a challenge to the table, leaving only reduced possibilities of identifying PE during CPR. Right heart mobile thrombus could be seen during CPR, suggesting the presence of PE [88]. A second finding, deep vein thrombosis (DVT), can be detected in about 30–50% of patients with PE by compression ultrasound [90].

While the need for emergent ultrasound diagnostics is not given in shockable rhythms, it may provide valuable information in peri-arrest situations or following ROSC, if a 12-lead electrocardiogram is inconclusive. Regional wall motion abnormalities can be seen even in patients without significant repolarisation abnormalities.

Tension pneumothorax: Ultrasound is not only faster than conventional chest X-rays or CT—it also offers better sensitivity and specificity than chest X-rays. In addition, it can be performed directly at the site of emergency [91] if the "classical" diagnostic means are uncertain.

Pericardial tamponade: A pericardial effusion was previously considered only a suspected diagnosis in the out-of-hospital setting, which could not be ruled out with certainty. With the increasing availability of portable ultrasound equipment, even users with little experience can answer the question of the presence of a pericardial effusion using the eFAST or FEEL protocol in the field [92].

3.5. Resuscitative Endovascular Balloon Occlusion of the Aorta (REBOA)

The principle of intra-aorta balloon catheter tamponade dates back to the 1950s and has first been described in soldiers with battle-related severe abdominal and pelvic bleeding during the Korean War [93].

In order to determinate the target area where the aortic occlusion balloon is supposed to be deployed, the REBOA concept defines specific "landing zones" (Figure 2) depending on the indication [94].

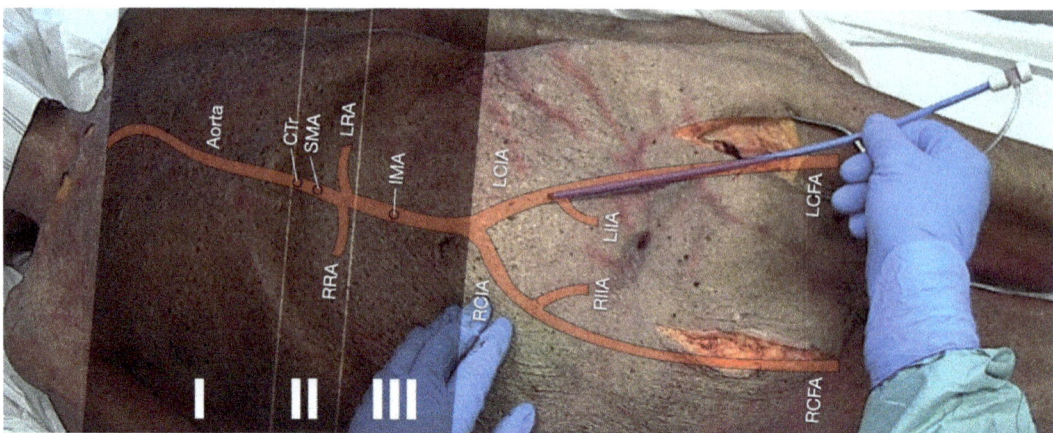

Figure 2. Schematic topographic projection of the aorta and its major branches on a cadaveric model: REBOA landing zones (**I**) (preferred in non-traumatic cardiac arrest), (**II**) (contraindicated), and (**III**) (preferred in pelvic trauma) are highlighted. Both femoral arteries have been prepared via a cutdown approach. Abbreviations: CTr = coeliac trunk, SMA = superior mesenteric artery, RRA = right renal artery, LRA = left renal artery, IMA = inferior mesenteric artery, RCIA = right common iliac artery, LCIA = left common iliac artery, RIIA = right internal iliac artery, LIIA = left internal iliac artery, RCFA = right common femoral artery, and LCFA = left common femoral artery.

(1) The ascendant aorta with the aortic arch is occasionally referred to as "Zone 0". Due to the branches of the carotid arteries supplying the brain with blood, balloon deployment is contraindicated in this zone.
(2) Zone I: The left subclavian artery to the celiac trunk. This position is preferred in non-traumatic cardiac arrest to enhance coronary and cerebral perfusion. Among other scopes of application, there may be aortic dissection or uncontrollable thoracic or visceral bleeding.
(3) Zone II: The coeliac trunk to the lowest renal artery supplying major intra- and retroperitoneal organs with blood. Balloon deployment is contraindicated in this zone.
(4) Zone III: The lowest renal artery to the aortic bifurcation. This position is preferred in uncontrollable sub-/pelvic or groin bleeding.

3.5.1. Achieving Hemostasis in Severe Trauma and Traumatic Cardiac Arrest (TCA)

As previously stated, REBOA is used to control bleeding from non-compressible injuries in critically injured casualties with uncontrolled hemorrhagic shock unresponsive to volume therapy [93]. Depending on the underlying trauma, the balloon occlusion may be deployed either in landing zone I (thoracic and upper abdominal bleeding and aortic dissection) or III (sub-/pelvic or grain bleeding) (Figure 2) [94].

As this special issue's focus is on sudden cardiac death rather than TCA, the application of REBOA in catastrophic bleeding is only briefly mentioned due to historic and didactic reasons. Pertinent literature might be of interest for further reading [93–95].

3.5.2. Improving Coronary Perfusion during CPR

When applied in trauma patients, the aortic occlusion substantially increased blood pressure which was expected to result in increased cerebral and coronary perfusion. Consistently, it is alleged that the REBOA procedure might have an epinephrine-like effect on aortic and subsequently coronary pressures [10]. As previously stated, those are associated with improved rates of ROSC and survival [17]. In order to enhance cardiac and cerebral perfusion pressures during CPR, the REBOA catheter should be placed in landing zone I (Figure 2).

As a matter of fact, the first experimental studies confirmed enhanced coronary and cerebral perfusion after performing the REBOA procedure in a porcine cardiac arrest model [96]. On this occasion, the effects on both perfusion pressures and ROSC are comparable to those achieved from the application of epinephrine [96]. For a long time, merely case reports and observational studies were published reporting that REBOA is feasible and effective in non-trauma cardiac arrest [97–104]. The clinical studies predominantly lack control groups and are limited to surrogate outcomes, but support the physiological considerations on perfusion as previously described [102–105]. Hence, REBOA is increasingly seen as an adjunct to non-trauma advanced cardiac life support (Table 4). If performed rapidly by a highly skilled team from an experienced center, enabling a short collapse-to-balloon time, it might serve as a bridge to treatment until PCI or ECMO [106].

Table 4. Overview of selected studies on REBOA in non-TCA.

Trial Abbreviation and Quotation	Design and Inclusion Criteria	Main Findings and Limitations
(a) RCTs on REBOA in non-traumatic cardiac arrest		
REBOARREST [107]	ALS an REBOA vs. standard ALS; RCT, multi-center (Norway); out-of-hospital; 2022-ongoing; calculated enrollment 200 patientsInclusion criteria: age 18–80, OHCA, non-TCA, witnessed or <10 min from the debut of arrest, and commenced ALS established and can be continued	Study currently recruiting
(b) observational trials on REBOA in non-traumatic cardiac arrest		
Feasibility of Pre-Hospital REBOA [98]	ALS an REBOA vs. standard ALS; RCT, single-center (Norway); out-of-hospital, helicopter; 2018–2019; 10 patientsInclusion criteria: age 18–75, OHCA, non-TCA, and witnessed or <10 min from the debut of arrest	The attempt was 100% successful (80% first attempt), 60% ROSC, 30% admission to hospital, 10% survival (30 days), procedural time 11.7 ± 3.2 min, and etCO$_2$ + 1.75 kPa after 1 minLimitations: feasibility study, a decision by study group, single-center, a small number of researchers and patients, and no autopsies (adverse effects)
NEURESCUE® Device as an Adjunct to Cardiac Arrest [NCT05146661]	REBOA device; interventional open-label single group study, single-center (Germany); in hospital emergency department; 2022-ongoing; calculated enrollment 10 patientsInclusion criteria: age 18–75, witnessed, CPR initiated ≤ 7 min of presumed arrest, not responding to standard ALS, and total CPR time ≤ 40 min at enrollment	Study currently recruiting

Legend: $\pm$ = equal, comparable and no statistically significant difference; ↑ = more, higher, better, and superior; ↓ = less, lower, worse, and inferior. Abbreviations: REBOA = resuscitative endovascular balloon occlusion of the aorta, TCA = traumatic cardiac arrest, OHCA = out-of-hospital cardiac arrest, RCT = randomized controlled trial, CPR = cardiopulmonary resuscitation, ALS = advanced life support, and etCO$_2$ = end-tidal carbon dioxide partial pressure.

In a randomized controlled feasibility study, a team from Heidelberg University Hospital examines the value of a REBOA device in non-trauma cardiac arrest. In addition to its safety and performance, secondary outcome measures and surrogate parameters such as blood pressure, CPR time intervals, and ROSC are of the investigators' particular interest [NCT05146661]. The currently ongoing multi-center randomized controlled REBOARREST trial is supposed to provide insight into survival, hemodynamics, organ function, and adverse events [107].

3.6. Arterial Blood Gas (ABG) Analysis

Point-of-care testing (POCT), similar to ABG analysis, is widely used in both intensive care medicine and emergency departments, as the knowledge of particular blood parameters may require further therapeutic procedures in the treatment of life-threatening conditions. Therefore, it is considered a common adjunct to the treatment of in-hospital cardiac arrest [5,54]. Beyond differentiating respiratory disorders, further, potentially reversible causes of cardiac arrest may be detected and treated by means of ABG analysis; for example, metabolic disorders, such as acidosis and alkalosis, as well as electrolyte abnormalities, such as hypo or hyperkalemia. The measurement results may trigger interventions such as the optimization of artificial respiration, the correction of acidosis (ventilatory or sodium bicarbonate), antidote, vasoactive, or fluid therapy, or may accelerate admission to the hospital for resuscitative hemodialysis [108,109].

Due to the size, energy demand, and characteristics of the analytical equipment, even if measured at the "point of care", most POCT applications had been restricted to health care facilities. With the advent of portable devices, blood gas analyzers have become available in the field [110,111]. Meanwhile, technological advances have enabled a rapid and reliable application in the prehospital environment [108].

The parameters obtained may support the responsible team in diagnosis and treatment decision-making [108,109]. While survival data from RCTs are still missing, it seems obvious that patients might profit from the earliest possible recognition and treatment of reversible causes during OHCA [112].

3.7. Thoracic Decompression

In addition to chest trauma as a main cause, pulmonary diseases, such as acute exacerbation of chronic obstructive pulmonary disease with consecutive pneumothorax, may be accompanied by progressive ventilatory and/or cardiocirculatory distress [113]. There is a risk of developing a life-threatening tension pneumothorax, which can be fatal if left untreated. Needle decompression and thoracostomy with or without drainage insertion are, therefore, life-saving interventions. The relief of tension pneumothorax by means of pleural puncture or minithoracostomy is an established invasive procedure. It is one of the basic techniques in the care of critically ill patients and every doctor working in emergency medicine must be able to perform it [92,114].

In highly dynamic situations with foudroyant shock, needle decompression is useful, as it is quick and easy to perform. Classically, it is performed in the Monaldi position in the second or third intercostal space of the midclavicular line. The indwelling venous cannulae often used for needle decompression are too short to reach the pleural space for a relevant proportion of patients [115,116]. For this reason, relevant course formats alternatively recommend needle decompression in the Bülau position in the fourth or fifth intercostal space between the anterior and midaxillary line (Figure 3) [117,118].

A tension pneumothorax can usually only be relieved for a short time with the puncture, so it seems sensible to always perform a minithoracostomy afterward [119]. The minithoracostomy is performed in the Bülau position. The life-saving intervention is the opening of the pleural space, not the insertion of a drain. Whether a chest drain should be inserted at the scene or in the hospital remains the subject of ongoing debate. Recent retrospective data suggest that there could be an increased risk of recurrent tension physiology if thoracostomy is not followed by the placement of a drain [120].

3.8. Pericardiocentesis

While chronic pericardial effusion, for example, due to infectious, inflammatory, or malignant disease, usually develops slowly, rapid accumulation in the event of a disease flare-up can lead to subacute cardiocirculatory decompensation. In the event of aortic dissection, after thoracic trauma or iatrogenic perforation (for example, PCI, aortic, or cardiac surgery), the development is dramatic. Even small amounts of blood can lead to a significant increase in intrapericardial pressure within a few minutes and clinically manifest pericardial tamponade [121].

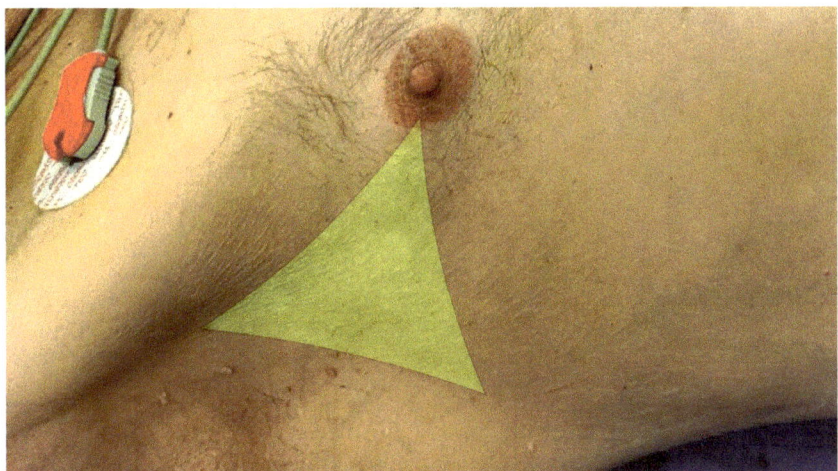

Figure 3. Projection of the Triangle of Safety formed by the posterior border of the pectoralis major muscle, the anterior border of the latissimus dorsi muscle, and the intermammillary line.

Clinical diagnosis of pericardial tamponade (Beck's Triad: hypotension with a narrowed pulse pressure, jugular venous distention, and muffled heart sounds) is difficult and unreliable, especially in a peri-arrest situation. As acute tamponade is not associated with a large effusion volume, a rather small effusion of 50 mL can cause cardiac tamponade in a hypovolemic state and lead to cardiac arrest. This reversible cause has to be treated immediately in order to restore perfusion. In this case, prehospital emergency ultrasonography is essential [121,122]. Furthermore, the integration of ultrasound reduces the time until relief of the pericardial tamponade (Figure 4a,b) [123].

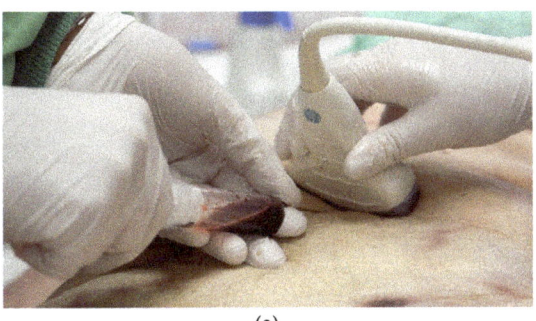
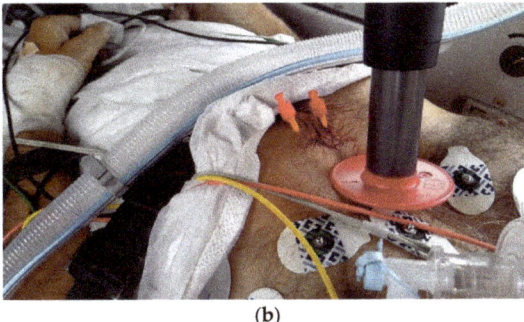

(a)   (b)

Figure 4. (**a**) Ultrasound-guided pericardiocentesis in a cadaveric model: The convex-array transducer is placed subxiphoidal to obtain a subcostal window 4-chamber view (S4CH) in order to guide the needle precisely under sight and thus achieve higher success rates; (**b**) Helicopter transport of a patient in sustained return of spontaneous circulation (ROSC) after ultrasound-guided relief of pericardial effusion in the field by the catheter-over-needle technique. Catheters have been left in place. An automated mechanical cardiopulmonary resuscitation (mCPR) device has been applied precautionarily.

In principle, two phenotypes of tamponade can be distinguished sonographically. On the one hand, a liquid tamponade is easily accessible for puncture; on the other hand, extensive clot formation can occur in the case of a hemopericardium. In the latter case, relief by pericardiocentesis is not promising and relief must be achieved by thoracotomy, as described below [54,119,121].

It must be mentioned restrictively that, to date, there is no systematic data available regarding the cause of cardiac tamponade in non-traumatic cardiac arrest. If the cardiac arrest was caused by aortic dissection or ventricular rupture, simply relieving tamponade could not solve the problem, as the underlying pathology cannot be treated with the options available in an out-of-hospital setting.

3.9. Resuscitative Thoracotomy

The resuscitative opening of the chest by means of a clamshell thoracotomy provides a quick overview and allows control of intrathoracic bleeding, proximal aortic compression, and access to the pericardium in cases of suspected or ultrasound-confirmed tamponade [92,124,125]. Therefore, it is indicated in traumatic cardiac arrest rather than sudden cardiac death. Nevertheless, this procedure is supposed to be discussed here as an advanced invasive resuscitation technique for the sake of completeness. As an invasive emergency technique, thoracotomy is firmly established in the current guidelines for cardiopulmonary resuscitation and polytrauma care, although the indication must be restrictive. According to the "4 E" rule, clamshell thoracotomy is only indicated if certain conditions concerning expertise, equipment, environment, and elapsed time are met [54].

Compared to left anterolateral thoracotomy, clamshell thoracotomy is more suitable for potentially reversible causes of trauma-induced cardiovascular arrest (Figure 5a,b). It allows an excellent overview of the intrathoracic organs and thus a wide range of interventions [124].

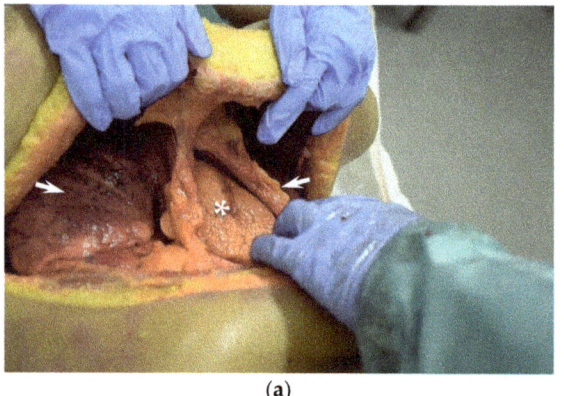
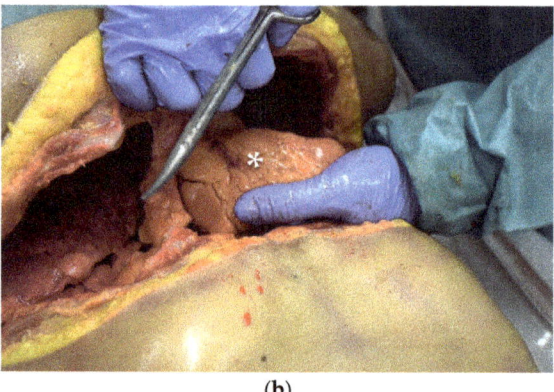

Figure 5. Clamshell thoracotomy in a cadaveric model: (**a**) Situs after thoracotomy, the chest is lifted by one rescuer to allow a good overview of the heart (asterisk) and lungs (arrowheads); (**b**) The second rescuer luxates the heart (asterisk) in order to be able to perform interventions.

The pericardium is incised in a T-shape to relieve pericardial tamponade and to inspect the heart for treatable injuries. Pericardial tamponade can be cleared manually. Relevant injuries to the lung can be treated by clamping or hilum twists as a last resort. Subdiaphragmatic bleeding can be reduced by manual compression of the aorta against the spine [92]. If internal cardiac massage is required, the heart should be taken between both hands and compressed in a walking motion from the apex to the base about 80 times per minute. However, resuscitative thoracotomy does not make sense to perform a thoracotomy in order to be able to resuscitate an open heart [126]. Despite numerous impressive case reports from highly experienced centers, evidence for this highly invasive procedure from clinical trials under routine care conditions is lacking.

4. Discussion of Concepts and Strategies

With the increasing establishment of advanced and invasive techniques in ALS, procedures may now potentially be considered in medical circulatory arrest whose applications were previously limited to traumatic cardiac arrest or trauma life support. This could make the boundaries of indications appear increasingly blurred (Figure 6).

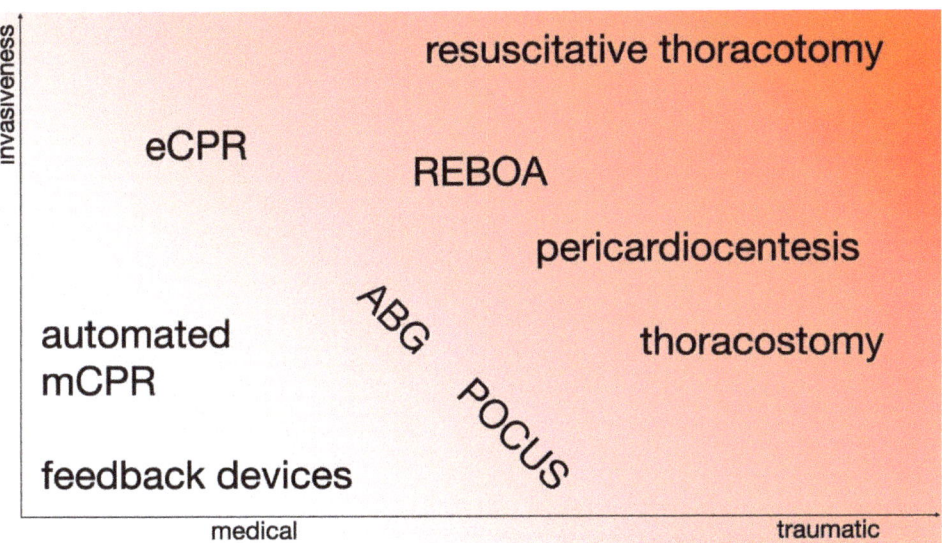

Figure 6. Advanced and invasive techniques may be considered in medical and traumatic cardiac arrest. Abbreviations: CPR = cardiopulmonary resuscitation, eCPR = extracorporeal CPR, mCPR = (automated) mechanical CPR, REBOA = resuscitative endovascular balloon occlusion of the aorta, ABG = arterial blood gas, and POCUS = point-of-care ultrasound.

4.1. Decision-Making and Timing

Advanced and invasive techniques may have a positive impact on survival but can be fraught with technical, social, situational, and organizational hurdles. Therefore, it is important that the emergency crew knows the infrastructure, with its highly qualified and skilled teams, and can deploy resources that can respond to this time-critical emergency within minutes. Here, the geographical and health characteristics of the different urban and rural areas must also be considered [127].

Time plays a major role in the context of OHCA. Ideally, and in terms of survival with good neurological outcome, the low-flow time should not be greater than 60 min [128,129]. This presents a major challenge to emergency teams. A lot of information has to be filtered in a short time and a decision has to be made for or against a resource-intensive attempt to help. Even if the local conditions provide all technical and personnel resources, the process is significantly influenced by the decisions of the team on site. A predefined decision point or mental model can have a major impact on the stressful teamwork, the further course of resuscitation, and the survival of the patient.

For teamwork to succeed resiliently and function efficiently, mental models can be helpful. Emergency teams should use and implement mental models even before the emergency. This can establish a clear decision tree, streamline processes, and expedite decisions (for example, a mental model for refractory cardiopulmonary resuscitation in OHCA) [130].

The decision point is a formal team time-out to plan the next 60 min, maximize the use of team resources, and anticipate procedures. At this point, brief considerations should be verbalized in the scenario, decided interprofessionally, and initiated immediately.

Taking eCPR as an example, after the second rhythm analysis, or after intubation, the team decides loudly and unanimously that, based on the information available, eCPR is indicated and the cannulation team can be dispatched. As Tonna and colleagues conclude, due to limited data, much of the current practice is based on expert opinion and institutional knowledge, rather than scientific evidence [127]. Depending on the local strategy, whether the cannulation is in- or out-of-hospital, once reversible causes have been ruled out, preparation for cannulation or transport to the hospital follows. If the cannulation is attempted in-hospital, the decision to proceed with eCPR must be reconsidered by the receiving team [131]. As a result of rapid decision making, time-intensive steps can be taken early and conditions can be created for eCPR to begin in less than 60 min [132]. This example highlights the importance of timing in this process and how decision-making impacts patient survival.

Awareness of the right timing and early activation of advanced procedures are imperative to lead to the reduction in low-flow times and should be included in local standard operating procedures (SOPs). Mental models for rare events and a decision point as a trigger in the resuscitation algorithm could support the processes.

Before highly invasive techniques are carried out, a short team briefing should take place in order to give all those involved in the operation the opportunity to "take themselves out of the situation" if they fear that they will be too emotionally burdened by the procedures. After the response, a structured team debriefing is a valuable educational strategy to improve team performance [133]. While the effect of debriefing on long-term patient outcomes is uncertain, there is evidence that structured debriefing improves clinical education, the efficiency of work, team climate, and patient safety [134–136]. Teams with alternating compositions, which is typical for emergency medicine, benefit most from structured debriefing [136]. Especially after stressful emergency responses, a structured and—if necessary, moderated—reappraisal and debriefing should also be offered for all personnel involved in a protected setting [137]. Early signs and support for stress reactions should also be made a subject of discussion.

4.2. Emergency Response and Continuing Care Structures

A promising approach to bring the therapeutic options previously described to the roadside is rapid response vehicles staffed with an experienced emergency physician. There are some proven concepts, such as London's air ambulance, which operates an advanced trauma team helicopter and a rapid response car during night time or in adverse weather or rather flight conditions [18]. Heidelberg University Hospital also operates a rapid response vehicle providing devices and experienced staff for invasive interventions, the "medical intervention car (MIC)" [19]. Utilizing both modes, rapid response cars and rescue helicopters, appears reasonable, as this concept will combine the advantages of a highly flexible system within the narrow spaces of a city with a system that allows for the deploying of the techniques quickly over long distances to rural areas.

Invasive procedures may be associated with relevant blood loss due to the intervention itself (e.g., ECMO and thoracotomy) or the underlying mechanism (e.g., trauma or aortic dissection) leading to cardiac arrest. In addition to bleeding control, volume replacement plays a central role. It is questionable whether a patient can be stabilized with crystalloid or colloid infusion solutions alone in the case of massive blood loss. While blood transfusion in an out-of-hospital setting was unimaginable in large parts of the world until recently, blood products are now increasingly available on the scene [19,54,138–141].

Embedding the algorithm on advanced and invasive procedures in local care structures is essential to ensure adequate continuing care for critically ill patients. This begins with raising public awareness programs for lay resuscitation. Receiving hospitals must have the necessary human, medical, and technical resources to ensure a seamless continuation of treatment and manage any complications that may arise, which is the case with cardiac arrest centers (CAC).

5. Conclusions

Despite all innovations, situation awareness, continuous training of technical and non-technical skills, and proper (effective and continuous) chest compressions, the earliest possible defibrillation and artificial respiration remain the basic framework of CPR.

Ultrasound under CPR is increasingly becoming a key skill for the evaluation of reversible causes of cardiac arrest, optimizing chest compressions and evaluating the hemodynamic situation after obtaining sustained ROSC.

For selected patient groups, under certain circumstances and, in particular, fields of application, advanced and invasive techniques may be an option to ensure sufficient organ (in particular, coronary and cerebral) perfusion. There is a lack of clear evidence regarding solid endpoints, such as survival. Hence, these techniques should only be conducted with clear therapeutic conceptions as a bridge to treatment by a specialist team.

This should be part of a larger treatment concept that requires appropriate emergency response systems, as well as definitive treatment in centers with established continuing care structures.

The decisions and timing made by the emergency team have a major impact on the time-critical scenario. Therefore, it is essential that emergency teams know and use local resources, establish mental models for rare emergencies, and set decision points as triggers that initiate processes early.

Supplementary Materials: The following supporting information can be downloaded at https://www.mdpi.com/article/10.3390/jcm11247315/s1, Video S1: Identification of the area of maximal compression (AMC) during ongoing manual chest compressions. Table S1: Searched literature sources; Table S2: Search terms.

Author Contributions: Writing—original draft preparation, M.O., S.K. and O.K.; writing—review and editing, E.P. and F.W.; visualization, M.O.; supervision, E.P. and F.W.; All authors have read and agreed to the published version of the manuscript.

Funding: This research received no external funding.

Institutional Review Board Statement: Not applicable.

Informed Consent Statement: Not applicable.

Data Availability Statement: Not applicable.

Acknowledgments: Some illustrations show the performance of invasive procedures in cadaveric models. The persons gave their informed consent during their lifetime and bequeathed their mortal remains to the Ruprecht Karls University of Heidelberg for scientific purposes. The authors are deeply grateful to the body donors and their surviving relatives for their valuable contribution to research and education.

Conflicts of Interest: The authors declare no conflict of interest.

Abbreviations

ABG	arterial blood gas
ALS	advanced life support
AMC	area of maximal compression
CAC	cardiac arrest center
CI	confidence interval
COI	conflict of interest
CPC	Glasgow–Pittsburgh cerebral performance category
CPR	cardiopulmonary resuscitation
CT	computed tomography
CTr	coeliac trunk
DSMB	data and safety monitoring board
DVT	deep vein thrombosis

ECLS	extracorporeal life support
ECMO	extracorporeal membrane oxygenation
eCPR	extracorporeal cardiopulmonary resuscitation (CPR)
eFAST	extended focused assessment with sonography for trauma
EMS	emergency medical service
etCO$_2$	end-tidal carbon dioxide partial pressure
FDA	US Food and Drug Administration
FEEL	focused echocardiographic evaluation in life support
ICU	intensive care unit
IHCA	in-hospital cardiac arrest
IMA	inferior mesenteric artery
IVC	inferior vena cava
LCFA	left common femoral artery
LCIA	left common iliac artery
LIIA	left internal iliac artery
LRA	left renal artery
LV	left ventricle
LVOT	left ventricular outflow tract
mCPR	(automated) mechanical cardiopulmonary resuscitation (CPR)
ME Bicaval	midoesophageal bicaval view
ME4CH	midoesophageal 4-chamber view
MELAX	midoesophageal long axis view
MIC	medical intervention car, a physician-staffed rapid response vehicle
mRS	modified Rankin Scale
OHCA	out-of-hospital cardiac arrest
OR	odds ratio
PCI	percutaneous coronary intervention
PE	pulmonary embolism
PEA	pulseless electrical activity
PLAX	parasternal long-axis view
POCT	point-of-care testing
POCUS	point-of-care ultrasound
RACA	return of spontaneous circulation (ROSC) after cardiac arrest
RCFA	right common femoral artery
RCIA	right common iliac artery
RCT	randomized controlled trial
REBOA	resuscitative endovascular balloon occlusion of the aorta
RIIA	right internal iliac artery
ROSC	return of spontaneous circulation
RRA	right renal artery
RV	right ventricle
S4CH	subcostal window 4-chamber view
SMA	superior mesenteric artery
SOP	standard operating procedure
TAVI	transcatheter aortic valve implantation
TCA	traumatic cardiac arrest
TGSAX	transgastric short axis view
TOE	trans-oesophageal echocardiography
TTE	trans-thoracic echocardiography
VF	ventricular fibrillation

References

1. Kouwenhoven, W.B.; Jude, J.R.; Knickerbocker, G.G. Closed-chest cardiac massage. *JAMA* **1960**, *173*, 1064–1067. [CrossRef] [PubMed]
2. Safar, P. Artificial Respitation. *Anesthesiology* **1960**, *21*, 570. [CrossRef]
3. Gräsner, J.-T.; Herlitz, J.; Tjelmeland, I.B.M.; Wnent, J.; Masterson, S.; Lilja, G.; Bein, B.; Böttiger, B.W.; Rosell-Ortiz, F.; Nolan, J.P.; et al. European Resuscitation Council Guidelines 2021: Epidemiology of cardiac arrest in Europe. *Resuscitation* **2021**, *161*, 61–79. [CrossRef]
4. Chamberlain, D. Never Quite There: A tale of Resuscitation Medicine. *Resuscitation* **2004**, *60*, 3–11. [CrossRef]
5. Soar, J.; Bottiger, B.W.; Carli, P.; Couper, K.; Deakin, C.D.; Djarv, T.; Lott, C.; Olasveengen, T.; Paal, P.; Pellis, T.; et al. European Resuscitation Council Guidelines 2021: Adult advanced life support. *Resuscitation* **2021**, *161*, 115–151. [CrossRef]
6. Rott, N.; Bottiger, B.W.; Lockey, A. The World Restart a Heart Initiative: How to save hundreds of thousands of lives worldwide. *Curr. Opin. Crit. Care* **2021**, *27*, 663–667. [CrossRef]
7. Bělohlávek, J.; Smalcova, J.; Rob, D.; Franek, O.; Smid, O.; Pokorna, M.; Horak, J.; Mrazek, V.; Kovarnik, T.; Zemanek, D.; et al. Effect of Intra-arrest Transport, Extracorporeal Cardiopulmonary Resuscitation, and Immediate Invasive Assessment and Treatment on Functional Neurologic Outcome in Refractory Out-of-Hospital Cardiac Arrest: A Randomized Clinical Trial. *JAMA* **2022**, *327*, 737–747. [CrossRef]
8. Bouhemad, B.; Brisson, H.; Le-Guen, M.; Arbelot, C.; Lu, Q.; Rouby, J.J. Bedside ultrasound assessment of positive end-expiratory pressure-induced lung recruitment. *Am. J. Respir. Crit. Care Med.* **2011**, *183*, 341–347. [CrossRef]
9. O'Brien, C.E.; Santos, P.T.; Reyes, M.; Adams, S.; Hopkins, C.D.; Kulikowicz, E.; Hamrick, J.L.; Hamrick, J.T.; Lee, J.K.; Kudchadkar, S.R.; et al. Association of diastolic blood pressure with survival during paediatric cardiopulmonary resuscitation. *Resuscitation* **2019**, *143*, 50–56. [CrossRef]
10. Brede, J.R. Aortic occlusion during cardiac arrest-mechanical adrenaline? *Resuscitation* **2022**, *179*, 94–96. [CrossRef]
11. Olasveengen, T.M.; Semeraro, F.; Ristagno, G.; Castren, M.; Handley, A.; Kuzovlev, A.; Monsieurs, K.G.; Raffay, V.; Smyth, M.; Soar, J.; et al. European Resuscitation Council Guidelines 2021: Basic Life Support. *Resuscitation* **2021**, *161*, 98–114. [CrossRef] [PubMed]
12. Nichol, G.; Thomas, E.; Callaway, C.W.; Hedges, J.; Powell, J.L.; Aufderheide, T.P.; Rea, T.; Lowe, R.; Brown, T.; Dreyer, J.; et al. Regional variation in out-of-hospital cardiac arrest incidence and outcome. *JAMA* **2008**, *300*, 1423–1431. [CrossRef]
13. Valenzuela, T.D.; Kern, K.B.; Clark, L.L.; Berg, R.A.; Berg, M.D.; Berg, D.D.; Hilwig, R.W.; Otto, C.W.; Newburn, D.; Ewy, G.A. Interruptions of chest compressions during emergency medical systems resuscitation. *Circulation* **2005**, *112*, 1259–1265. [CrossRef] [PubMed]
14. Ochoa, F.J.; Ramalle-Gomara, E.; Lisa, V.; Saralegui, I. The effect of rescuer fatigue on the quality of chest compressions. *Resuscitation* **1998**, *37*, 149–152. [CrossRef]
15. Eftestol, T.; Sunde, K.; Steen, P.A. Effects of interrupting precordial compressions on the calculated probability of defibrillation success during out-of-hospital cardiac arrest. *Circulation* **2002**, *105*, 2270–2273. [CrossRef]
16. Christenson, J.; Andrusiek, D.; Everson-Stewart, S.; Kudenchuk, P.; Hostler, D.; Powell, J.; Callaway, C.W.; Bishop, D.; Vaillancourt, C.; Davis, D.; et al. Chest compression fraction determines survival in patients with out-of-hospital ventricular fibrillation. *Circulation* **2009**, *120*, 1241–1247. [CrossRef]
17. Paradis, N.A.; Martin, G.B.; Rivers, E.P.; Goetting, M.G.; Appleton, T.J.; Feingold, M.; Nowak, R.M. Coronary perfusion pressure and the return of spontaneous circulation in human cardiopulmonary resuscitation. *JAMA* **1990**, *263*, 1106–1113. [CrossRef]
18. Rehn, M.; Davies, G.; Smith, P.; Lockey, D.J. Structure of Rapid Response Car Operations in an Urban Trauma Service. *Air Med. J.* **2016**, *35*, 143–147. [CrossRef]
19. Obermaier, M.; Fiedler, M.O.; Göring, M.; Hochreiter, M.; Küßner, T.; Mohr, S.; Popp, E.; Schmitt, F.C.F.; Weigand, M.A.; Weilbacher, F.; et al. Medical Intervention Car: Projekt zur Verbesserung der außerklinischen Notfallversorgung. In *Elsevier Emergency: Innovative Konzepte*; Gollwitzer, J., Grusnick, H.-M., Klausmeier, M., Eds.; Elsevier: Amsterdam, The Netherlands, 2020; pp. 18–24.
20. Richardson, A.S.C.; Tonna, J.E.; Nanjayya, V.; Nixon, P.; Abrams, D.C.; Raman, L.; Bernard, S.; Finney, S.J.; Grunau, B.; Youngquist, S.T.; et al. Extracorporeal Cardiopulmonary Resuscitation in Adults. Interim Guideline Consensus Statement From the Extracorporeal Life Support Organization. *Asaio J.* **2021**, *67*, 221–228. [CrossRef]
21. Bernhard, M.; Friedmann, C.; Aul, A.; Helm, M.; Mutzbauer, T.S.; Doll, S.; Völkl, A.; Gries, A. Praxisorientiertes Ausbildungskonzept für invasive Notfalltechniken. *Notf. Rett. Med.* **2010**, *14*, 475–482. [CrossRef]
22. Schneider, N.R.E.; Küßner, T.; Weilbacher, F.; Göring, M.; Mohr, S.; Rudolph, M.; Popp, E. Invasive Notfalltechniken – INTECH Advanced. *Notf. Rett. Med.* **2018**, *22*, 87–99. [CrossRef]
23. Trummer, G.; Muller, T.; Muellenbach, R.M.; Markewitz, A.; Pilarczyk, K.; Bittner, S.; Boeken, U.; Benk, C.; Baumgartel, M.; Bauer, A.; et al. Training module extracorporeal life support (ECLS): Consensus statement of the DIVI, DGTHG, DGfK, DGAI, DGIIN, DGF, GRC and DGK. *Anaesthesist* **2021**, *70*, 603–606. [CrossRef]
24. Eismann, H.; Schild, S.; Neuhaus, C.; Baus, J.; Happel, O.; Heller, A.R.; Richter, T.; Weinert, M.; Sedlmayr, B.; Sedlmayr, M.; et al. Cognitive aids for crisis management in anaesthesiology: Principles and applications. *Anästhesth. Intensivmed.* **2020**, *61*, 239–247. [CrossRef]
25. Lukas, R.P.; Gräsner, J.T.; Seewald, S.; Lefering, R.; Weber, T.P.; Van Aken, H.; Fischer, M.; Bohn, A. Chest compression quality management and return of spontaneous circulation: A matched-pair registry study. *Resuscitation* **2012**, *83*, 1212–1218. [CrossRef]

26. Brouwer, T.F.; Walker, R.G.; Chapman, F.W.; Koster, R.W. Association Between Chest Compression Interruptions and Clinical Outcomes of Ventricular Fibrillation Out-of-Hospital Cardiac Arrest. *Circulation* **2015**, *132*, 1030–1037. [CrossRef]
27. Gugelmin-Almeida, D.; Tobase, L.; Polastri, T.F.; Peres, H.H.C.; Timerman, S. Do automated real-time feedback devices improve CPR quality? A systematic review of literature. *Resusc. Plus* **2021**, *6*, 100108. [CrossRef]
28. Wang, S.A.; Su, C.P.; Fan, H.Y.; Hou, W.H.; Chen, Y.C. Effects of real-time feedback on cardiopulmonary resuscitation quality on outcomes in adult patients with cardiac arrest: A systematic review and meta-analysis. *Resuscitation* **2020**, *155*, 82–90. [CrossRef]
29. Goharani, R.; Vahedian-Azimi, A.; Farzanegan, B.; Bashar, F.R.; Hajiesmaeili, M.; Shojaei, S.; Madani, S.J.; Gohari-Moghaddam, K.; Hatamian, S.; Mosavinasab, S.M.M.; et al. Real-time compression feedback for patients with in-hospital cardiac arrest: A multi-center randomized controlled clinical trial. *J. Intensive Care* **2019**, *7*, 5. [CrossRef]
30. Goharani, R.; Vahedian-Azimi, A.; Pourhoseingholi, M.A.; Amanpour, F.; Rosano, G.M.C.; Sahebkar, A. Survival to intensive care unit discharge among in-hospital cardiac arrest patients by applying audiovisual feedback device. *ESC Heart Fail.* **2021**, *8*, 4652–4660. [CrossRef]
31. Hostler, D.; Everson-Stewart, S.; Rea, T.D.; Stiell, I.G.; Callaway, C.W.; Kudenchuk, P.J.; Sears, G.K.; Emerson, S.S.; Nichol, G.; Resuscitation Outcomes Consortium, I. Effect of real-time feedback during cardiopulmonary resuscitation outside hospital: Prospective, cluster-randomised trial. *Br. Med. J.* **2011**, *342*, d512. [CrossRef]
32. Wyckoff, M.H.; Greif, R.; Morley, P.T.; Ng, K.C.; Olasveengen, T.M.; Singletary, E.M.; Soar, J.; Cheng, A.; Drennan, I.R.; Liley, H.G.; et al. 2022 International Consensus on Cardiopulmonary Resuscitation and Emergency Cardiovascular Care Science With Treatment Recommendations: Summary From the Basic Life Support; Advanced Life Support; Pediatric Life Support; Neonatal Life Support; Education, Implementation, and Teams; and First Aid Task Forces. *Resuscitation* **2022**. [CrossRef]
33. Hallstrom, A.; Rea, T.D.; Sayre, M.R.; Christenson, J.; Anton, A.R.; Mosesso, V.N., Jr.; Van Ottingham, L.; Olsufka, M.; Pennington, S.; White, L.J.; et al. Manual chest compression vs use of an automated chest compression device during resuscitation following out-of-hospital cardiac arrest: A randomized trial. *JAMA* **2006**, *295*, 2620–2628. [CrossRef] [PubMed]
34. Wik, L.; Olsen, J.A.; Persse, D.; Sterz, F.; Lozano, M., Jr.; Brouwer, M.A.; Westfall, M.; Souders, C.M.; Malzer, R.; van Grunsven, P.M.; et al. Manual vs. integrated automatic load-distributing band CPR with equal survival after out of hospital cardiac arrest. The randomized CIRC trial. *Resuscitation* **2014**, *85*, 741–748. [CrossRef] [PubMed]
35. Rubertsson, S.; Lindgren, E.; Smekal, D.; Ostlund, O.; Silfverstolpe, J.; Lichtveld, R.A.; Boomars, R.; Ahlstedt, B.; Skoog, G.; Kastberg, R.; et al. Mechanical chest compressions and simultaneous defibrillation vs conventional cardiopulmonary resuscitation in out-of-hospital cardiac arrest: The LINC randomized trial. *JAMA* **2014**, *311*, 53–61. [CrossRef] [PubMed]
36. Perkins, G.D.; Lall, R.; Quinn, T.; Deakin, C.D.; Cooke, M.W.; Horton, J.; Lamb, S.E.; Slowther, A.M.; Woollard, M.; Carson, A.; et al. Mechanical versus manual chest compression for out-of-hospital cardiac arrest (PARAMEDIC): A pragmatic, cluster randomised controlled trial. *Lancet* **2015**, *385*, 947–955. [CrossRef]
37. Anantharaman, V.; Ng, B.L.; Ang, S.H.; Lee, C.Y.; Leong, S.H.; Ong, M.E.; Chua, S.J.; Rabind, A.C.; Anjali, N.B.; Hao, Y. Prompt use of mechanical cardiopulmonary resuscitation in out-of-hospital cardiac arrest: The MECCA study report. *Singapore Med. J.* **2017**, *58*, 424–431. [CrossRef]
38. Obermaier, M. Stellenwert von Kardiokompressionssystemen in der außer- und innerklinischen Reanimation: Eine retrospektive Registeranalyse und prospektive Metaanalyse. Ph.D. Thesis, Medizinische Fakultät, Universität Ulm, Open Access Repositorium of Ulm University (OPARU), Ulm, Germany, 2018.
39. Wang, P.L.; Brooks, S.C. Mechanical versus manual chest compressions for cardiac arrest. *Cochrane Database Syst. Rev.* **2018**, *8*, CD007260. [CrossRef]
40. Seewald, S.; Obermaier, M.; Lefering, R.; Bohn, A.; Georgieff, M.; Muth, C.-M.; Gräsner, J.-T.; Masterson, S.; Scholz, J.; Wnent, J. Application of mechanical cardiopulmonary resuscitation devices and their value in out-of-hospital cardiac arrest: A retrospective analysis of the German Resuscitation Registry. *PLoS ONE* **2019**, *14*, e0208113. [CrossRef]
41. Obermaier, M.; Seewald, S.; Muth, C.-M.; Gräsner, J.-T. Präklinischer Einsatz von Kardiokompressionssystemen und deren Rolle in der präklinischen Reanimation: Eine retrospektive Analyse des Deutschen Reanimationsregisters. *Anästhesiologie Intensivmed.* **2014**, *55*, S13–S14.
42. Wik, L.; Olsen, J.A.; Persse, D.; Sterz, F.; Lozano, M.; Brouwer, M.A.; Westfall, M.; Souders, C.M.; Malzer, R.; van Grunsven, P.M.; et al. Integrated autopulse CPR improves survival from out-of hospital cardiac arrests compared to manual CPR after controlling for EMS response times. *Circulation* **2013**, *128*, S1.
43. Ong, M.E.H.; Ornato, J.P.; Edwards, D.P.; Dhindsa, H.S.; Best, A.M.; Ines, C.S.; Hickey, S.; Clark, B.; Williams, D.C.; Powell, R.G.; et al. Use of an automated, load-distributing band chest compression device for out-of-hospital cardiac arrest resuscitation. *JAMA* **2006**, *295*, 2629–2637. [CrossRef] [PubMed]
44. Obermaier, M.; Zimmermann, J.B.; Popp, E.; Weigand, M.A.; Weiterer, S.; Dinse-Lambracht, A.; Muth, C.-M.; Nußbaum, B.L.; Gräsner, J.-T.; Seewald, S.; et al. Automated mechanical cardiopulmonary resuscitation devices versus manual chest compression in the treatment of cardiac arrest: Protocol of a systematic review and meta-analysis comparing machine to human. *BMJ Open* **2021**, *11*, e042062. [CrossRef] [PubMed]
45. Chiang, C.Y.; Lim, K.C.; Lai, P.C.; Tsai, T.Y.; Huang, Y.T.; Tsai, M.J. Comparison between Prehospital Mechanical Cardiopulmonary Resuscitation (CPR) Devices and Manual CPR for Out-of-Hospital Cardiac Arrest: A Systematic Review, Meta-Analysis, and Trial Sequential Analysis. *J. Clin. Med.* **2022**, *11*, 1448. [CrossRef] [PubMed]

46. Obermaier, M.; Schramm, C. LUCAS® leaving its footprints during cardiopulmonary resuscitation. *Vis. J. Emerg. Med.* **2019**, *17*, 100666. [CrossRef]
47. Obermaier, M.; Do, T.D. Hemodynamically Relevant Intrathoracic Bleeding Following CPR: Case Report on Resuscitation-associated Injury to Intercostal Arteries with the Need for Transcatheter Arterial Embolization. *Notarzt.* **2022**. [CrossRef]
48. Ondruschka, B.; Baier, C.; Bayer, R.; Hammer, N.; Dressler, J.; Bernhard, M. Chest compression-associated injuries in cardiac arrest patients treated with manual chest compressions versus automated chest compression devices (LUCAS II) - a forensic autopsy-based comparison. *Forensic Sci. Med. Pathol.* **2018**, *14*, 515–525. [CrossRef]
49. Ondruschka, B.; Baier, C.; Bernhard, M.; Buschmann, C.; Dressler, J.; Schlote, J.; Zwirner, J.; Hammer, N. Frequency and intensity of pulmonary bone marrow and fat embolism due to manual or automated chest compressions during cardiopulmonary resuscitation. *Forensic Sci. Med. Pathol.* **2019**, *15*, 48–55. [CrossRef]
50. Risom, M.; Jorgensen, H.; Rasmussen, L.S.; Sorensen, A.M. Resuscitation, prolonged cardiac arrest, and an automated chest compression device. *J. Emerg. Med.* **2010**, *38*, 481–483. [CrossRef]
51. Paal, P.; Brugger, H.; Boyd, J. Accidental hypothermia. *N. Engl. J. Med.* **2013**, *368*, 682. [CrossRef]
52. Holmstrom, P.; Boyd, J.; Sorsa, M.; Kuisma, M. A case of hypothermic cardiac arrest treated with an external chest compression device (LUCAS) during transport to re-warming. *Resuscitation* **2005**, *67*, 139–141. [CrossRef]
53. Wik, L.; Kiil, S. Use of an automatic mechanical chest compression device (LUCAS) as a bridge to establishing cardiopulmonary bypass for a patient with hypothermic cardiac arrest. *Resuscitation* **2005**, *66*, 391–394. [CrossRef] [PubMed]
54. Lott, C.; Truhlar, A.; Alfonzo, A.; Barelli, A.; Gonzalez-Salvado, V.; Hinkelbein, J.; Nolan, J.P.; Paal, P.; Perkins, G.D.; Thies, K.C.; et al. European Resuscitation Council Guidelines 2021: Cardiac arrest in special circumstances. *Resuscitation* **2021**, *161*, 152–219. [CrossRef]
55. Gässler, H.; Ventzke, M.M.; Lampl, L.; Helm, M. Transport with ongoing resuscitation: A comparison between manual and mechanical compression. *Emerg. Med. J.* **2013**, *30*, 589–592. [CrossRef] [PubMed]
56. Ventzke, M.M.; Gassler, H.; Lampl, L.; Helm, M. Cardio pump reloaded: In-hospital resuscitation during transport. *Intern Emerg. Med.* **2013**, *8*, 621–626. [CrossRef]
57. Gässler, H.; Kümmerle, S.; Ventzke, M.M.; Lampl, L.; Helm, M. Mechanical chest compression: An alternative in helicopter emergency medical services? *Intern Emerg. Med.* **2015**, *10*, 715–720. [CrossRef] [PubMed]
58. Bonnemeier, H.; Simonis, G.; Olivecrona, G.; Weidtmann, B.; Gotberg, M.; Weitz, G.; Gerling, I.; Strasser, R.; Frey, N. Continuous mechanical chest compression during in-hospital cardiopulmonary resuscitation of patients with pulseless electrical activity. *Resuscitation* **2011**, *82*, 155–159. [CrossRef]
59. Wirth, S.; Korner, M.; Treitl, M.; Linsenmaier, U.; Leidel, B.A.; Jaschkowitz, T.; Reiser, M.F.; Kanz, K.G. Computed tomography during cardiopulmonary resuscitation using automated chest compression devices—An initial study. *Eur. Radiol.* **2009**, *19*, 1857–1866. [CrossRef]
60. Schubert, E.C.; Kanz, K.G.; Linsenmaier, U.; Bogner, V.; Wirth, S.; Angstwurm, M. Use of computed tomography and mechanical CPR in cardiac arrest to confirm pulmonary embolism: A case study. *CJEM* **2016**, *18*, 66–69. [CrossRef]
61. Agarwala, R.; Barber, R. A pitfall of Autopulse. *Anaesthesia* **2011**, *66*, 142–143. [CrossRef]
62. Wagner, H.; Terkelsen, C.J.; Friberg, H.; Harnek, J.; Kern, K.; Lassen, J.F.; Olivecrona, G.K. Cardiac arrest in the catheterisation laboratory: A 5-year experience of using mechanical chest compressions to facilitate PCI during prolonged resuscitation efforts. *Resuscitation* **2010**, *81*, 383–387. [CrossRef]
63. Weiss, A.; Frisch, C.; Hornung, R.; Baubin, M.; Lederer, W. A retrospective analysis of fibrinolytic and adjunctive antithrombotic treatment during cardiopulmonary resuscitation. *Sci. Rep.* **2021**, *11*, 24095. [CrossRef]
64. Satler, L.F.; Pichard, A.D. The use of automated chest compression for arrest during TAVI. *Catheter. Cardiovasc. Interv.* **2013**, *82*, 849–850. [CrossRef]
65. Vatsgar, T.T.; Ingebrigtsen, O.; Fjose, L.O.; Wikstrom, B.; Nilsen, J.E.; Wik, L. Cardiac arrest and resuscitation with an automatic mechanical chest compression device (LUCAS) due to anaphylaxis of a woman receiving caesarean section because of pre-eclampsia. *Resuscitation* **2006**, *68*, 155–159. [CrossRef] [PubMed]
66. Dumans-Nizard, V.; Fischler, M. Intraoperative use of an automated chest compression device. *Anesthesiology* **2011**, *114*, 1253–1255. [CrossRef] [PubMed]
67. Wind, J.; Hoogland, E.R.; van Heurn, L.W. Preservation techniques for donors after cardiac death kidneys. *Curr. Opin. Organ. Transplant.* **2011**, *16*, 157–161. [CrossRef]
68. Gräsner, J.-T.; Jantzen, T.; Cavus, E.; Gries, A.; Breckwoldt, J.; Böttiger, B.W.; Bein, B.; Dörges, V.; Fischer, M.; Messelken, M.; et al. Neuheiten aus Ausbildung und Lehre, Grundlagenforschung, klinischen Studien und Qualitätsmanagement. 4. Wissenschafttliche Arbeitstage Notfallmedizin 2008 in Kiel. *Anästhesiologie Intensivmed.* **2008**, *49*, 679.
69. FDA. U.S. Food & Drug Administration Website. Available online: www.fda.gov (accessed on 27 July 2022).
70. Yannopoulos, D.; Bartos, J.; Raveendran, G.; Walser, E.; Connett, J.; Murray, T.A.; Collins, G.; Zhang, L.; Kalra, R.; Kosmopoulos, M.; et al. Advanced reperfusion strategies for patients with out-of-hospital cardiac arrest and refractory ventricular fibrillation (ARREST): A phase 2, single centre, open-label, randomised controlled trial. *Lancet* **2020**, *396*, 1807–1816. [CrossRef]
71. Rob, D.; Smalcova, J.; Smid, O.; Kral, A.; Kovarnik, T.; Zemanek, D.; Kavalkova, P.; Huptych, M.; Komarek, A.; Franek, O.; et al. Extracorporeal versus conventional cardiopulmonary resuscitation for refractory out-of-hospital cardiac arrest: A secondary analysis of the Prague OHCA trial. *Crit. Care* **2022**, *26*, 330. [CrossRef]

72. Grasner, J.T.; Wnent, J.; Herlitz, J.; Perkins, G.D.; Lefering, R.; Tjelmeland, I.; Koster, R.W.; Masterson, S.; Rossell-Ortiz, F.; Maurer, H.; et al. Survival after out-of-hospital cardiac arrest in Europe - Results of the EuReCa TWO study. *Resuscitation* **2020**, *148*, 218–226. [CrossRef]
73. Wengenmayer, T.; Rombach, S.; Ramshorn, F.; Biever, P.; Bode, C.; Duerschmied, D.; Staudacher, D.L. Influence of low-flow time on survival after extracorporeal cardiopulmonary resuscitation (eCPR). *Crit. Care* **2017**, *21*, 157. [CrossRef]
74. Mørk, S.R.; Bøtker, M.T.; Christensen, S.; Tang, M.; Terkelsen, C.J. Survival and neurological outcome after out-of-hospital cardiac arrest treated with and without mechanical circulatory support. *Resusc. Plus* **2022**, *10*, 100230. [CrossRef]
75. AWMF. *S3-Leitlinie 011/021: Einsatz der extrakorporalen Zirkulation (ECLS/ECMO) bei Herz- und Kreislaufversagen*; Arbeitsgemeinschaft der Wissenschaftlichen Medizinischen Fachgesellschaften (AWMF): Berlin, Germany, 2020.
76. Debaty, G.; Lamhaut, L.; Aubert, R.; Nicol, M.; Sanchez, C.; Chavanon, O.; Bouzat, P.; Durand, M.; Vanzetto, G.; Hutin, A.; et al. Prognostic value of signs of life throughout cardiopulmonary resuscitation for refractory out-of-hospital cardiac arrest. *Resuscitation* **2021**, *162*, 163–170. [CrossRef] [PubMed]
77. Kashiura, M.; Sugiyama, K.; Tanabe, T.; Akashi, A.; Hamabe, Y. Effect of ultrasonography and fluoroscopic guidance on the incidence of complications of cannulation in extracorporeal cardiopulmonary resuscitation in out-of-hospital cardiac arrest: A retrospective observational study. *BMC Anesthesiol.* **2017**, *17*, 4. [CrossRef] [PubMed]
78. Lamhaut, L.; Hutin, A.; Dagron, C.; Baud, F.; An, K.; Carli, P. A new hybrid technique for extracorporeal cardiopulmonary resuscitation for use by nonsurgeons. *Emergencias* **2021**, *33*, 156–157.
79. Danial, P.; Hajage, D.; Nguyen, L.S.; Mastroianni, C.; Demondion, P.; Schmidt, M.; Bougle, A.; Amour, J.; Leprince, P.; Combes, A.; et al. Percutaneous versus surgical femoro-femoral veno-arterial ECMO: A propensity score matched study. *Intensive Care Med.* **2018**, *44*, 2153–2161. [CrossRef] [PubMed]
80. Kirkpatrick, A.W.; Sirois, M.; Laupland, K.B.; Liu, D.; Rowan, K.; Ball, C.G.; Hameed, S.M.; Brown, R.; Simons, R.; Dulchavsky, S.A.; et al. Hand-held thoracic sonography for detecting post-traumatic pneumothoraces: The Extended Focused Assessment with Sonography for Trauma (EFAST). *J. Trauma* **2004**, *57*, 288–295. [CrossRef] [PubMed]
81. Breitkreutz, R.; Price, S.; Steiger, H.V.; Seeger, F.H.; Ilper, H.; Ackermann, H.; Rudolph, M.; Uddin, S.; Weigand, M.A.; Muller, E.; et al. Focused echocardiographic evaluation in life support and peri-resuscitation of emergency patients: A prospective trial. *Resuscitation* **2010**, *81*, 1527–1533. [CrossRef]
82. Nestaas, S.; Stensæth, K.H.; Rosseland, V.; Kramer-Johansen, J. Radiological assessment of chest compression point and achievable compression depth in cardiac patients. *Scand. J. Trauma Resusc. Emerg. Med.* **2016**, *24*, 54. [CrossRef]
83. Pickard, A.; Darby, M.; Soar, J. Radiological assessment of the adult chest: Implications for chest compressions. *Resuscitation* **2006**, *71*, 387–390. [CrossRef]
84. Shin, J.; Rhee, J.E.; Kim, K. Is the inter-nipple line the correct hand position for effective chest compression in adult cardiopulmonary resuscitation? *Resuscitation* **2007**, *75*, 305–310. [CrossRef]
85. Blaivas, M. Transesophageal echocardiography during cardiopulmonary arrest in the emergency department. *Resuscitation* **2008**, *78*, 135–140. [CrossRef]
86. Teran, F.; Dean, A.J.; Centeno, C.; Panebianco, N.L.; Zeidan, A.J.; Chan, W.; Abella, B.S. Evaluation of out-of-hospital cardiac arrest using transesophageal echocardiography in the emergency department. *Resuscitation* **2019**, *137*, 140–147. [CrossRef]
87. Pruszczyk, P.; Goliszek, S.; Lichodziejewska, B.; Kostrubiec, M.; Ciurzynski, M.; Kurnicka, K.; Dzikowska-Diduch, O.; Palczewski, P.; Wyzgal, A. Prognostic value of echocardiography in normotensive patients with acute pulmonary embolism. *JACC Cardiovasc. Imaging* **2014**, *7*, 553–560. [CrossRef]
88. Konstantinides, S.V.; Meyer, G.; Becattini, C.; Bueno, H.; Geersing, G.J.; Harjola, V.P.; Huisman, M.V.; Humbert, M.; Jennings, C.S.; Jimenez, D.; et al. 2019 ESC Guidelines for the diagnosis and management of acute pulmonary embolism developed in collaboration with the European Respiratory Society (ERS). *Eur. Heart J.* **2020**, *41*, 543–603. [CrossRef] [PubMed]
89. Wardi, G.; Blanchard, D.; Dittrich, T.; Kaushal, K.; Sell, R. Right ventricle dysfunction and echocardiographic parameters in the first 24h following resuscitation in the post-cardiac arrest patient: A retrospective cohort study. *Resuscitation* **2016**, *103*, 71–74. [CrossRef] [PubMed]
90. Righini, M.; Le Gal, G.; Aujesky, D.; Roy, P.-M.; Sanchez, O.; Verschuren, F.; Rutschmann, O.; Nonent, M.; Cornuz, J.; Thys, F.; et al. Diagnosis of pulmonary embolism by multidetector CT alone or combined with venous ultrasonography of the leg: A randomised non-inferiority trial. *Lancet* **2008**, *371*, 1343–1352. [CrossRef] [PubMed]
91. Alrajab, S.; Youssef, A.M.; Akkus, N.I.; Caldito, G. Pleural ultrasonography versus chest radiography for the diagnosis of pneumothorax: Review of the literature and meta-analysis. *Crit. Care* **2013**, *17*, R208. [CrossRef]
92. Obermaier, M.; Katzenschlager, S.; Schneider, N.R.E. Diagnostik und invasive Maßnahmen beim Thoraxtrauma. *AINS-Anästhesiologie Intensivmed. Notf. Schmerzther.* **2020**, *55*, 620–633. [CrossRef]
93. Hughes, C.W. Use of an intra-aortic balloon catheter tamponade for controlling intra-abdominal hemorrhage in man. *Surgery* **1954**, *36*, 65–68. [CrossRef]
94. King, D.R. Initial Care of the Severely Injured Patient. *N. Engl. J. Med.* **2019**, *380*, 763–770. [CrossRef]
95. Castellini, G.; Gianola, S.; Biffi, A.; Porcu, G.; Fabbri, A.; Ruggieri, M.P.; Coniglio, C.; Napoletano, A.; Coclite, D.; D'Angelo, D.; et al. Resuscitative endovascular balloon occlusion of the aorta (REBOA) in patients with major trauma and uncontrolled haemorrhagic shock: A systematic review with meta-analysis. *World J. Emerg. Surg.* **2021**, *16*, 41. [CrossRef] [PubMed]

96. Hutin, A.; Levy, Y.; Lidouren, F.; Kohlhauer, M.; Carli, P.; Ghaleh, B.; Lamhaut, L.; Tissier, R. Resuscitative endovascular balloon occlusion of the aorta vs epinephrine in the treatment of non-traumatic cardiac arrest in swine. *Ann. Intensive Care* **2021**, *11*, 81. [CrossRef] [PubMed]
97. Deakin, C.D.; Barron, D.J. Haemodynamic effects of descending aortic occlusion during cardiopulmonary resuscitation. *Resuscitation* **1996**, *33*, 49–52. [CrossRef] [PubMed]
98. Brede, J.R.; Lafrenz, T.; Klepstad, P.; Skjaerseth, E.A.; Nordseth, T.; Sovik, E.; Kruger, A.J. Feasibility of Pre-Hospital Resuscitative Endovascular Balloon Occlusion of the Aorta in Non-Traumatic Out-of-Hospital Cardiac Arrest. *J. Am. Heart Assoc.* **2019**, *8*, e014394. [CrossRef]
99. McGreevy, D.; Dogan, E.; Toivola, A.; Bilos, L.; Pirouzran, A.; Nilsson, K.; Hörer, T. Endovascular resuscitation with aortic balloon occlusion in non-trauma cases: First use of ER-REBOA in Europe. *J. Endovasc. Resusc. Trauma Manag.* **2017**, *1*, 42–49. [CrossRef]
100. Drumheller, B.C.; Pinizzotto, J.; Overberger, R.C.; Sabolick, E.E. Goal-directed cardiopulmonary resuscitation for refractory out-of-hospital cardiac arrest in the emergency Department: A feasibility study. *Resusc. Plus* **2021**, *7*, 100159. [CrossRef]
101. Levis, A.; Greif, R.; Hautz, W.E.; Lehmann, L.E.; Hunziker, L.; Fehr, T.; Haenggi, M. Resuscitative endovascular balloon occlusion of the aorta (REBOA) during cardiopulmonary resuscitation: A pilot study. *Resuscitation* **2020**, *156*, 27–34. [CrossRef]
102. Gamberini, L.; Coniglio, C.; Lupi, C.; Tartaglione, M.; Mazzoli, C.A.; Baldazzi, M.; Cecchi, A.; Ferri, E.; Chiarini, V.; Semeraro, F.; et al. Resuscitative endovascular occlusion of the aorta (REBOA) for refractory out of hospital cardiac arrest. An Utstein-based case series. *Resuscitation* **2021**, *165*, 161–169. [CrossRef]
103. Brede, J.R.; Skjaerseth, E.; Klepstad, P.; Nordseth, T.; Kruger, A.J. Changes in peripheral arterial blood pressure after resuscitative endovascular balloon occlusion of the aorta (REBOA) in non-traumatic cardiac arrest patients. *BMC Emerg. Med.* **2021**, *21*, 157. [CrossRef]
104. Jang, D.H.; Lee, D.K.; Jo, Y.H.; Park, S.M.; Oh, Y.T.; Im, C.W. Resuscitative endovascular occlusion of the aorta (REBOA) as a mechanical method for increasing the coronary perfusion pressure in non-traumatic out-of-hospital cardiac arrest patients. *Resuscitation* **2022**. [CrossRef]
105. Daley, J.; Buckley, R.; Kisken, K.C.; Barber, D.; Ayyagari, R.; Wira, C.; Aydin, A.; Latich, I.; Lozada, J.C.P.; Joseph, D.; et al. Emergency department initiated resuscitative endovascular balloon occlusion of the aorta (REBOA) for out-of-hospital cardiac arrest is feasible and associated with improvements in end-tidal carbon dioxide. *J. Am. Coll. Emerg. Physicians Open* **2022**, *3*, e12791. [CrossRef] [PubMed]
106. Daley, J.; Morrison, J.J.; Sather, J.; Hile, L. The role of resuscitative endovascular balloon occlusion of the aorta (REBOA) as an adjunct to ACLS in non-traumatic cardiac arrest. *Am. J. Emerg. Med.* **2017**, *35*, 731–736. [CrossRef] [PubMed]
107. Brede, J.R.; Skulberg, A.K.; Rehn, M.; Thorsen, K.; Klepstad, P.; Tylleskar, I.; Farbu, B.; Dale, J.; Nordseth, T.; Wiseth, R.; et al. REBOARREST, resuscitative endovascular balloon occlusion of the aorta in non-traumatic out-of-hospital cardiac arrest: A study protocol for a randomised, parallel group, clinical multicentre trial. *Trials* **2021**, *22*, 511. [CrossRef] [PubMed]
108. Wildner, G.; Pauker, N.; Archan, S.; Gemes, G.; Rigaud, M.; Pocivalnik, M.; Prause, G. Arterial line in prehospital emergency settings - A feasibility study in four physician-staffed emergency medical systems. *Resuscitation* **2011**, *82*, 1198–1201. [CrossRef]
109. Zwisler, S.T.; Zincuk, Y.; Bering, C.B.; Zincuk, A.; Nybo, M.; Mikkelsen, S. Diagnostic value of prehospital arterial blood gas measurements - a randomised controlled trial. *Scand. J. Trauma Resusc. Emerg. Med.* **2019**, *27*, 32. [CrossRef]
110. Gilbert, H.C.; Vender, J.S. Arterial Blood Gas Monitoring. *Crit. Care Clin.* **1995**, *11*, 233–248. [CrossRef] [PubMed]
111. Prause, G.; Ratzenhofer-Komenda, B.; Offner, A.; Lauda, P.; Voit, H.; Pojer, H. Prehospital point of care testing of blood gases and electrolytes - an evaluation of IRMA. *Crit. Care* **1997**, *1*, 79–83. [CrossRef]
112. Spindelboeck, W.; Gemes, G.; Strasser, C.; Toescher, K.; Kores, B.; Metnitz, P.; Haas, J.; Prause, G. Arterial blood gases during and their dynamic changes after cardiopulmonary resuscitation: A prospective clinical study. *Resuscitation* **2016**, *106*, 24–29. [CrossRef]
113. Spindelboeck, W.; Moser, A. Spontaneous tension pneumothorax and CO_2 narcosis in a near fatal episode of chronic obstructive pulmonary disease exacerbation. *Am. J. Emerg. Med.* **2012**, *30*, 1664.e3. [CrossRef]
114. Kleber, C.; Giesecke, M.T.; Tsokos, M.; Haas, N.P.; Buschmann, C.T. Trauma-related preventable deaths in Berlin 2010: Need to change prehospital management strategies and trauma management education. *World J. Surg.* **2013**, *37*, 1154–1161. [CrossRef]
115. Laan, D.V.; Vu, T.D.N.; Thiels, C.A.; Pandian, T.K.; Schiller, H.J.; Murad, M.H.; Aho, J.M. Chest wall thickness and decompression failure: A systematic review and meta-analysis comparing anatomic locations in needle thoracostomy. *Injury* **2016**, *47*, 797–804. [CrossRef] [PubMed]
116. Inaba, K.; Branco, B.C.; Eckstein, M.; Shatz, D.V.; Martin, M.J.; Green, D.J.; Noguchi, T.T.; Demetriades, D. Optimal positioning for emergent needle thoracostomy: A cadaver-based study. *J. Trauma* **2011**, *71*, 1099–1103. [CrossRef] [PubMed]
117. Advanced Trauma Life Support. *ATLS®10th Edition Compendium of Change*; American College of Surgeons: Chicago, IL, USA, 2018.
118. Joint Trauma System's (JTS) Committee on Tactical Combat Casualty Care (CoTCCC). Tactical Combat Casualty Care (TCCC) Guidelines for Medical Personnel. *J. Spec. Oper. Med.* **2022**, *22*, 11–17. [CrossRef]
119. Martin, M.; Satterly, S.; Inaba, K.; Blair, K. Does needle thoracostomy provide adequate and effective decompression of tension pneumothorax? *J. Trauma Acute Care Surg.* **2012**, *73*, 1412–1417. [CrossRef] [PubMed]
120. Garner, A.; Poynter, E.; Parsell, R.; Weatherall, A.; Morgan, M.; Lee, A. Association between three prehospital thoracic decompression techniques by physicians and complications: A retrospective, multicentre study in adults. *Eur. J. Trauma Emerg. Surg.* **2022**. [CrossRef]

121. Adler, Y.; Charron, P.; Imazio, M.; Badano, L.; Baron-Esquivias, G.; Bogaert, J.; Brucato, A.; Gueret, P.; Klingel, K.; Lionis, C.; et al. 2015 ESC Guidelines for the diagnosis and management of pericardial diseases: The Task Force for the Diagnosis and Management of Pericardial Diseases of the European Society of Cardiology (ESC)Endorsed by: The European Association for Cardio-Thoracic Surgery (EACTS). *Eur. Heart J.* **2015**, *36*, 2921–2964. [CrossRef]
122. Alerhand, S.; Carter, J.M. What echocardiographic findings suggest a pericardial effusion is causing tamponade? *Am. J. Emerg. Med.* **2019**, *37*, 321–326. [CrossRef]
123. Alpert, E.A.; Amit, U.; Guranda, L.; Mahagna, R.; Grossman, S.A.; Bentancur, A. Emergency department point-of-care ultrasonography improves time to pericardiocentesis for clinically significant effusions. *Clin. Exp. Emerg. Med.* **2017**, *4*, 128–132. [CrossRef]
124. Flaris, A.N.; Simms, E.R.; Prat, N.; Reynard, F.; Caillot, J.L.; Voiglio, E.J. Clamshell incision versus left anterolateral thoracotomy. Which one is faster when performing a resuscitative thoracotomy? The tortoise and the hare revisited. *World J. Surg.* **2015**, *39*, 1306–1311. [CrossRef]
125. Davies, G.E.; Lockey, D.J. Thirteen survivors of prehospital thoracotomy for penetrating trauma: A prehospital physician-performed resuscitation procedure that can yield good results. *J. Trauma* **2011**, *70*, E75–E78. [CrossRef]
126. Endo, A.; Shiraishi, A.; Otomo, Y.; Tomita, M.; Matsui, H.; Murata, K. Open-chest versus closed-chest cardiopulmonary resuscitation in blunt trauma: Analysis of a nationwide trauma registry. *Crit. Care* **2017**, *21*, 169. [CrossRef]
127. Tonna, J.E.; Keenan, H.T.; Weir, C. A qualitative analysis of physician decision making in the use of extracorporeal cardiopulmonary resuscitation for refractory cardiac arrest. *Resusc. Plus* **2022**, *11*, 100278. [CrossRef]
128. Tonna, J.E.; Becker, L.B.; Girotra, S.; Selzman, C.; Thiagarajan, R.R.; Presson, A.P.; Zhang, C.; Keenan, H.T. Resuscitation Using eCPR to Predict Survival After In-Hospital Cardiac Arrest (Rescue-IHCA Score) Survival Prediction Model–An Analysis of the American Heart Association Get With the Guidelines–Resuscitation Registry. *Circulation* **2019**, *140*, A205. [CrossRef]
129. Otani, T.; Sawano, H.; Natsukawa, T.; Nakashima, T.; Oku, H.; Gon, C.; Takahagi, M.; Hayashi, Y. Low-flow time is associated with a favorable neurological outcome in out-of-hospital cardiac arrest patients resuscitated with extracorporeal cardiopulmonary resuscitation. *J. Crit. Care* **2018**, *48*, 15–20. [CrossRef] [PubMed]
130. Al-Azri, N.H. How to think like an emergency care provider: A conceptual mental model for decision making in emergency care. *Int. J. Emerg. Med.* **2020**, *13*, 17. [CrossRef]
131. Alm-Kruse, K.; Sorensen, G.; Osbakk, S.A.; Sunde, K.; Bendz, B.; Andersen, G.O.; Fiane, A.; Hagen, O.A.; Kramer-Johansen, J. Outcome in refractory out-of-hospital cardiac arrest before and after implementation of an ECPR protocol. *Resuscitation* **2021**, *162*, 35–42. [CrossRef]
132. Michels, G.; Wengenmayer, T.; Hagl, C.; Dohmen, C.; Bottiger, B.W.; Bauersachs, J.; Markewitz, A.; Bauer, A.; Grasner, J.T.; Pfister, R.; et al. Recommendations for extracorporeal cardiopulmonary resuscitation (eCPR): Consensus statement of DGIIN, DGK, DGTHG, DGfK, DGNI, DGAI, DIVI and GRC. *Clin. Res. Cardiol.* **2019**, *108*, 455–464. [CrossRef] [PubMed]
133. Lacerenza, C.N.; Marlow, S.L.; Tannenbaum, S.I.; Salas, E. Team development interventions: Evidence-based approaches for improving teamwork. *Am. Psychol.* **2018**, *73*, 517–531. [CrossRef]
134. Couper, K.; Salman, B.; Soar, J.; Finn, J.; Perkins, G.D. Debriefing to improve outcomes from critical illness: A systematic review and meta-analysis. *Intensive Care Med.* **2013**, *39*, 1513–1523. [CrossRef]
135. Rudolph, J.W.; Simon, R.; Raemer, D.B.; Eppich, W.J. Debriefing as formative assessment: Closing performance gaps in medical education. *Acad. Emerg. Med.* **2008**, *15*, 1010–1016. [CrossRef]
136. Leong, K.; Hanskamp-Sebregts, M.; van der Wal, R.A.; Wolff, A.P. Effects of perioperative briefing and debriefing on patient safety: A prospective intervention study. *BMJ Open* **2017**, *7*, e018367. [CrossRef]
137. Johnson, T.J.; Millinchamp, F.J.; Kelly, F.E. Use of a team immediate debrief tool to improve staff well-being after potentially traumatic events. *Anaesthesia* **2021**, *76*, 1001–1002. [CrossRef]
138. Roehl, A.; Grottke, O. Prehospital administration of blood and plasma products. *Curr. Opin. Anaesthesiol.* **2021**, *34*, 507–513. [CrossRef] [PubMed]
139. Crombie, N.; Doughty, H.A.; Bishop, J.R.B.; Desai, A.; Dixon, E.F.; Hancox, J.M.; Herbert, M.J.; Leech, C.; Lewis, S.J.; Nash, M.R.; et al. Resuscitation with blood products in patients with trauma-related haemorrhagic shock receiving prehospital care (RePHILL): A multicentre, open-label, randomised, controlled, phase 3 trial. *Lancet Haematol.* **2022**, *9*, e250–e261. [CrossRef] [PubMed]
140. Thiels, C.A.; Aho, J.M.; Fahy, A.S.; Parker, M.E.; Glasgow, A.E.; Berns, K.S.; Habermann, E.B.; Zietlow, S.P.; Zielinski, M.D. Prehospital Blood Transfusions in Non-Trauma Patients. *World J. Surg.* **2016**, *40*, 2297–2304. [CrossRef] [PubMed]
141. Thies, K.C.; Truhlar, A.; Keene, D.; Hinkelbein, J.; Rutzler, K.; Brazzi, L.; Vivien, B. Pre-hospital blood transfusion—An ESA survey of European practice. *Scand. J. Trauma Resusc. Emerg. Med.* **2020**, *28*, 79. [CrossRef]

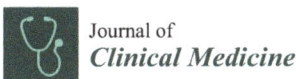

Article

Effect of a Targeted Ambulance Treatment Quality Improvement Programme on Outcomes from Out-of-Hospital Cardiac Arrest: A Metropolitan Citywide Intervention Study

Xuejie Dong [1,2,†], Liang Wang [3,†], Hanbing Xu [1], Yingfang Ye [3], Zhenxiang Zhou [3,*] and Lin Zhang [1,4,*]

1. School of Public Health, Shanghai Jiao Tong University, Shanghai 200025, China
2. Department of Global Health, Peking University School of Public Health, Beijing 100191, China
3. Suzhou Emergency Center, Suzhou 215002, China
4. School of Nursing, Shanghai Jiao Tong University, Shanghai 200025, China
* Correspondence: szjjzx120@163.com (Z.Z.); zhanglynn@sjtu.edu.cn (L.Z.); Tel.: +86-512-69352136 (Z.Z.); +86-21-63846590 (L.Z.)
† These authors contributed equally to this work.

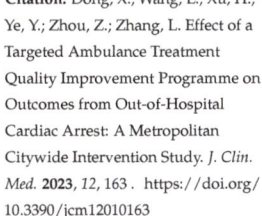

Citation: Dong, X.; Wang, L.; Xu, H.; Ye, Y.; Zhou, Z.; Zhang, L. Effect of a Targeted Ambulance Treatment Quality Improvement Programme on Outcomes from Out-of-Hospital Cardiac Arrest: A Metropolitan Citywide Intervention Study. *J. Clin. Med.* **2023**, *12*, 163. https://doi.org/10.3390/jcm12010163

Academic Editors: Michael Behnes and Tobias Schupp

Received: 31 October 2022
Revised: 18 December 2022
Accepted: 20 December 2022
Published: 25 December 2022

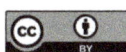

Copyright: © 2022 by the authors. Licensee MDPI, Basel, Switzerland. This article is an open access article distributed under the terms and conditions of the Creative Commons Attribution (CC BY) license (https://creativecommons.org/licenses/by/4.0/).

Abstract: The performance of ambulance crew affects the quality of pre-hospital treatment, which is vital to the survival for out-of-hospital cardiac arrest (OHCA) patients, yet remains suboptimal in China. In this retrospective analysis study, we aimed to examine the effect of a citywide quality improvement programme on provision of prehospital advanced life support (ALS) by emergency medical service (EMS) system. EMS-treated adult OHCA patients after the implementation of the programme (1 January 2021 to 30 June 2022) were compared with historical controls (1 June 2019 to 31 August 2020) in Suzhou. Multivariable logistic regression analysis and propensity score matching procedures were applied to compare the outcomes between two periods for total OHCA cases and subgroup of cases treated by fixed or non-fixed ambulance crews. A total of 1465 patients (pre-period/post-period: 610/855) were included. In the 1:1 matched analysis of 591 cases for each period, significant improvement ($p < 0.05$) was observed for the proportion of intravenous (IV) access (23.4% vs. 68.2%), advanced airway management (49.2% vs. 57.0%), and return of spontaneous circulation (ROSC) at handover (5.4% vs. 9.0%). The fixed ambulance crews performed better than non-fixed group in IV access and advanced airway management for both periods. There were significant increases in IV access (AOR 12.66, 95%CI 9.02–18.10, $p < 0.001$), advanced airway management (AOR 1.67, 95% CI 1.30–2.16, $p < 0.001$) and ROSC at handover (AOR 2.37, 95%CI 1.38–4.23, $p = 0.002$) after intervention in unfixed group, while no significant improvement was observed in fixed group except for IV access (AOR 7.65, 95%CI 9.02–18.10, $p < 0.001$). In conclusion, the quality improvement program was positively associated with the provision of prehospital ALS interventions and prehospital ROSC following OHCA. The fixed ambulance crews performed better in critical care provision and prehospital outcome, yet increased protocol adherence and targeted training could fill the underperformance of non-fixed crews efficaciously.

Keywords: out-of-hospital cardiac arrest; quality improvement; advanced life support; ROSC; ambulance crew

1. Introduction

Out-of-hospital cardiac arrest (OHCA) is a major public health problem globally with high mortality, high morbidity, and large variation in survival between communities [1]. In China, the incidence of cardiac arrest was estimated to be 550,000 cases per year and the survival was only 1–2% [2,3]. The survival outcome of OHCA is largely determined by the timelines and performance of pre-hospital interventions, known as the "chain of survival", and could be affected by patient factors, event factors, and system factors of the emergency medical service (EMS) system [4]. The EMS is not only the first healthcare encounter providing advanced life support (ALS) to OHCA patients, but also works its way through monitoring of all the prehospital links in the chain of survival [5,6]. Hence, enhancing EMS performance and quality is fundamental for improving OHCA outcomes.

Various systemic attempts have been made to optimize the timelines and quality of EMS performance [7,8]. Studies have shown improved patient outcomes with higher adherence to guideline components within EMS systems, including EMS performed high-quality cardiopulmonary resuscitation (CPR), team-based training, structured resuscitation choreography, training, feedback, and profiling [9–13]. Quality improvement programmes focusing on above components have been shown to be associated with improved EMS performance and increased patient survival [10,14].

The performance of EMS personnel is a modifiable factor that may also influence patient outcome. Studies have found that ambulance crew staffing models and numbers [15,16], staffing patterns [17], level of training or individual experience [18,19] all affect the ambulance crew performance and outcome. The EMS in China has adopted a supplementary physician or physician-paramedic model for ambulance advanced care: the prehospital medical crew of the urban EMS typically consists of one physician, one nurse, one stretcher-bearer, and one driver [20,21]. The crew configuration and the number of personnel on the ambulance are always the same. It was hypothesized that a fixed ambulance crew (i.e., the crew members remain the same) would perform better than the unfixed one (i.e., the crew members would be changed) with more tacit understanding of each other and better team coordination. However, there is relatively little evidence to address the differences in the quality of care and patient outcomes performed by fixed or unfixed ambulance crew.

In China, the survival rate of OHCA remains poor for years, and new interventions are needed for further optimization. Suzhou EMS first employed the dispatcher-assisted CPR (DA-CPR) protocols in China from 2010, and equipped itself with improved information technology [22]. In 2020, based on evidence that higher adherence to guidelines, targeted training, monitoring and feedback, and coordinated ambulance crews improve OHCA outcomes, Suzhou EMS implemented a 4-month (from 1 September 2020 to 30 December 2020) citywide quality improvement programme, including a standardization of ambulance treatment protocol, targeted training of ambulance crew combined with quality monitoring and feedback throughout the whole process.

The purpose of this study was to examine the impact of this quality improvement programme on provision of prehospital ALS for OHCA patients and prehospital return of spontaneous circulation (ROSC). Moreover, we tested the hypothesis that fixed ambulance crew would be correlated with better performance and patient outcome.

2. Materials and Methods

2.1. Study Design

This was a retrospective analysis of prospectively collected EMS registry data of Suzhou EMS from 1 July 2019 to 30 June 2022, to investigate the effects of quality improvement interventions on ALS treatment and outcome of OHCA patients. Adult OHCA patients (aged $\geq$ 18 years) receiving EMS treatment after the implementation of the quality improvement programme between 1 January 2021 and 30 June 2022 were compared with historical controls between 1 July 2019 and 31 August 2020. Cases during the COVID-19 epidemic periods (1 February 2020 to 30 April 2020, and 1 February 2022 to 30 April 2022) were excluded.

2.2. Setting

Suzhou EMS center services a population of about 6.7 million people across 2996 square kilometers in 6 urban districts with an annual emergency call volume of $\approx$412,000 and annual ambulance dispatch volume of $\approx$144,000. The EMS center consists of 157 physicians, 176 nurses, 83 stretcher-bearers, and 171 drivers responding from 45 stations (1 directly affiliated station and 44 network stations), and works its way through dispatching, prehospital transport, and treatment of patients. The Medical Priority Dispatch System (MPDS) protocol is used by Suzhou EMS since 2011. For suspected cardiac arrests, DA-CPR is delivered and the nearest available ambulance unit is dispatched to perform ALS care.

Each ambulance unit consists of one physician, one nurse, one stretcher-bearer, and one driver. According to the way physician and nurse are partnered, the ambulance units were classified into two types: fixed and unfixed. In a fixed unit, one physician would always work with the same nurse, and they may cooperate with specific stretcher-bearer/driver or not. In an unfixed unit, there is no specific partnership between physician and nurse, one physician would work with different nurses on every duty, and they may cooperate with specific stretcher-bearer/driver or not. It should be mentioned that the physician in a fixed unit is a dedicated prehospital personnel who only works on ambulance, while in an unfixed unit, the physician could be dedicated prehospital personnel or rotated from in-hospital emergency department or other in-hospital departments. During the study period, there were 11 fixed ambulance crew stations and 34 unfixed stations in Suzhou EMS.

2.3. Intervention

In 2020, Suzhou EMS implemented a 4-month (from 1 September 2020 to 31 December 2020) citywide quality improvement programme consisting of the following: (1) standardized ambulance treatment protocol adopted, (2) ambulance crew targeted training, (3) quality monitoring, feedback, and post-event debriefing.

2.3.1. Standardized Ambulance Treatment Protocol Adopted

On 1 September 2020, Suzhou EMS launched a prehospital standardized ambulance treatment protocol for OHCA patients, as shown in Figure 1, which was the first ALS treatment protocol for ambulance crews. Previously, although the ambulance crews performed according to the treatment guidelines, there was no unified ALS team choreography, and each team mainly operated according to their own experience. It was usual that the physician on the ambulance dictated the treatment measures, which could lead to a large variation in ALS treatment quality. The standardized treatment protocol was developed in line with the updated ALS guidelines (further modified based on the 2020 American Heart Association (AHA) guideline in October 2020), combined with the best practices of well-performing local EMS stations. The standardized treatment protocol highlighted the flow of ALS interventions, the specific role for each member of ambulance crews, and the timing for hospital transfer or termination of resuscitation. Consistent with the indeterminate evidence regarding duration of resuscitative efforts, no time limit was given for field attempts, but it was suggested that all appropriate resuscitation efforts be made and that efforts should continue until (1) the patient be transported if good prognostic signs were present after field efforts; (2) the declaration of death; or (3) strong demand for transfer from the patient's families.

2.3.2. Ambulance Crew Targeted Training

All personnel of EMS stations were instructed in the standardized protocol using lectures and simulated practices over a 4-month period. They underwent live didactic training on the updated AHA guidelines, the standardized protocol, and its key indicators measures. Experiences from the best-performing EMS stations were shared. An adding lecture was held after the 2020 AHA ALS guideline update released in October 2020. In the practice sessions, all ambulance crews performed hands-on simulated resuscitations using mannequins with feedback function, supervised by the medical director and medical division officers.

2.3.3. Quality Monitoring, Feedback, and Post-Event Debriefing

The EMS medical director (L. Wang) performed a post-incident review of all cardiac arrests. A monthly feedback report was sent to each EMS stations and every ambulance crew involved in the resuscitation at the end of each month. Direct feedback was provided to the ambulance crew in person if any corrective action was needed.

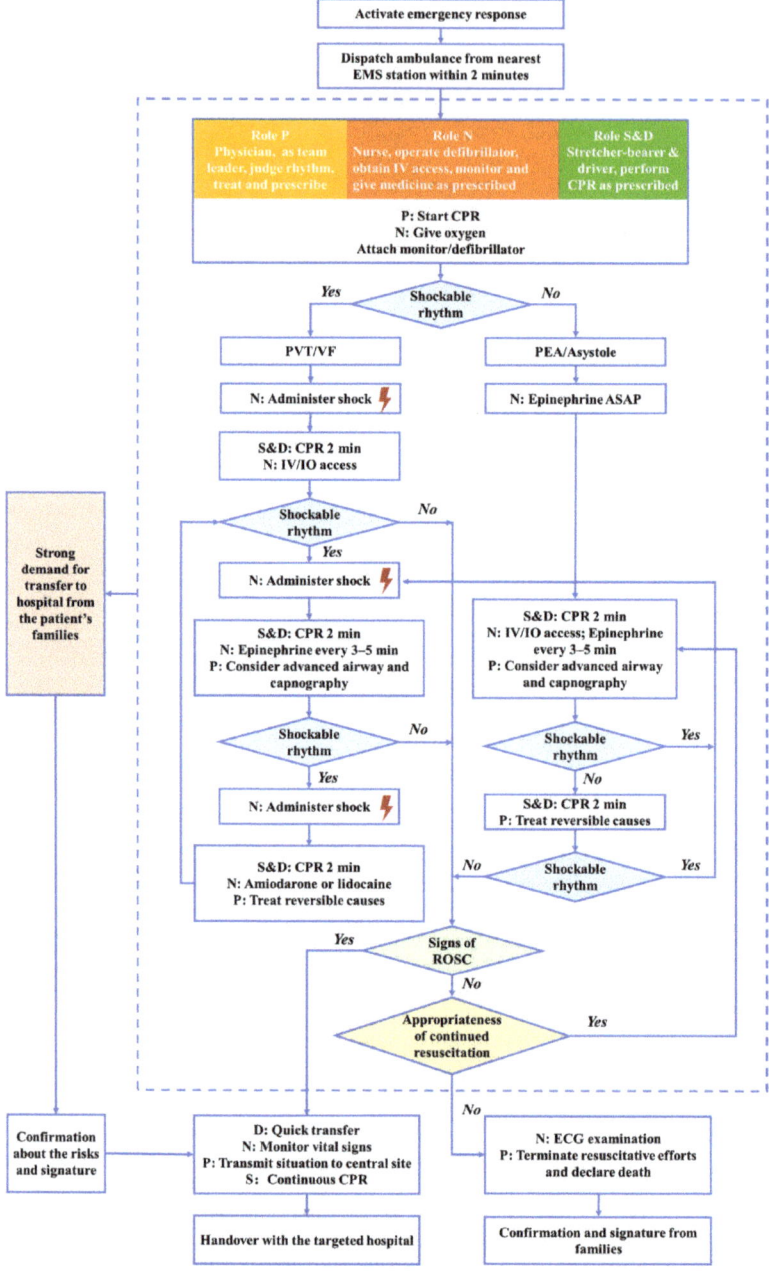

Figure 1. The standardized ambulance treatment protocol for OHCA patients. EMS, emergency medical services; OHCA, out-of-hospital cardiac arrest; CPR, cardiopulmonary resuscitation; PVT, pulseless ventricular tachycardia; VF, ventricular fibrillation; PEA, pulseless electrical activity; IV, intravenous; IO, intraosseous; ROSC, return of spontaneous circulation; ECG, electrocardiograph.

2.4. Data Source

This study used data from the MPDS system registry and pre-hospital electronic medical record system of Suzhou EMS. The MPDS system registry is generated automatically along with the dispatching process and recorded the patient's age, gender, location, chief complaint, dispatcher suspected disease, and the duration of each phase of the dispatch instructions. The pre-hospital electronic medical record is filled by ambulance physicians at the field using a tablet computer, and completed after transporting the patients to in-hospital emergency department, which contains patient's symptoms, field diagnosis, disease history, treatment measures, pre-hospital outcome, time intervals, EMS station and ambulance personnel.

2.5. Study Population

All EMS-treated patients with OHCA between 1 July 2019 and 30 June 2022 were included. Patients who were confirmed dead at scene, whose resuscitation was not initiated or refused, who were only transferred from one hospital to another, pediatric patients younger than 18 years of age, and those cases in which time variables were missing or treated by stations built after the quality improvement programme were excluded. There were two COVID-19 epidemic periods in Suzhou: 1 February 2020 to 30 April 2020 and 1 February 2022 to 30 April 2022, respectively. The ambulance treatment protocol during epidemic was different from that of epidemic-free period, thus OHCA cases occurring in these two periods were excluded (Figure 2).

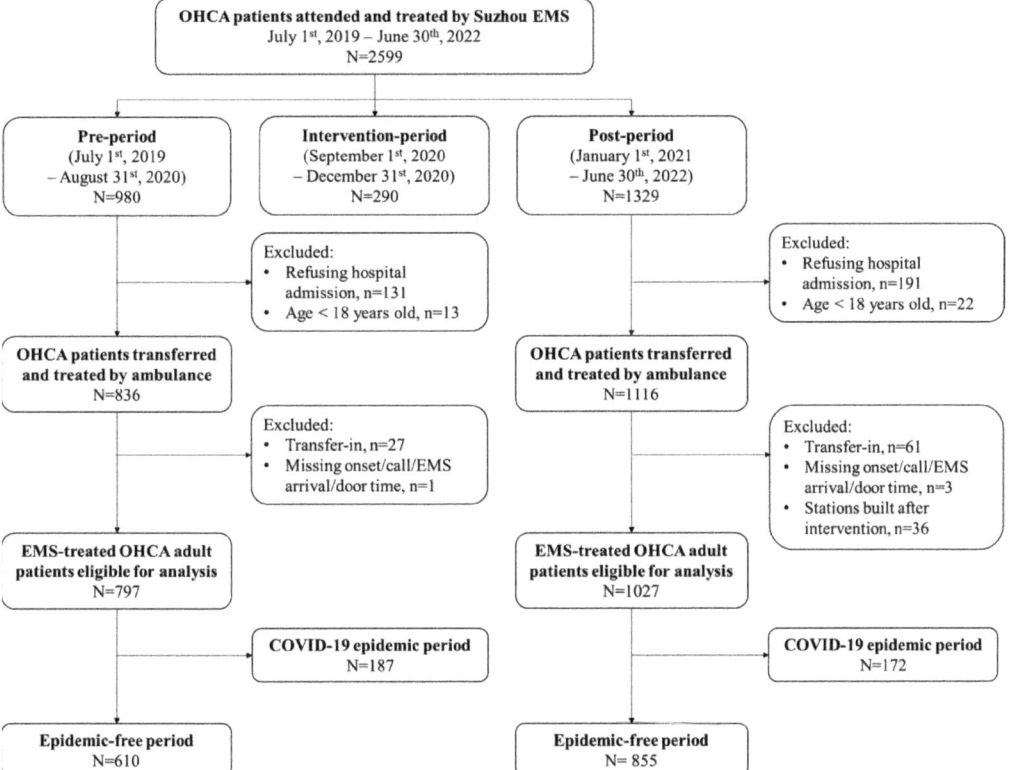

Figure 2. Patient flowchart. OHCA, out-of-hospital cardiac arrest; EMS, emergency medical services. There were 2 COVID-19 epidemic periods in Suzhou: 1 February 2020 to 30 April 2020 of pre-period, and 1 February 2022 to 30 April 2022 of post-period, respectively.

2.6. Data Collection and Outcome Measures

The primary outcome was the proportion of ROSC at handover at hospital. The secondary outcomes were prehospital ALS interventions by ambulance crews, including defibrillation, intravenous (IV) access, IV epinephrine administration, and advanced airway management. Outcomes were obtained from the pre-hospital electronic medical record system.

The following variables of interests were collected: patient demographics (age, gender), event characteristics (location of arrest, date and time of arrest, cardiovascular disease (CVD) history, etiology, onset-to-call time [from symptom onset to call receiving time]), EMS system factors (response interval [from call receiving time to scene arrival time of the ambulance crew], scene interval [from scene arrival time of the ambulance crew to departure time from the scene], transport interval [from the departure time from the scene to emergency department (ED) arrival time], prehospital interval [from call receiving time to ED arrival time], ambulance crew type), prehospital ALS interventions (EMS defibrillation, IV access, IV epinephrine administration, advanced airway management), intervention period (pre- and post-intervention period), prehospital ROSC (ROSC at handover).

2.7. Statistical Analysis

The patient demographics, event characteristic, EMS system factors, prehospital ALS interventions, and prehospital ROSC were compared between pre-intervention and post-intervention period. Normal distribution was confirmed using the Kolmogorov–Smirnov test. Continuous variables with normal distribution were shown as mean (standard deviation, SD), and compared by student t test. Continuous variables with non-normal distribution were shown as median (interquartile range, IQR), and compared using Wilcoxon test. Categorical variables were presented as the number (percentage), and compared using chi square test.

To compare the proportions of prehospital ALS interventions and ROSC at handover at hospital between two groups, both propensity score-matching analysis and logistic regression analysis were conducted to adjust for selection bias. In propensity score-matching analysis, we calculate estimated propensity score by fitting a logistic regression model that included age, gender, location, onset on weekend, call time of the day, CVD history, etiology, onset-to-call-time, call-to-arrival time, on-scene time, scene-to-hospital time, call-to-hospital time, ambulance crew type. We performed 1:1 matching without replacement for each patient, using a nearest-neighbor matching algorithm with a caliper width of 0.02. Matched patients were compared to assess balance in covariates (i.e., standardized differences for each covariate were <10%). For total OHCA cases and subgroup of fixed and non-fixed ambulance crew, a multivariable logistic regression model adjusted for age, gender, location, onset on weekend, call time of the day, CVD history, etiology, onset-to-call time, call-to-arrive time was used to compare the proportions of prehospital ALS interventions between the two groups to calculate the adjusted odds ratio (AOR) and 95% confidence interval (95% CI). Another multivariable logistic regression model adjusted for age, gender, location, onset on weekend, call time of the day, CVD history, etiology, onset-to-call time, call-to-arrive time, on-scene time, scene-to-hospital time was used to compare the proportion of ROSC at handover at hospital.

A two-sided significance level of less than 0.05 was considered statistically significant. All statistical analyses were performed using R software version 4.0.4.

3. Results

3.1. Patient Characteristics

A total of 2599 OHCA patients were treated by Suzhou EMS during the study period. The EMS attended and treated OHCA incidence rates of urban districts in Suzhou were 11.8, 13.0, 13.2, 13.2 per 100,000 population per year from 2019 to 2022. After exclusion of patients during the intervention-period and COVID-19 epidemic periods, 1465 patients were included as total study population. Of these, 610 (41.6%) and 855 (58.4%) occurred during the pre- and post-intervention periods, respectively. All included patients were witnessed and called for help by bystanders, attended and treated by EMS, all received CPR by EMS on-scene and during transport.

The patient demographics and event factors were similar between two periods. The post-period group showed longer scene interval [5.6 (3.0, 9.2) > 5.2 (2.6, 8.5) min, $p = 0.033$], longer transport interval [8.8 (5.3, 14.2) > 7.1 (4.4, 10.3) min, $p < 0.001$], longer prehospital interval [28.7 (22.0, 36.2) > 25.7 (20.8, 33.4) min, $p < 0.001$], and higher proportion of non-fixed ambulance crew (74.5% vs. 69.3%, $p = 0.033$) than the pre-period (Table 1).

Table 1. Demographics, prognostic factors, and outcomes of OHCA patients during the pre-period and post-period in total cases and propensity score matched cases.

	Total Cases (N = 1465)			Propensity Score-Matched Cases [a] (N = 1206)			
	Pre-Period (N = 610)	Post-Period (N = 855)	p	Pre-Period (N = 591)	Post-Period (N = 591)	p	SMD
Gender = female, n (%)	154 (25.2)	221 (25.8)	0.81	150 (25.4)	148 (25.0)	0.95	0.008
Age, mean (SD)	60.88 (17.85)	62.31 (16.65)	0.12	60.83 (17.88)	60.72 (16.84)	0.91	0.006
Location = home, n (%)	372 (61.0)	530 (62.0)	0.70	360 (60.9)	358 (60.6)	0.95	0.007
Onset on weekend, n (%)	190 (31.1)	243 (28.4)	0.27	183 (31.0)	178 (30.1)	0.80	0.018
Call time of day, n (%)			0.91			0.95	0.034
0:00–5:59	84 (13.8)	114 (13.3)		82 (13.9)	78 (13.2)		
6:00–11:59	198 (32.5)	266 (31.1)		189 (32.0)	191 (32.3)		
12:00–17:59	176 (28.9)	260 (30.4)		174 (29.4)	181 (30.6)		
18:00–23:59	152 (24.9)	215 (25.1)		146 (24.7)	141 (23.9)		
CVD history, n (%)	190 (31.1)	302 (35.3)	0.10	188 (31.8)	181 (30.6)	0.71	0.026
Presumed cardiac etiology, n (%)	444 (72.8)	655 (76.6)	0.10	435 (73.6)	432 (73.1)	0.89	0.011
Onset-to-call time, min, Median (IQR)	15.0 (10.0, 20.0)	15.0 (10.0, 20.0)	0.35	15.0 (10.0, 20.0)	15.00 (10.0, 20.0)	0.26	0.046
Response interval, min, Median (IQR)	11.8 (9.1, 15.5)	11.4 (8.6, 15.2)	0.07	11.8 (9.0, 15.5)	12.0 (8.8, 15.9)	0.88	0.004
Scene interval, min, Median (IQR)	5.2 (2.6, 8.5)	5.6 (3.0, 9.2)	0.033	5.2 (2.7, 8.5)	5.1 (2.8, 8.3)	0.84	0.038
Transport interval, min, Median (IQR)	7.1 (4.4, 10.3)	8.8 (5.3, 14.2)	<0.001	7.0 (4.4, 10.3)	7.6 (4.6, 11.9)	0.23	0.069
Prehospital interval, min, Median (IQR)	25.7 (20.8, 33.4)	28.7 (22.0, 36.2)	<0.001	25.7 (20.8, 33.3)	27.4 (20.9, 34.7)	0.13	0.031
Ambulance crew type, n (%)			0.033			1	0.004
Fixed	187 (30.7)	218 (25.5)		186 (31.5)	185 (31.3)		
Non-fixed	423 (69.3)	637 (74.5)		405 (68.5)	406 (68.7)		
Treatment-EMS defibrillation, n (%)	34 (5.6)	42 (4.9)	0.63	34 (5.8)	18 (3.0)	0.032	/
Treatment-IV access, n (%)	139 (22.8)	580 (67.8)	<0.001	138 (23.4)	403 (68.2)	<0.001	/
Treatment-IV epinephrine use, n (%)	5 (0.8)	15 (1.8)	0.17	5 (0.8)	10 (1.7)	0.29	/
Treatment-airway, n (%)	296 (48.5)	492 (57.5)	0.001	291 (49.2)	337 (57.0)	0.009	/
ROSC at handover at hospital, n (%)	32 (5.2)	77 (9.0)	0.008	32 (5.4)	53 (9.0)	0.024	/

[a] Propensity score matched for: gender, age, location, onset on weekend, call time of the day, CVD history, etiology, onset-to-call time, call-to-arrive time, on-scene time, scene-to-hospital time, call-to-hospital time, ambulance crew type. OHCA, out–of-hospital cardiac arrest; CVD, cardiovascular disease; EMS, emergency medical services; ROSC, return of spontaneous circulation; IV, intravenous; SD, standard deviation; IQR, interquartile range; SMD, standardized mean differences.

3.2. Main Analysis

After propensity score matching, 591 patients of both groups were matched, the post-matching standardized mean differences were <10% for all matching covariates. In matched cases, the post-intervention group showed higher proportion of IV access (68.2% vs. 23.4%, $p < 0.001$) and advanced airway management (57.0% vs. 49.2%, $p = 0.009$), lower proportion of EMS defibrillation (3.0% vs. 5.8%, $p = 0.032$). The ROSC rate at handover at hospital was significantly improved after the intervention (9.0% vs. 5.4%, $p = 0.024$) (Table 1).

In the multivariable logistic regression model of total cases, the intervention was associated with higher proportion of IV access (AOR: 7.23; 95%CI: 5.69–9.24, $p < 0.001$), advanced airway management (AOR: 1.41; 95%CI: 1.14–1.75, $p = 0.002$), and ROSC at handover at hospital (AOR: 1.81, 95%CI: 1.18–2.84, $p = 0.008$) (Figure 3).

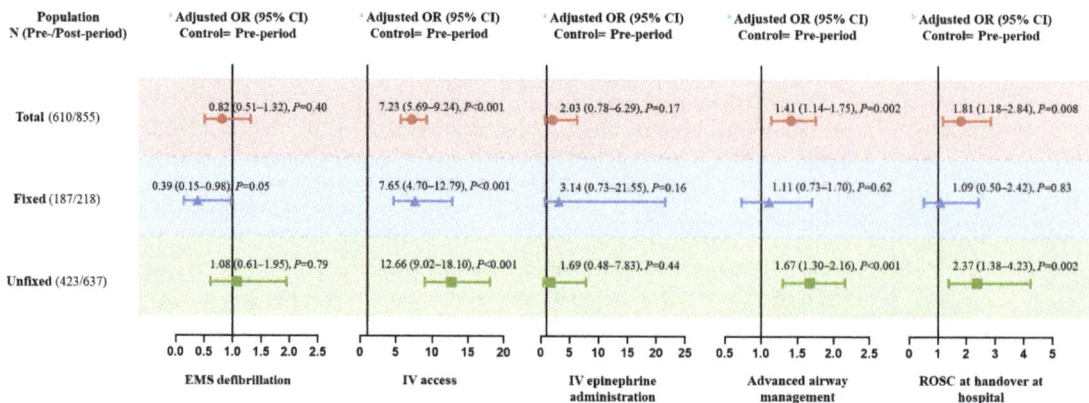

Figure 3. Adjusted logistic regression analysis of the effect of the improvement intervention on outcomes in EMS-treated OHCA patients by the type of ambulance crew. (ORs were calculated for post-period vs. pre-period; [a] Adjusted for gender, age, location, onset on weekend, call time of the day, CVD history, etiology, onset-to-call time, call-to-arrive time; [b] Adjusted for gender, age, location, onset on weekend, call time of the day, CVD history, etiology, onset-to-call time, call-to-arrive time, on-scene time, scene-to-hospital time.). EMS, emergency medical services; OHCA, out-of-hospital cardiac arrest; CVD, cardiovascular disease; IV, intravenous; ROSC, return of spontaneous circulation; OR, odds ratio; CI, confidence interval.

3.3. Subgroup Analysis by Types of Ambulance Crew

Table 2 and Figure 3 showed the results of subgroup analysis by types of ambulance crew. For prehospital ALS interventions, the proportions of IV access and advanced airway management were significantly higher in fixed group than non-fixed group both in pre-period and post-period. The multivariable logistic regression results suggested a significant increase in the proportion of IV access in fixed group (AOR: 7.65; 95% CI: 4.70–12.79, $p < 0.001$), proportions of IV access (AOR: 12.66; 95%CI: 9.02–18.10, $p < 0.001$) and advanced airway management (AOR: 1.67; 95%CI: 1.30–2.16, $p < 0.001$) in non-fixed group.

Table 2. Demographics, prognostic factors, and outcomes of OHCA patients treated by fixed or non-fixed EMS stations during the pre-period and post-period.

	Pre-Period (N = 610)			Post-Period (N = 855)		
	Fixed Crew (N = 187)	Non-Fixed Crew (N = 423)	p	Fixed Crew (N = 218)	Non-Fixed Crew (N = 637)	p
Gender = female, n (%)	47 (25.1)	107 (25.3)	1.0	53 (24.3)	168 (26.4)	0.59
Age, mean (SD)	61.19 (18.04)	60.74 (17.79)	0.78	64.18 (16.13)	61.67 (16.79)	0.06
Location = home, n (%)	114 (61.0)	258 (61.0)	1.0	136 (62.4)	394 (61.9)	0.94
Onset on weekend, n (%)	63 (33.7)	127 (30.0)	0.39	67 (30.7)	176 (27.6)	0.39
Call time of day, n (%)			0.45			0.66
0:00–5:59	23 (12.3)	61 (14.4)		26 (11.9)	88 (13.8)	
6:00–11:59	69 (36.9)	129 (30.5)		71 (32.6)	195 (30.6)	
12:00–17:59	49 (26.2)	127 (30.0)		71 (32.6)	189 (29.7)	
18:00–23:59	46 (24.6)	106 (25.1)		50 (22.9)	165 (25.9)	
CVD history, n (%)	57 (30.5)	133 (31.4)	0.85	79 (36.2)	223 (35.0)	0.74
Presumed cardiac etiology, n (%)	144 (77.0)	300 (70.9)	0.14	179 (82.1)	476 (74.7)	0.026
Onset-to-call time, min, Median (IQR)	20.00 (10.00, 20.00)	15.00 (10.00, 20.00)	0.018	20.00 (10.00, 20.00)	15.00 (10.00, 20.00)	0.034
Response interval, min, Median (IQR)	11.03 (8.63, 13.96)	12.45 (9.50, 16.21)	<0.001	11.80 (9.07, 15.21)	11.28 (8.47, 15.18)	0.49
Scene interval, min, Median (IQR)	5.27 (2.69, 7.74)	5.08 (2.48, 8.79)	0.93	4.94 (2.78, 7.82)	5.82 (3.03, 9.60)	0.024
Transport interval, min, Median (IQR)	7.60 (5.03, 10.38)	6.73 (4.28, 10.25)	0.049	9.47 (6.13, 13.37)	8.58 (4.98, 14.72)	0.27

Table 2. *Cont.*

	Pre-Period (N = 610)			Post-Period (N = 855)		
	Fixed Crew (N = 187)	Non-Fixed Crew (N = 423)	p	Fixed Crew (N = 218)	Non-Fixed Crew (N = 637)	p
Prehospital interval, min, Median (IQR)	24.80 (21.15, 32.27)	26.18 (20.74, 34.51)	0.25	28.55 (21.97, 35.14)	28.76 (22.06, 36.96)	0.33
Treatment-EMS defibrillation, n (%)	14 (7.5)	20 (4.7)	0.13	8 (3.7)	34 (5.3)	0.37
Treatment-IV access, n (%)	90 (48.1)	49 (11.6)	<0.001	189 (86.7)	391 (61.4)	<0.001
Treatment-epinephrine use, n (%)	2 (1.1)	3 (0.7)	0.65	7 (3.2)	8 (1.3)	0.07
Treatment-airway, n (%)	122 (65.2)	174 (41.1)	<0.001	149 (68.3)	343 (53.8)	<0.001
ROSC at handover at hospital, n (%)	14 (7.5)	18 (4.3)	0.12	17 (7.8)	60 (9.4)	0.58

OHCA, out-of-hospital cardiac arrest; CVD, cardiovascular disease; EMS, emergency medical services; ROSC, return of spontaneous circulation; IV, intravenous; SD, standard deviation; IQR, interquartile range.

In terms of ROSC at handover at hospital, though it was not statistically significant, higher ROSC rate was achieved in fixed group in pre-period (7.5% vs. 4.3%, p = 0.12), and in non-fixed group in the post-period (7.8% vs. 9.4%, p = 0.58). The intervention significantly improved the prehospital ROSC rate in the non-fixed group (AOR: 2.37; 95%CI: 1.38–4.23, p = 0.002), while showed no obvious effect in the fixed group (AOR: 1.09; 95%CI: 0.50–2.42, p = 0.83).

4. Discussion

In this metropolitan citywide intervention study, the implementation of a quality improvement programme, including a standardization of ambulance treatment protocol, targeted training of ambulance crew, and quality monitoring and feedback, improved the prehospital outcome of OHCA patients. Specifically, the intervention was associated with higher prehospital ROSC rate, and more prehospital ALS interventions such as IV access and advanced airway management. Subgroup analysis indicated that, compared with non-fixed crews, the fixed ambulance crew performed better in prehospital ALS interventions. The quality improvement programme increased the proportion of prehospital IV access, advanced airway management, and ROSC in non-fixed ambulance crew, while a non-significant improvement was seen in the fixed group.

The implementation of continuous quality improvement is an alternative approach to improving OHCA survival, which has been advocated and proved by many EMS systems [7,8,14]. Our findings added to the existing evidence that guideline adherence, coordination of tasks, team-focused resuscitation, and feedback are all instrumental in helping the EMS crews with improved treatment quality [9–11]. The adoption of standardized protocol is important as it provides a highly organized team treatment guide for chaotic resuscitation effort in most underperforming crews. Comparing with the proportions of pre-hospital drug administration and defibrillation in countries of high ROSC rates, such as Australia (40.4%/60.9%) [14], Germany (54.0%/25.1%) [23], and Japan (22.3%/59.2%) [24], the proportions of epinephrine administration (0.8% vs. 1.8%) and defibrillation (5.6% vs. 4.9%) remain comparatively low in China. As a result, continuous emphasizing, and training on implementing reasonable resuscitation interventions should be improved.

Another vital contributor of our interventions is that the protocol requires ambulance crews to provide on-scene resuscitation until either ROSC or termination of efforts. Despite the requirement, the on-scene time in Suzhou was only about 5 min, which was 20–40 min shorter than that reported in high ROSC countries such as North America [25], Korea [17], Germany [26] or Australia [27]. Previous studies suggested to stabilize patients on-scene before transport to hospital to avoid the fraction of time without intervention during transport [10,28]. In this sense, the marked difference of on-scene interval would explain why the ALS interventions were less used and prehospital ROSC was less often achieved in Suzhou. This lack of implementation of protocol was led by several issues: first, in most cases the patient's family showed strong demand for transfer to hospital due to an inherent public perception that fast-transfer is the best; second, ambulance crews held the idea of fast-transfer under the pressure of insufficient ambulance resources; third, there was no clear requirement or limit of the on-scene interval during quality monitoring and feedback. It was needed to further optimize the protocol, emphasize quality monitoring, and conduct targeted community education for public.

It has been underlined by studies that the timing of ALS was more important than the provision of ALS interventions [25,29,30]. In this study, though we found increased proportion of ALS interventions as well as prehospital ROSC after the quality improvement programme, the results of subgroups showed that a higher proportion of ALS did not necessarily mean a higher proportion of ROSC. The more decisive factor in Suzhou may be the timing of treatment: the prehospital interval of about 28 min was comparable to other published data, however the response time of more than 10 min was much longer than that of North America (5–6 min) [25], Australia (7–8 min) [14], Korea (7–8 min) [17], or Japan (6–9 min) [31]. More critically, though the interval from symptom onset to call was shortened than what we reported in 2015 (30 min) [22], it was still 15–20 min. Considering the probability of survival following cardiac arrest drops 10% per minute with no intervention [32], this 15–20 min delay means that most patients lost their chance of survival during waiting, and any effort to improve on-scene ALS measures will be of no help. Our findings, along with others [8,33,34], indicate that each link in the chain of survival should be strengthened, and that efforts to involve every individual in the whole community to save patients are always warranted.

The size, pattern, level of specialty and training of ambulance crews are considered to influence the outcomes of patients with OHCA [15–17]. In Suzhou, the physician in a fixed crew is a dedicated prehospital personnel who only works on ambulance, while the physician in a non-fixed unit could be rotated from in-hospital emergency department or other in-hospital departments. The proportions of prehospital ALS interventions were higher in the fixed ambulance crews, which might be due to by the higher level of team coordination, and the more experience of physicians to deal with OHCA cases. In a recent systematic review, researchers emphasized that higher exposure to attempted resuscitation cases, but not years of clinical EMS experience, was associated with improved patient outcome [18]. Although the baseline difference did exist, the performance of non-fixed crews could be largely improved after use of standardized protocol and team-based training, which increased their "exposure" to simulated OHCA treatment. We suggested that, instead of finding a perfect "fixedness" of ambulance crews, the protocol adherence and targeted training are needed.

This paper reported the process and result of Suzhou's first citywide quality improvement programme. The effectiveness of our results should be interpreted in the context of some limitations. First, because multiple interventions were simultaneously adopted, it is impossible to identify the components responsible for the observed improvement of outcomes. Second, this study used a before-and-after analytic design, which may have been affected by temporal trends in OHCA survival. Third, this was a retrospective study, which increased the risk of residual confounding. Although we eliminated imbalance using propensity score-matching analysis, unmeasured confounding factors may have influenced the outcomes. Fourth, due to limited variables in the database, the in-hospital outcomes, the quality, and time interval for each prehospital ALS interventions could not be obtained. Fifth, it was recorded in our database that all the cases had received DA-CPR and ambulance CPR, but whether any individual received bystander CPR is unknown. Last, the impact of the COVID-19 pandemic has significantly changed systems-of-care for OHCA in Suzhou, though we simply excluded cases occurring in two epidemic periods, we were unable to rule it out completely.

5. Conclusions

The implementation of a citywide quality improvement programme with a standardization of ambulance treatment protocol, targeted training of ambulance crew, and quality monitoring and feedback, was associated with higher prehospital ROSC rates and improved prehospital ALS interventions by ambulance crews. Though the fixed ambulance crews performed better than non-fixed crews in critical care provision and prehospital outcome, protocol adherence and targeted training could fill the underperformance of non-fixed crews efficaciously. Further improvements are needed to strengthen each link in the survival chain with a focus on ambulance treatment protocol and education.

Author Contributions: Conceptualization, L.Z. and Z.Z.; data curation, X.D. and L.W.; formal analysis, X.D. and H.X.; project administration, L.Z. and Z.Z.; resources, L.W., Y.Y. and Z.Z.; supervision, L.Z. and L.W.; visualization, H.X. and Y.Y.; validation, L.W.; writing—original draft preparation, X.D., H.X. and L.W.; writing—review and editing, L.Z. and Z.Z. All authors have read and agreed to the published version of the manuscript.

Funding: This research was funded by National Natural Science Foundation of China, grant number 72074144, the Program of "science, education and health promotion" for youth in Suzhou, grant number KJXW2019055, and Innovative Research Team of High-level Local Universities in Shanghai, grant number SHSMU-ZDCX20212801.

Institutional Review Board Statement: Not applicable.

Informed Consent Statement: Informed consent was waived due to the retrospective nature of the study.

Data Availability Statement: Data are available from the corresponding author on reasonable request.

Conflicts of Interest: The authors declare no conflict of interest.

Abbreviations

OHCA—out-of-hospital cardiac arrest; EMS—emergency medical services; ALS—advanced life support; CPR—cardiopulmonary resuscitation; DA-CPR—dispatcher-assisted CPR; ROSC—return of spontaneous circulation; MPDS—Medical Priority Dispatch System; AHA—American Heart Association; IV—intravenous; IO—intraosseous; ECG—electrocardiograph; CVD—cardiovascular disease; ED—emergency department; SD—standard deviation; IQR—interquartile range; AOR—adjusted odds ratio; CI—confidence interval; SMD—standardized mean differences.

References

1. Kiguchi, T.; Okubo, M.; Nishiyama, C.; Maconochie, I.; Ong, M.E.H.; Kern, K.B.; Wyckoff, M.H.; McNally, B.; Christensen, E.F.; Tjelmeland, I.; et al. Out-of-hospital cardiac arrest across the world: First report from the international liaison committee on resuscitation (ilcor). *Resuscitation* **2020**, *152*, 39–49. [CrossRef] [PubMed]
2. Xu, F.; Zhang, Y.; Chen, Y. Cardiopulmonary resuscitation training in china: Current situation and future development. *JAMA Cardiol.* **2017**, *2*, 469–470. [CrossRef] [PubMed]
3. Hou, L.; Wang, Y.; Wang, W. Optimization of the pre-hospital rescue system for out-of-hospital cardiac arrest in China. *China CDC Wkly.* **2022**, *4*, 52–55. [CrossRef] [PubMed]
4. Ong, M.E.H.; Perkins, G.D.; Cariou, A. Out-of-hospital cardiac arrest: Prehospital management. *Lancet* **2018**, *391*, 980–988. [CrossRef]
5. Berg, K.M.; Cheng, A.; Panchal, A.R.; Topjian, A.A.; Aziz, K.; Bhanji, F.; Bigham, B.L.; Hirsch, K.G.; Hoover, A.V.; Kurz, M.C.; et al. Part 7: Systems of care: 2020 american heart association guidelines for cardiopulmonary resuscitation and emergency cardiovascular care. *Circulation* **2020**, *142*, S580–S604. [CrossRef]
6. Semeraro, F.; Greif, R.; Böttiger, B.; Burkart, R.; Cimpoesu, D.; Georgiou, M.; Yeung, J.; Lippert, F.; Lockey, A.S.; Olasveengen, T.; et al. European resuscitation council guidelines 2021: Systems saving lives. *Resuscitation* **2021**, *161*, 80–97. [CrossRef]
7. Sporer, K.; Jacobs, M.; Derevin, L.; Duval, S.; Pointer, J. Continuous quality improvement efforts increase survival with favorable neurologic outcome after out-of-hospital cardiac arrest. *Prehosp. Emerg. Care* **2017**, *21*, 1–6. [CrossRef]
8. Hwang, W.S.; Park, J.S.; Kim, S.J.; Hong, Y.S.; Moon, S.W.; Lee, S.W. A system-wide approach from the community to the hospital for improving neurologic outcomes in out-of-hospital cardiac arrest patients. *Eur. J. Emerg. Med.* **2017**, *24*, 87–95. [CrossRef]
9. Chen, T.T.; Ma, M.H.; Chen, F.J.; Hu, F.C.; Lu, Y.C.; Chiang, W.C.; Ko, P.C. The relationship between survival after out-of-hospital cardiac arrest and process measures for emergency medical service ambulance team performance. *Resuscitation* **2015**, *97*, 55–60. [CrossRef]

10. Hopkins, C.L.; Burk, C.; Moser, S.; Meersman, J.; Baldwin, C.; Youngquist, S.T. Implementation of pit crew approach and cardiopulmonary resuscitation metrics for out-of-hospital cardiac arrest improves patient survival and neurological outcome. *J. Am. Heart Assoc.* **2016**, *5*, e002892. [CrossRef]
11. Pearson, D.A.; Nelson, R.D.; Monk, L.; Tyson, C.; Jollis, J.G.; Granger, C.B.; Corbett, C.; Garvey, L.; Runyon, M.S. Comparison of team-focused cpr vs standard cpr in resuscitation from out-of-hospital cardiac arrest: Results from a statewide quality improvement initiative. *Resuscitation* **2016**, *105*, 165–172. [CrossRef] [PubMed]
12. GRA. Acting on the Call. 2018. Available online: https://www.globalresuscitationalliance.org/wp-content/pdf/acting_on_the_call.pdf (accessed on 16 August 2022).
13. Park, S.Y.; Lim, D.; Kim, S.C.; Ryu, J.H.; Kim, Y.H.; Choi, B.; Kim, S.H. Effect of prehospital epinephrine use on survival from out-of-hospital cardiac arrest and on emergency medical services. *J. Clin. Med.* **2021**, *11*, 190. [CrossRef] [PubMed]
14. Nehme, Z.; Ball, J.; Stephenson, M.; Walker, T.; Stub, D.; Smith, K. Effect of a resuscitation quality improvement programme on outcomes from out-of-hospital cardiac arrest. *Resuscitation* **2021**, *162*, 236–244. [CrossRef] [PubMed]
15. Fang, P.H.; Lin, Y.Y.; Lu, C.H.; Lee, C.C.; Lin, C.H. Impacts of emergency medical technician configurations on outcomes of patients with out-of-hospital cardiac arrest. *Int. J. Environ. Res. Public Health* **2020**, *17*, 1930. [CrossRef] [PubMed]
16. Warren, S.A.; Prince, D.K.; Huszti, E.; Rea, T.D.; Fitzpatrick, A.L.; Andrusiek, D.L.; Darling, S.; Morrison, L.J.; Vilke, G.M.; Nichol, G. Volume versus outcome: More emergency medical services personnel on-scene and increased survival after out-of-hospital cardiac arrest. *Resuscitation* **2015**, *94*, 40–48. [CrossRef] [PubMed]
17. Lee, S.H.; Lee, S.Y.; Park, J.H.; Song, K.J.; Shin, S.D. Effects of a designated ambulance team response on prehospital return of spontaneous circulation and advanced cardiac life support of out-of-hospital cardiac arrest: A nationwide natural experimental study. *Prehosp. Emerg. Care* **2022**, *26*, 1–8. [CrossRef] [PubMed]
18. Bray, J.; Nehme, Z.; Nguyen, A.; Lockey, A.; Finn, J. A systematic review of the impact of emergency medical service practitioner experience and exposure to out of hospital cardiac arrest on patient outcomes. *Resuscitation* **2020**, *155*, 134–142. [CrossRef]
19. Kim, K.H.; Ro, Y.S.; Park, J.H.; Kim, T.H.; Jeong, J.; Hong, K.J.; Song, K.J.; Shin, S.D. Association between case volume of ambulance stations and clinical outcomes of out-of-hospital cardiac arrest: A nationwide multilevel analysis. *Resuscitation* **2021**, *163*, 71–77. [CrossRef]
20. Wilson, M.H.; Habig, K.; Wright, C.; Hughes, A.; Davies, G.; Imray, C.H. Pre-hospital emergency medicine. *Lancet* **2015**, *386*, 2526–2534. [CrossRef]
21. Shao, F.; Li, H.; Ma, S.; Li, D.; Li, C. Outcomes of out-of-hospital cardiac arrest in beijing: A 5-year cross-sectional study. *BMJ Open* **2021**, *11*, e041917. [CrossRef]
22. Zhang, L.; Luo, M.; Myklebust, H.; Pan, C.; Wang, L.; Zhou, Z.; Yang, Q.; Lin, Q.; Zheng, Z.J. When dispatcher assistance is not saving lives: Assessment of process compliance, barriers and outcomes in out-of-hospital cardiac arrest in a metropolitan city in china. *Emerg. Med. J.* **2021**, *38*, 252–257. [CrossRef] [PubMed]
23. Stroop, R.; Kerner, T.; Strickmann, B.; Hensel, M. Mobile phone-based alerting of cpr-trained volunteers simultaneously with the ambulance can reduce the resuscitation-free interval and improve outcome after out-of-hospital cardiac arrest: A german, population-based cohort study. *Resuscitation* **2020**, *147*, 57–64. [CrossRef] [PubMed]
24. Hasegawa, M.; Abe, T.; Nagata, T.; Onozuka, D.; Hagihara, A. The number of prehospital defibrillation shocks and 1-month survival in patients with out-of-hospital cardiac arrest. *Scand. J. Trauma Resusc. Emerg. Med.* **2015**, *23*, 34. [CrossRef] [PubMed]
25. Okubo, M.; Komukai, S.; Callaway, C.W.; Izawa, J. Association of timing of epinephrine administration with outcomes in adults with out-of-hospital cardiac arrest. *JAMA Network Open* **2021**, *4*, e2120176. [CrossRef]
26. Bürger, A.; Wnent, J.; Bohn, A.; Jantzen, T.; Brenner, S.; Lefering, R.; Seewald, S.; Gräsner, J.T.; Fischer, M. The effect of ambulance response time on survival following out-of-hospital cardiac arrest. *Dtsch. Arztebl. Int.* **2018**, *115*, 541–548. [CrossRef]
27. Beck, B.; Bray, J.E.; Smith, K.; Walker, T.; Grantham, H.; Hein, C.; Thorrowgood, M.; Smith, A.; Inoue, M.; Smith, T.; et al. Description of the ambulance services participating in the aus-roc australian and new zealand out-of-hospital cardiac arrest epistry. *Emerg. Med. Australas* **2016**, *28*, 673–683. [CrossRef]
28. Lee, S.G.W.; Hong, K.J.; Kim, T.H.; Choi, S.; Shin, S.D.; Song, K.J.; Ro, Y.S.; Jeong, J.; Park, Y.J.; Park, J.H. Quality of chest compressions during prehospital resuscitation phase from scene arrival to ambulance transport in out-of-hospital cardiac arrest. *Resuscitation* **2022**, *180*, 1–7. [CrossRef]
29. Izawa, J.; Iwami, T.; Gibo, K.; Okubo, M.; Kajino, K.; Kiyohara, K.; Nishiyama, C.; Nishiuchi, T.; Hayashi, Y.; Kiguchi, T.; et al. Timing of advanced airway management by emergency medical services personnel following out-of-hospital cardiac arrest: A population-based cohort study. *Resuscitation* **2018**, *128*, 16–23. [CrossRef]
30. Hosomi, S.; Kitamura, T.; Sobue, T.; Zha, L.; Kiyohara, K.; Matsuyama, T.; Oda, J. Association between timing of epinephrine administration and outcomes of traumatic out-of-hospital cardiac arrest following traffic collisions. *J. Clin. Med.* **2022**, *11*, 3564. [CrossRef]
31. Shibahashi, K.; Kato, T.; Hikone, M.; Sugiyama, K. Fifteen-year secular changes in the care and outcomes of patients with out-of-hospital cardiac arrest in japan: A nationwide, population-based study. *Eur. Heart J. Qual. Care Clin. Outcomes* **2022**. *ahead of print*. [CrossRef]
32. Weisfeldt, M.L.; Becker, L.B. Resuscitation after cardiac arrest: A 3-phase time-sensitive model. *JAMA* **2002**, *288*, 3035–3038. [CrossRef] [PubMed]

33. Del Rios, M.; Weber, J.; Pugach, O.; Nguyen, H.; Campbell, T.; Islam, S.; Spencer, L.S.; Markul, E.; Bunney, E.B.; Vanden Hoek, T. Large urban center improves out-of-hospital cardiac arrest survival. *Resuscitation* **2019**, *139*, 234–240. [CrossRef] [PubMed]
34. Scapigliati, A.; Zace, D.; Matsuyama, T.; Pisapia, L.; Saviani, M.; Semeraro, F.; Ristagno, G.; Laurenti, P.; Bray, J.E.; Greif, R.; et al. Community initiatives to promote basic life support implementation-a scoping review. *J. Clin. Med.* **2021**, *10*, 5719. [CrossRef] [PubMed]

Disclaimer/Publisher's Note: The statements, opinions and data contained in all publications are solely those of the individual author(s) and contributor(s) and not of MDPI and/or the editor(s). MDPI and/or the editor(s) disclaim responsibility for any injury to people or property resulting from any ideas, methods, instructions or products referred to in the content.

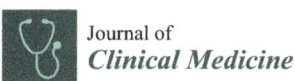

Article

Being Underweight Is Associated with Increased Risk of Sudden Cardiac Death in People with Diabetes Mellitus

Yun Gi Kim [1], Kyung-Do Han [2], Seung-Young Roh [3], Joo Hee Jeong [1], Yun Young Choi [1], Kyongjin Min [4], Jaemin Shim [1], Jong-Il Choi [1,*] and Young-Hoon Kim [1]

1. Division of Cardiology, Department of Internal Medicine, Korea University College of Medicine, Korea University Anam Hospital, Seoul 02841, Republic of Korea
2. Department of Statistics and Actuarial Science, Soongsil University, Seoul 06978, Republic of Korea
3. Division of Cardiology, Department of Internal Medicine, Korea University College of Medicine, Korea University Guro Hospital, Seoul 08308, Republic of Korea
4. Division of Cardiology, Department of Internal Medicine, Sanggye Paik Hospital, Inje University College of Medicine, Seoul 01757, Republic of Korea
* Correspondence: jongilchoi@korea.ac.kr; Tel.: +82-2-920-5445; Fax: +82-2-927-1478

Abstract: Background: Diabetes mellitus (DM) can cause various atherosclerotic cardiovascular disease including sudden cardiac death (SCD). The impact of being underweight on the risk of SCD in people with DM remains to be revealed. We aimed to evaluate the risk of SCD according to body-mass index (BMI; kg/m^2) level in DM population. Methods: We used a nationwide healthcare insurance database to conduct this study. We identified people with DM among those who underwent nationwide health screening during 2009 to 2012. Medical follow-up data was available until December 2018. Results: A total of 2,602,577 people with DM with a 17,851,797 person*year follow-up were analyzed. The underweight group (BMI < 18.5) showed 2.4-fold increased risk of SCD during follow-up (adjusted-hazard ratio [HR] = 2.40; 95% confidence interval [CI] = 2.26–2.56; p < 0.001). When normal-BMI group (18.5 $\leq$ BMI < 23) was set as a reference, underweight group (adjusted-HR = 2.01; 95% CI = 1.88–2.14) showed even higher risk of SCD compared with the obesity group (BMI $\geq$ 30; adjusted-HR = 0.89; 95% CI = 0.84–0.94). When BMI was stratified by one unit, BMI and SCD risk showed a U-curve association with the highest risk observed at low BMI levels. The lowest risk was observed in 27 $\leq$ BMI < 28 group. The association between being underweight and increased SCD risk in DM people was maintained throughout various subgroups. Conclusions: Being underweight is significantly associated with an increased risk of SCD in the DM population. A steep rise in the risk of SCD was observed as the BMI level decreased below 23. The lowest risk of SCD was observed in 27 $\leq$ BMI < 28 group.

Keywords: underweight; diabetes mellitus; sudden cardiac death

1. Introduction

Significant social and economic losses occur every day due to sudden cardiac death (SCD) [1,2]. Despite substantial improvements in the overall management of SCD victims, survival and especially neurologically intact survival after SCD is still not satisfactory [3–7]. An intrinsic obstacle for SCD management is the narrow window of timely intervention and adequate cardiopulmonary resuscitation immediately after an SCD event, which is critical for survival of victims [3–5,8,9].

Diabetes mellitus (DM) is a known risk factor for SCD and prior studies demonstrated a robust association between fasting blood glucose and risk of SCD [10–12]. A recent study based on the Korean nationwide healthcare database revealed an 80% increased risk of SCD in DM patients, and even higher risk (three-fold) in uncontrolled DM patients, despite improvements in oral antidiabetic medications and coronary revascularization capabilities [12]. Despite the strong association between DM and SCD, identification of

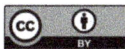

specific subgroups such as uncontrolled DM patients who are subject to substantially increased risk of SCD will be essential for primary prevention of SCD in DM patients.

Prior studies reported that obesity is a significant predictor for occurrence of SCD in the general population (including those with and without diabetes) [13–16]. However, the association between being underweight and SCD is not fully understood. Jee et al. revealed that high body-mass index (BMI) is associated with a significantly increased risk of cardiovascular death in the general population of South Korea. However, low BMI did not show any significant association with cardiovascular death [14]. Another study conducted with 2.3 million of the general population of Israel with 40 years of follow-up also reported a considerably increased risk of SCD in obese people but not in people who are underweight [15]. In contrast, Chang et al. reported in their meta-analysis that there was a 59% increased risk of all-cause mortality in diabetic people who were underweight [17].

Both under- and overweight conditions are important risk factors for DM and adequate weight control is recommended for DM patients to prevent cardiovascular complications [18]. In this study, we aimed to evaluate the risk of SCD in DM patients who are underweight. Due to the low incidence of SCD, we utilized nationwide health screening data to analyze a sufficient number of SCD events and to enable various subgroup analyses.

2. Patients and Methods

2.1. Nationwide Database

This study was based on the Korean National Health Insurance Service (K-NHIS) database. All citizens of South Korea are mandatory subscribers of the K-NHIS and medical data stored in the K-NHIS can represent the entire people of South Korea. Claims of various diagnostic codes based on International Classification of Disease, tenth edition (ICD-10) such as hypertension, DM, dyslipidemia, atrial fibrillation, or heart failure, and a prescription history of various drugs are recorded in the K-NHIS database. The K-NHIS offers a biennial health screening program to its subscribers who are $\geq$20 years old. Body weight and height are directly measured during health screening, enabling classification of participants according to BMI value. Additional medical data such as blood pressure, waist circumference, amount of alcohol consumption, smoking status, physical activity level, various laboratory tests such as complete blood cell count, liver function, renal function, fasting blood glucose (FBG), and lipid profile are measured during health screening.

2.2. Participants

Among people who underwent nationwide health screening during 2009 to 2012, those with a prior diagnosis of DM were enrolled. Only people with type 2 DM was screened and people with type 1 DM was not included in this study. Those with prior diagnosis of SCD and age < 20 years at health screening were excluded from the study. Baseline medical history such as hypertension, DM, or prior SCD event was identified by the data obtained during January 2002 to December 2008. Medical data gathered until December 2018 were analyzed. The nature of subscription to the K-NHIS is mandatory and exclusive and therefore, no follow-up losses exist except for migration.

The Institutional Review Board of Korea University Medicine Anam Hospital and the official review committee of the K-NHIS approved this study. Written informed consent was waived considering the retrospective nature of the study. The ethical guidelines of the 2013 Declaration of Helsinki and legal regulations of South Korea were strictly observed throughout the study.

2.3. Sudden Cardiac Death

The main outcome of this study was the occurrence of SCD. In this study, we intended to identify death events that occurred unexpectedly and suddenly which are assumed to originate from cardiac problems. We first identified sudden death events with ICD-10 codes. Subsequently, we excluded potential non-cardiac sudden death events to exclusively identify SCD among sudden death events. Aborted SCD events were also included as SCD.

Performance of cardiopulmonary resuscitation without ICD-10 codes for SCD was also classified as SCD events.

The identification of occurrence of an SCD event was based on the ICD-10 codes claimed from emergency departments throughout South Korea. Only claims accompanied by cardiopulmonary resuscitation or a declaration of death were considered as SCD. In-hospital claim of ICD-10 codes for SCD was not included in this analysis. The ICD-10 codes used to identify SCD were as follows: I46.0 (cardiac arrest with successful resuscitation), I46.1 (sudden cardiac arrest), I46.9 (cardiac arrest, cause unspecified), I49.0 (ventricular fibrillation and flutter), R96.0 (instantaneous death), and R96.1 (death occurring less than 24 h from symptom onset). Both aborted and non-aborted SCD were included as a main outcome.

The incidence of SCD was defined as the number of events per 1000 person*year follow-up. Due to ICD-10 coding-based detection of main outcomes, the claims for SCD or death that occurred within one year after health screening were not counted as a main outcome. For example, claims of SCD codes immediately after health screening can be actual SCD events after health screening or just repeat claims of SCD which happened before health screening. The robustness of our coding strategy for SCD and other medical conditions was validated in prior studies [12,19–25].

If the participants had a prior diagnosis of asphyxia, suffocation, drowning, gastrointestinal bleeding, cerebral hemorrhage, ischemic stroke, sepsis, anaphylaxis, trauma, lightning strike, electric shock, or burn within 6 months (including those claimed simultaneously with ICD-10 codes for SCD) of the diagnosis of SCD, the event was not counted as a SCD event.

2.4. Definitions

Underweight was defined as BMI < 18.5 kg/m^2. Normal body weight, high-normal body weight, pre-obesity, and obesity were defined as $18.5 \leq$ BMI < 23.0, $23.0 \leq$ BMI < 25.0, $25.0 \leq$ BMI < 30.0, and BMI $\geq$ 30.0, respectively.

Either FBG (FBG $\geq$ 126 mg/dL for DM and FBG 100–125 mg/dL for impaired fasting glucose (IFG)) or a claim of ICD-10 codes for DM or IFG by a physician was used for the diagnosis of DM or IFG. Hypertension was diagnosed based on ICD-10 codes for hypertension or measured blood pressure during nationwide health screening. The Modification of Diet in Renal Disease equation was used to define chronic kidney disease (estimated glomerular filtration rate < 60 mL/min/1.73 m^2). A self-questionnaire acquired during health screening was used to define smoking status (current-smoker: $\geq$100 cigarettes in their lifetime; ex-smoker: $\geq$100 cigarettes in their lifetime, but had not smoked within one month of health screening; never-smoker: <100 cigarettes in their lifetime) and alcohol consumption (nondrinker: 0 g of alcohol per week; mild- to moderate-drinker: <210 g of alcohol per week; heavy-drinker, $\geq$210 g of alcohol per week). Regular physical activity was defined as having one or more sessions of high (such as running, climbing, or intense bicycle activities) or moderate physical activity (such as walking fast, tennis, or moderate bicycle activities) in a week.

2.5. Statistical Analysis

The Student's t-test was used to compare continuous variables which were expressed as mean $\pm$ standard deviation. Categorical variables were compared using the chi-square test or Fisher's exact test, as appropriate. Cox-regression analysis was used to calculate raw and adjusted hazard ratios with 95% confidence intervals (CIs). People with missing data were excluded from the study and no imputation was done. Statistical significance was defined as p values $\leq$ 0.05 in two-tailed tests. All statistical analyses were performed with SAS version 9.2 (SAS Institute, Cary, NC, USA).

2.6. Data Availability Statement

The data underlying this article are available in the article and in its online Supplementary Material.

3. Results

3.1. Study Population

We identified a total of 2,746,079 people with DM who underwent nationwide health screening during 2009 to 2012. People were excluded from the analysis if they were under 20 years ($n = 390$), had missing data (117,446), had a prior diagnosis of SCD during the screening period (2002 to 2008; $n = 934$), or had a death or SCD event within one year after health screening ($n = 24,732$). People were followed until December 2018 with a total of 17,851,797 person*year follow-up duration. Mean follow-up period per person was 6.86 years and a total of 26,341 SCD events were detected. The flow of this study is summarized in Figure 1.

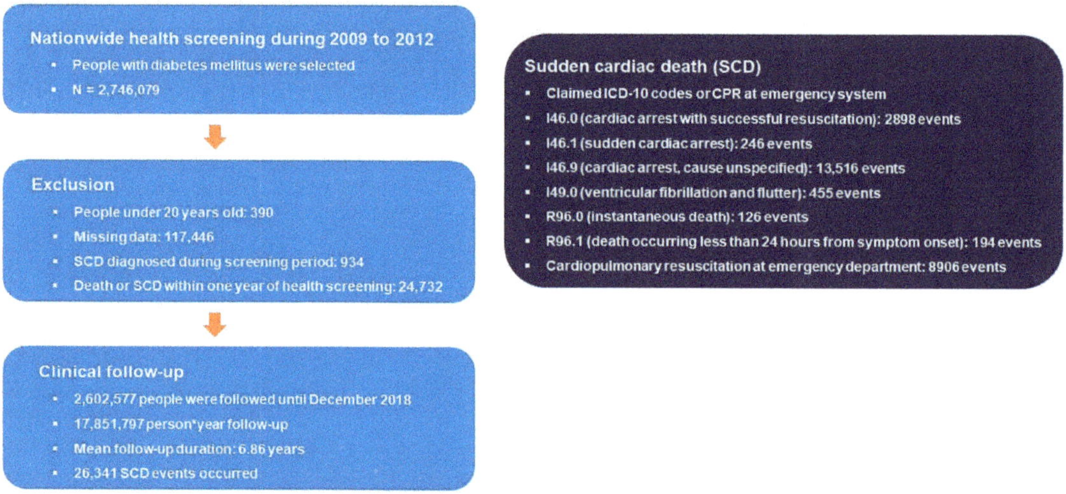

Figure 1. Flow of the study. ICD-10: International Classification of Disease, tenth edition; SCD: sudden cardiac death.

Baseline demographics according to BMI value are described in Table 1. A significant difference was observed throughout various parameters such as age, sex, smoking status, alcohol consumption, income level, and prevalence of various medical diseases such as hypertension or dyslipidemia. People who were underweight (BMI < 18.5) were significantly older (59.7 years vs. 57.4 years; $p < 0.001$); were more likely to be women (42.9% vs. 39.9%; $p < 0.001$), current smokers (34.0% vs. 25.7%; $p < 0.001$), non-drinkers (63.7% vs. 57.2%; $p < 0.001$), and lowest income quartile (25.0% vs. 20.9%; $p < 0.001$); were less likely to have regular exercise (14.6% vs. 20.7%; $p < 0.001$); had lower prevalence of hypertension (38.4% vs. 57.1%; $p < 0.001$) and dyslipidemia (21.9% vs. 42.3%; $p < 0.001$). The prevalence of DM for five or more years (30.8% vs. 31.1%; $p = 0.156$) and prescription of three or more oral antidiabetic medications (14.8% vs. 14.5%; $p = 0.112$) were similar between underweight and non-underweight groups. However, the percentage of people on insulin therapy was significantly higher in the underweight group (14.4% vs. 8.7%; $p < 0.001$).

Table 1. Baseline characteristics of people according to BMI value.

	Body-Mass Index (BMI)					BMI ≥ 18.5	p Value (<18.5 vs. ≥18.5)
	BMI < 18.5	18.5 ≤ BMI < 23	23 ≤ BMI < 25	25 ≤ BMI < 30	BMI ≥ 30	p Value	
n	41,598	648,206	645,444	1,066,439	200,890		2,560,979	
Age, years	59.7 ± 16.1	58.6 ± 12.9	58.3 ± 11.7	57.0 ± 11.8	53.0 ± 13.0	<0.001	57.4 ± 12.3	<0.001
Age groups						<0.001		<0.001
<40	5172 (12.4%)	47,580 (7.3%)	35,757 (5.5%)	76,107 (7.1%)	32,037 (16.0%)		191,481 (7.5%)	
40 ≤ age < 65	18,663 (44.9%)	378,603 (58.4%)	406,130 (62.9%)	690,485 (64.8%)	126,645 (63.0%)		1,601,863 (62.6%)	
≥65	17,763 (42.7%)	222,023 (34.3%)	203,557 (31.5%)	299,847 (28.1%)	42,208 (21.0%)		767,635 (30.0%)	
Sex						<0.001		<0.001
Male	23,765 (57.1%)	382,404 (59.0%)	403,135 (62.5%)	653,020 (61.2%)	99,974 (49.8%)		1,538,533 (60.1%)	
Female	17,833 (42.9%)	265,802 (41.0%)	242,309 (37.5%)	413,419 (38.8%)	100,916 (50.2%)		1,022,446 (39.9%)	
Income (lowest quartile)	10,377 (25.0%)	142,184 (21.9%)	132,778 (20.6%)	217,179 (20.4%)	43,936 (21.9%)	<0.001	536,077 (20.9%)	<0.001
Smoking						<0.001		<0.001
Non	22,586 (54.3%)	360,640 (55.6%)	352,969 (54.7%)	589,443 (55.3%)	122,660 (61.1%)		1,425,712 (55.7%)	
Ex	4865 (11.7%)	103,684 (16.0%)	126,303 (19.6%)	215,921 (20.3%)	30,257 (15.1%)		476,165 (18.6%)	
Current	14,147 (34.0%)	183,882 (28.4%)	166,172 (25.8%)	261,075 (24.5%)	47,973 (23.9%)		659,102 (25.7%)	
Drinking						<0.001		<0.001
Non	26,504 (63.7%)	383,752 (59.2%)	365,192 (56.6%)	595,316 (55.8%)	120,730 (60.1%)		1,464,990 (57.2%)	
Mild	11,386 (27.4%)	205,557 (31.7%)	217,857 (33.8%)	357,372 (33.5%)	59,925 (29.8%)		840,711 (32.8%)	
Heavy	3708 (8.9%)	58,897 (9.1%)	62,395 (9.7%)	113,751 (10.7%)	20,235 (10.1%)		255,278 (10.0%)	
Regular exercise	6065 (14.6%)	134,781 (20.8%)	142,392 (22.1%)	219,627 (20.6%)	33,160 (16.5%)	<0.001	529,960 (20.7%)	<0.001
Hypertension	15,965 (38.4%)	301,988 (46.6%)	352,520 (54.6%)	664,559 (62.3%)	143,015 (71.2%)	<0.001	1,462,082 (57.1%)	<0.001
Dyslipidemia	9092 (21.9%)	223,499 (34.5%)	268,170 (41.6%)	490,648 (46.0%)	99,901 (49.7%)	<0.001	1,082,218 (42.3%)	<0.001
DM duration, ≥5 years	12,806 (30.8%)	227,952 (35.2%)	214,249 (33.2%)	307,177 (28.8%)	47,331 (23.6%)	<0.001	796,709 (31.1%)	0.156
On Insulin	5983 (14.4%)	68,633 (10.6%)	55,762 (8.6%)	82,799 (7.8%)	14,764 (7.4%)	<0.001	221,958 (8.7%)	<0.001
Oran antidiabetics, ≥3	6144 (14.8%)	102,545 (15.8%)	95,288 (14.8%)	146,073 (13.7%)	27,257 (13.6%)	<0.001	371,163 (14.5%)	0.112
BMI (kg/m^2)	17.4 ± 0.9	21.4 ± 1.2	24.0 ± 0.6	26.9 ± 1.3	32.3 ± 2.4	<0.001	25.2 ± 3.3	<0.001
Waist circumference (cm)	70.0 ± 6.4	78.0 ± 6.0	83.5 ± 5.4	89.2 ± 6.1	98.7 ± 7.8	<0.001	85.7 ± 8.5	<0.001
Systolic BP (mmHg)	122.3 ± 17.4	126.1 ± 16.1	128.5 ± 15.5	130.6 ± 15.3	133.7 ± 15.9	<0.001	129.2 ± 15.8	<0.001
Diastolic BP (mmHg)	75.3 ± 10.8	76.9 ± 10.2	78.5 ± 10.0	80.2 ± 10.1	82.6 ± 10.7	<0.001	79.1 ± 10.3	<0.001
Fasting glucose (mg/dL)	152.1 ± 65.5	146.4 ± 51.7	144.3 ± 46.4	143.6 ± 43.8	145.7 ± 45.2	<0.001	144.7 ± 46.7	<0.001
Total cholesterol (mg/dL)	183.0 ± 41.7	191.6 ± 41.9	196.2 ± 42.6	199.1 ± 43.0	202.6 ± 43.4	<0.001	196.7 ± 42.8	<0.001
HDL (mg/dL)	59.1 ± 28.5	54.6 ± 25.5	51.9 ± 23.5	50.6 ± 22.9	50.2 ± 22.0	<0.001	51.9 ± 23.7	<0.001
LDL (mg/dL)	101.4 ± 41.5	108.8 ± 40.2	111.4 ± 40.8	112.2 ± 41.6	114.0 ± 41.9	<0.001	111.3 ± 41.1	<0.001
Triglyceride (mg/dL)	101.5 (100.9–102.0)	123.6 (123.5–123.8)	144.8 (144.6–145.0)	160.7 (160.6–160.9)	171.4 (171.0–171.8)	<0.001	147.2 (147.1–147.3)	<0.001

BMI: body-mass index; BP: blood pressure; DM: diabetes mellitus; HDL: high-density lipoprotein; LDL: low-density lipoprotein.

3.2. Risk of Sudden Cardiac Death

The raw incidence of SCD was significantly higher in people who were underweight (4.38 vs. 1.43; HR = 3.11; 95% CI = 2.93–3.31; $p < 0.001$; Table 2). Kaplan–Meier curve analysis revealed a steady and continuous divergence of cumulative events of SCD between underweight and non-underweight group (log rank $p < 0.001$; Supplementary Figure S1). After adjustment of confounders (age, sex, income level, smoking history, alcohol consumption, regular physical activity, hypertension, dyslipidemia, fasting glucose, duration of DM, use of insulin, and number of oral antidiabetic medications), people who were underweight showed a 2.4-fold increased risk of SCD during follow-up (adjusted-HR = 2.40; 95% CI = 2.26–2.56; $p < 0.001$; Table 2). The risk of SCD differed across BMI value and with normal body weight (18.5 ≤ BMI < 23) as a reference, pre-obesity (25 ≤ BMI < 30; adjusted-HR 0.71; 95% CI = 0.69–0.74; $p < 0.001$) and being underweight (adjusted-HR = 2.01; 95% CI = 1.88–2.14; $p < 0.001$) had the lowest and highest risk, respectively (Table 2). When people were classified by one unit of BMI (kg/m^2), people with 27 ≤ BMI < 28 had the lowest risk of SCD and people with BMI < 17 experienced the highest risk (Figure 2 and Supplementary Table S1).

Table 2. Impact of underweight on SCD in DM patients.

	N	SCD	Follow-Up Duration (Person-Years)	Incidence	Hazard Ratio with 95% Confidence Interval		
					Non-Adjusted	Model 1	Model 2
Underweight							
No (BMI ≥ 18.5)	2,560,979	25,259	17,604,724	1.43	1 (reference)	1 (reference)	1 (reference)
Yes (BMI < 18.5)	41,598	1082	247,073	4.38	3.11 (2.93–3.31)	2.56 (2.41–2.72)	2.40 (2.26–2.56)
BMI value							
BMI < 18.5	41,598	1082	247,073	4.38	2.29 (2.15–2.44)	2.01 (1.94–2.20)	2.01 (1.88–2.14)
18.5 ≤ BMI < 23	648,206	8491	4,355,959	1.95	1 (reference)	1 (reference)	1 (reference)
23 ≤ BMI < 25	645,444	6401	4,457,801	1.44	0.73 (0.71–0.76)	0.75 (0.73–0.78)	0.77 (0.75–0.80)
25 ≤ BMI < 30	1,066,439	8844	7,408,578	1.19	0.61 (0.59–0.63)	0.69 (0.67–0.71)	0.71 (0.69–0.74)
BMI ≥ 30	200,890	1523	1,382,385	1.10	0.57 (0.54–0.60)	0.89 (0.84–0.94)	0.89 (0.84–0.94)

Incidence is per 1000 person-years of follow-up. BMI: body-mass index; DM: diabetes mellitus; SCD: sudden cardiac death. Model 1: adjusted for age and sex. Model 2: adjusted for age, sex, income level, smoking history, alcohol consumption, regular physical activity, hypertension, dyslipidemia, fasting glucose, duration of DM, use of insulin, and number of oral antidiabetic medications.

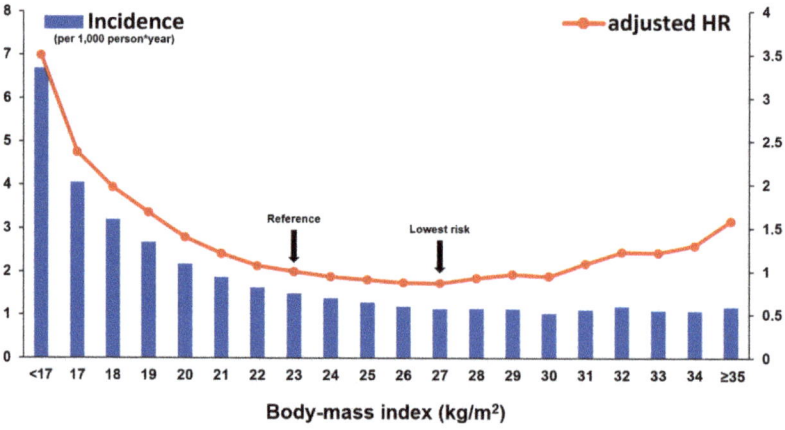

Figure 2. Risk of SCD according to BMI value. The raw incidence of SCD was higher in diabetic patients with low BMI. In the multivariate model, the risk of SCD and BMI showed a U-curve association; the risk was significantly higher in patients with low BMI than high BMI. The multivariate model is adjusted for age, sex, income level, smoking history, alcohol consumption, regular physical activity, hypertension, dyslipidemia, fasting glucose, duration of DM, use of insulin, and number of oral antidiabetic medications. HR: hazard ratio; SCD: sudden cardiac death.

3.3. Subgroup Analysis

The impact of being underweight was analyzed in various subgroups. Being underweight was associated with significantly increased risk of SCD regardless of age, sex, income level, smoking history, alcohol consumption, regular physical activity, hypertension, dyslipidemia, fasting glucose, duration of DM, use of insulin, and number of oral antidiabetic medications (Figure 3 and Supplementary Table S2). However, significant interactions were observed with age, alcohol consumption, presence of dyslipidemia, and insulin use. People in the age range $40 \leq$ age < 64 (adjusted-HR = 3.36; 95% CI = 3.06–3.70; p for interaction < 0.001), who were heavy-drinkers (adjusted-HR = 3.19; 95% CI = 2.67–3.82; p for interaction = 0.010), those without dyslipidemia (adjusted-HR = 2.50; 95% CI = 2.33–2.68; p for interaction = 0.015), and who were not on insulin therapy (adjusted-HR = 2.49; 95% CI = 2.32–2.67; p for interaction = 0.031) showed a stronger association between being underweight and SCD compared with their counterparts.

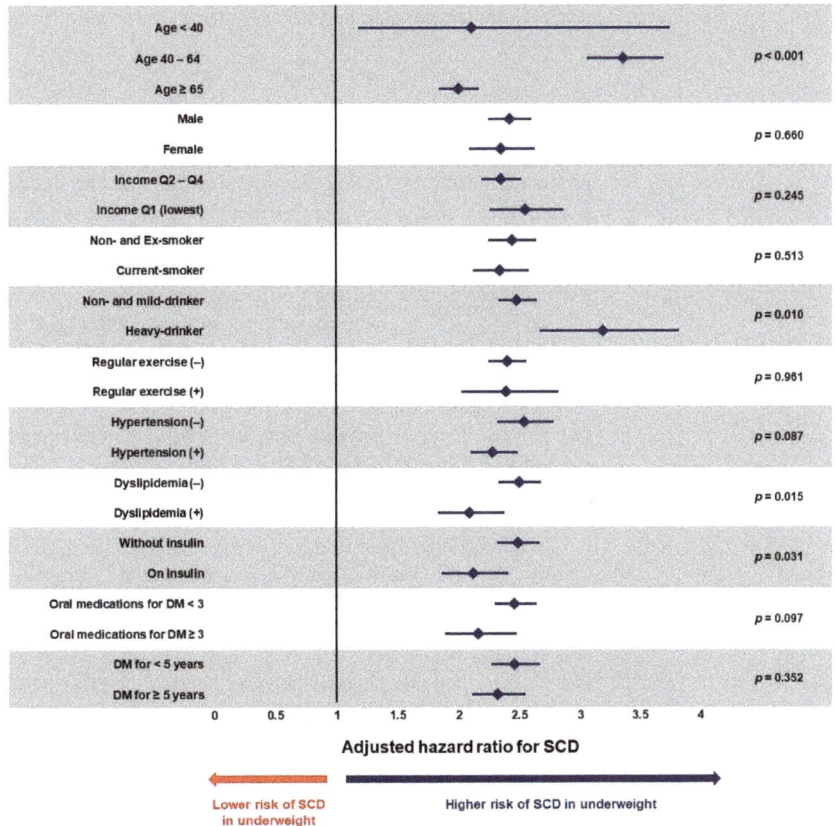

Figure 3. Subgroup analysis. DM: diabetes mellitus; SCD: sudden cardiac death. Despite significant interactions with age, alcohol consumption, dyslipidemia, and insulin use, being underweight was associated with a significantly increased risk of SCD in all subgroups. Underweight is defined as those with BMI less than 18.5 kg/m^2. Values are expressed as adjusted hazard ratio with 95% confidence interval. Hazard ratios are adjusted for age, sex, income level, smoking history, alcohol consumption, regular physical activity, hypertension, dyslipidemia, fasting glucose, duration of DM, use of insulin, and number of oral antidiabetic medications.

4. Discussion

The current study demonstrated that (i) being underweight was associated with a 2.4-fold increased risk of SCD in DM patients; (ii) DM patients who were pre-obese ($25 \leq BMI < 30$), and more specifically, $27 \leq BMI < 28$ showed the lowest risk of SCD; (iii) a stronger association between being underweight and the risk of SCD was observed in middle-aged people (40–65), heavy-drinkers, and those without dyslipidemia and insulin therapy. The strength of this study is its large sample size (n = 2,602,577), sufficient SCD events (n = 26,341), and long follow-up duration (mean 6.86 years per person) which enabled various subgroup analyses.

Diabetes mellitus is associated with various cardiovascular complications including SCD. Since SCD is associated with a low chance of survival and even lower chance of neurologically intact survival, prevention rather than treatment might be the appropriate strategy to reduce the socioeconomic burden [26–29]. The observed association between being underweight and SCD in DM patients indicates a specific subset of patients that might benefit from intensified monitoring and medical treatment for primary prevention of SCD.

4.1. Obesity and SCD

The cluster of glucose intolerance, central obesity, dyslipidemia, and elevated blood pressure is the hallmark of metabolic syndrome [30]. Our recent study revealed a significantly increased risk of SCD in people with metabolic syndrome which was in accordance with prior studies [25,31,32]. However, the current study revealed different results with DM people at the pre-obesity stage having the lowest risk of SCD. Obese DM patients also showed a 11% lower risk of SCD compared with normal weight DM patients in this study. The potential cause for a lack of association (or even inverse association) between obesity and SCD in DM population is not fully explained. However, the degree of obesity and ethnic difference can be important. When participants were stratified by one unit of BMI, people with BMI $\geq$ 35 showed a clear increase in the risk of SCD which suggests that extreme obesity can increase the risk of SCD. People with BMI $\geq$ 35 only comprised 0.89% of the entire cohort which is much less than in western populations. This ethnic difference might have diluted the association between obesity and SCD.

4.2. Being Underweight and SCD

Unlike obesity, being underweight was clearly associated with increased risk of SCD. A 2.4-fold increased risk of SCD after adjustment of confounders, steady divergence observed in Kaplan–Meier curve analysis, and linear increase in adjusted-HR per one unit decline in BMI within the underweight group all suggest a strong and robust association between being underweight and SCD in people with DM. Although the results of this study can only suggest an association and not causality, intensified monitoring of heart function or coronary artery disease might be justified in DM patients who are underweight, considering a significantly increased risk in comparison with non-underweight people and also the observed absolute incidence (4.38 SCD events per 1000 person*year).

The underlying pathophysiology of this association is not clear. One possible explanation is the genetic susceptibility of underweight DM patients. Those who develop DM despite being underweight might have been more genetically susceptible [33]. A study by Perry et al. revealed that a variant (rs8090011) in the *LAMA1* gene was associated with DM in the subset of underweight cases [33]. Several genetic variations leading to DM in underweight populations might exist and it could be possible that these genetic variations might make a substantial contribution to occurrence of SCD. Whether genetic characteristics unique to underweight DM patients can impact SCD risk is an area of future research. Another possible explanation is the severity of DM. The severity of DM might be more severe in underweight DM patients. However, the percentage of DM duration $\geq$ 5 years and prescription of $\geq$3 oral antidiabetic medications were similar between underweight vs. non-underweight groups. Although the prescription rate of insulin was significantly higher in the underweight group (14.4% vs. 8.7%), the difference was adjusted in our multivariate model. Despite significant interaction existed according to insulin use with those without insulin having higher adjusted-HR, the underweight group had a significantly higher risk of SCD in both without insulin and on insulin groups. Presence of undetected confounders might also explain the obesity paradox observed in this study. Although we adjusted various covariates such as age, sex, income, alcohol, smoking, physical activity, hypertension, dyslipidemia, and duration and treatment of DM, there can still be unmeasured covariates such as ongoing inflammation. People might have been already ill at the time of BMI measurement and this issue can contribute to obesity paradox. However, we solved this problem by excluding any SCD events or death within one year after nationwide health screening.

4.3. Limitations

Several limitations exist in this study. Despite validation of our coding strategy in various prior publications, coding inaccuracies can be problematic due to the retrospective nature of current study [19,23,24]. Generalizability is another limitation since this analysis was exclusively based on an East Asian population. We were not able to measure serial BMI value which limited additional analysis regarding the impact of temporal change of BMI on the risk of SCD. The observed higher risk of SCA in underweight people can be due to unmeasured confounders. Although we excluded potential non-cardiac causes of sudden death, some of them might have been included in primary events. Since this study was based on claim data of ICD-10 codes, we were not able to clarify specific cardiac causes of SCD. Finally, hemoglobin A1c level was not available although we had fasting blood glucose data.

5. Conclusions

Compared with normal weight, being underweight was significantly associated with increased risk of SCD in people with DM. In contrast, high normal weight, pre-obesity, and obesity was associated with a decreased risk of SCD in DM population. The BMI value associated with the lowest risk of SCD was 27 kg/m^2. Our study raises awareness of SCD risk in DM patients with accompanying underweight. Whether correction of underweight can decrease the risk of SCD remains to be explored.

Supplementary Materials: The following supporting information can be downloaded at: https://www.mdpi.com/article/10.3390/jcm12031045/s1, Figure S1: Cumulative incidence of SCD; Table S1: Risk of SCD according to BMI value (people and event numbers); Table S2: Subgroup analysis (people and event numbers).

Author Contributions: J.-I.C. had full access to all data in this study and takes responsibility for its integrity and analytical accuracy. The study concept and design were developed by Y.G.K., Y.Y.C., K.-D.H., J.-I.C. and Y.-H.K. The data analysis and interpretation were performed by Y.G.K., Y.Y.C., K.-D.H., K.M. and J.-I.C. The manuscript was drafted by Y.G.K., K.-D.H. and J.-I.C. The statistical analysis was performed by Y.G.K., K.-D.H. and J.-I.C. The data collection was performed by Y.G.K., S.-Y.R., K.-D.H., J.H.J., J.S. and J.-I.C. All authors have read and agreed to the published version of the manuscript.

Funding: This work was supported by a Korea University grant (J.-I.C.), a grant from Korea University Anam Hospital, Seoul, Republic of Korea (J.-I.C.), and in part by a National Research Foundation of Korea (NRF) grant funded by the Korean government (MSIT, Ministry of Science and ICT) (No. 2021R1A2C2011325 to J.-I.C.). The funders had no role in data collection, analysis, or interpretation; trial design; patient recruitment; or any other aspect pertinent to the study.

Institutional Review Board Statement: The current study was approved by the Institutional Review Board of Korea University Medicine Anam Hospital (IRB number: 2021AN0185) and official review committee of the K-NHIS

Informed Consent Statement: Considering the retrospective nature of this study, the requirement for written informed consent was waived

Data Availability Statement: The raw data underlying this article cannot be shared publicly due to privacy reasons and legal regulations of the Republic of Korea. The raw data is stored and analyzed only in the designated server managed by the K-NHIS

Conflicts of Interest: The authors declare no conflict of interest.

Abbreviations

BMI = body-mass index; CI = confidence interval; DM = diabetes mellitus; FBG: fasting blood glucose; ICD = International Classification of Disease; K-NHIS = Korean National Health Insurance Service; SCD = sudden cardiac death.

References

1. Ackerman, M.; Atkins, D.L.; Triedman, J.K. Sudden Cardiac Death in the Young. *Circulation* **2016**, *133*, 1006–1026. [CrossRef] [PubMed]
2. Hemingway, H.; Malik, M.; Marmot, M. Social and psychosocial influences on sudden cardiac death, ventricular arrhythmia and cardiac autonomic function. *Eur. Heart J.* **2001**, *22*, 1082–1101. [CrossRef] [PubMed]
3. Hasselqvist-Ax, I.; Riva, G.; Herlitz, J.; Rosenqvist, M.; Hollenberg, J.; Nordberg, P.; Ringh, M.; Jonsson, M.; Axelsson, C.; Lindqvist, J.; et al. Early cardiopulmonary resuscitation in out-of-hospital cardiac arrest. *N. Engl. J. Med.* **2015**, *372*, 2307–2315. [CrossRef] [PubMed]
4. Eisenberg, M.S.; Hallstrom, A.; Bergner, L. Long-term survival after out-of-hospital cardiac arrest. *N. Engl. J. Med.* **1982**, *306*, 1340–1343. [CrossRef]
5. Blewer, A.L.; Ho, A.F.W.; Shahidah, N.; White, A.E.; Pek, P.P.; Ng, Y.Y.; Mao, D.R.; Tiah, L.; Chia, M.Y.; Leong, B.S.; et al. Impact of bystander-focused public health interventions on cardiopulmonary resuscitation and survival: A cohort study. *Lancet Public Health* **2020**, *5*, e428–e436. [CrossRef]
6. Berdowski, J.; Berg, R.A.; Tijssen, J.G.; Koster, R.W. Global incidences of out-of-hospital cardiac arrest and survival rates: Systematic review of 67 prospective studies. *Resuscitation* **2010**, *81*, 1479–1487. [CrossRef]
7. El-Battrawy, I.; Pilsinger, C.; Liebe, V.; Lang, S.; Kuschyk, J.; Zhou, X.; Borggrefe, M.; Röger, S.; Akin, I. Impact of sacubitril/valsartan on the long-term incidence of ventricular arrhythmias in chronic heart failure patients. *J. Clin. Med.* **2019**, *8*, 1582. [CrossRef]
8. Myat, A.; Song, K.-J.; Rea, T. Out-of-hospital cardiac arrest: Current concepts. *Lancet* **2018**, *391*, 970–979. [CrossRef]
9. Pannone, L.; Falasconi, G.; Cianfanelli, L.; Baldetti, L.; Moroni, F.; Spoladore, R.; Vergara, P. Sudden cardiac death in patients with heart disease and preserved systolic function: Current options for risk stratification. *J. Clin. Med.* **2021**, *10*, 1823. [CrossRef]
10. Jouven, X.; Lemaître, R.N.; Rea, T.D.; Sotoodehnia, N.; Empana, J.-P.; Siscovick, D.S. Diabetes, glucose level, and risk of sudden cardiac death. *Eur. Heart J.* **2005**, *26*, 2142–2147. [CrossRef]
11. Lynge, T.H.; Svane, J.; Pedersen-Bjergaard, U.; Gislason, G.; Torp-Pedersen, C.; Banner, J.; Risgaard, B.; Winkel, B.G.; Tfelt-Hansen, J. Sudden cardiac death among persons with diabetes aged 1–49 years: A 10-year nationwide study of 14294 deaths in Denmark. *Eur. Heart J.* **2020**, *41*, 2699–2706. [CrossRef] [PubMed]
12. Kim, Y.G.; Roh, S.Y.; Han, K.-D.; Jeong, J.H.; Choi, Y.Y.; Min, K.; Shim, J.; Choi, J.-I.; Kim, Y.-H. Hypertension and diabetes including their earlier stage are associated with increased risk of sudden cardiac arrest. *Sci. Rep.* **2022**, *12*, 1–9. [CrossRef] [PubMed]
13. Calle, E.E.; Thun, M.J.; Petrelli, J.M.; Rodriguez, C.; Heath, C.W., Jr. Body-mass index and mortality in a prospective cohort of U.S. adults. *N. Engl. J. Med.* **1999**, *341*, 1097–1105. [CrossRef] [PubMed]
14. Jee, S.H.; Sull, J.W.; Park, J.; Lee, S.-Y.; Ohrr, H.; Guallar, E.; Samet, J.M. Body-mass index and mortality in Korean men and women. *N. Engl. J. Med.* **2006**, *355*, 779–787. [CrossRef] [PubMed]
15. Twig, G.; Yaniv, G.; Levine, H.; Leiba, A.; Goldberger, N.; Derazne, E.; Ben-Ami Shor, D.; Tzur, D.; Afek, A.; Shamiss, A. Body-mass index in 2.3 million adolescents and cardiovascular death in adulthood. *N. Engl. J. Med.* **2016**, *374*, 2430–2440. [CrossRef]
16. Rozen, G.; Elbaz-Greener, G.; Margolis, G.; Marai, I.; Heist, E.K.; Ruskin, J.N.; Carasso, S.; Roguin, A.; Birati, E.Y.; Amir, O. The Obesity Paradox in Real-World Nation-Wide Cohort of Patients Admitted for a Stroke in the US. *J. Clin. Med.* **2022**, *11*, 1678. [CrossRef] [PubMed]
17. Chang, H.-W.; Li, Y.-H.; Hsieh, C.-H.; Liu, P.-Y.; Lin, G.-M. Association of body mass index with all-cause mortality in patients with diabetes: A systemic review and meta-analysis. *Cardiovasc. Diagn. Ther.* **2016**, *6*, 109. [CrossRef]
18. Sairenchi, T.; Iso, H.; Irie, F.; Fukasawa, N.; Ota, H.; Muto, T. Underweight as a predictor of diabetes in older adults: A large cohort study. *Diabetes Care* **2008**, *31*, 583–584. [CrossRef]
19. Kim, Y.G.; Han, K.D.; Choi, J.I.; Choi, Y.Y.; Choi, H.Y.; Boo, K.Y.; Kim, D.Y.; Lee, K.N.; Shim, J.; Kim, J.S.; et al. Non-genetic risk factors for atrial fibrillation are equally important in both young and old age: A nationwide population-based study. *Eur. J. Prev. Cardiol.* **2021**, *28*, 666–676. [CrossRef]

20. Kim, Y.G.; Han, K.D.; Kim, D.Y.; Choi, Y.Y.; Choi, H.Y.; Roh, S.Y.; Shim, J.; Kim, J.S.; Choi, J.I.; Kim, Y.H. Different Influence of Blood Pressure on New-Onset Atrial Fibrillation in Pre- and Postmenopausal Women: A Nationwide Population-Based Study. *Hypertension* **2021**, *77*, 1500–1509. [CrossRef]
21. Kim, Y.G.; Han, K.D.; Choi, J.I.; Choi, Y.Y.; Choi, H.Y.; Shim, J.; Kim, Y.H. Premature ventricular contraction is associated with increased risk of atrial fibrillation: A nationwide population-based study. *Sci. Rep.* **2021**, *11*, 1601. [CrossRef]
22. Roh, S.Y.; Choi, J.I.; Kim, M.S.; Cho, E.Y.; Kim, Y.G.; Lee, K.N.; Shim, J.; Kim, J.S.; Kim, Y.H. Incidence and etiology of sudden cardiac arrest in Koreans: A cohort from the national health insurance service database. *PLoS ONE* **2020**, *15*, e0242769. [CrossRef]
23. Kim, Y.G.; Han, K.D.; Choi, J.I.; Yung Boo, K.; Kim, D.Y.; Oh, S.K.; Lee, K.N.; Shim, J.; Kim, J.S.; Kim, Y.H. Impact of the Duration and Degree of Hypertension and Body Weight on New-Onset Atrial Fibrillation: A Nationwide Population-Based Study. *Hypertension* **2019**, *74*, e45–e51. [CrossRef]
24. Kim, Y.G.; Oh, S.K.; Choi, H.Y.; Choi, J.I. Inherited arrhythmia syndrome predisposing to sudden cardiac death. *Korean J. Intern. Med.* **2021**, *36*, 527–538. [CrossRef]
25. Kim, Y.G.; Han, K.; Jeong, J.H.; Roh, S.Y.; Choi, Y.Y.; Min, K.; Shim, J.; Choi, J.I.; Kim, Y.H. Metabolic Syndrome, Gamma-Glutamyl Transferase, and Risk of Sudden Cardiac Death. *J. Clin. Med.* **2022**, *11*, 1781. [CrossRef]
26. Mild therapeutic hypothermia to improve the neurologic outcome after cardiac arrest. *N. Engl. J. Med.* **2002**, *346*, 549–556. [CrossRef]
27. de Vreede-Swagemakers, J.J.; Gorgels, A.P.; Dubois-Arbouw, W.I.; van Ree, J.W.; Daemen, M.J.; Houben, L.G.; Wellens, H.J. Out-of-hospital cardiac arrest in the 1990's: A population-based study in the Maastricht area on incidence, characteristics and survival. *J. Am. Coll. Cardiol.* **1997**, *30*, 1500–1505. [CrossRef]
28. Culley, L.L.; Rea, T.D.; Murray, J.A.; Welles, B.; Fahrenbruch, C.E.; Olsufka, M.; Eisenberg, M.S.; Copass, M.K. Public access defibrillation in out-of-hospital cardiac arrest: A community-based study. *Circulation* **2004**, *109*, 1859–1863. [CrossRef]
29. Kim, C.; Fahrenbruch, C.E.; Cobb, L.A.; Eisenberg, M.S. Out-of-hospital cardiac arrest in men and women. *Circulation* **2001**, *104*, 2699–2703. [CrossRef]
30. Haffner, S.; Taegtmeyer, H. Epidemic obesity and the metabolic syndrome. *Circulation* **2003**, *108*, 1541–1545. [CrossRef]
31. Empana, J.P.; Duciemetiere, P.; Balkau, B.; Jouven, X. Contribution of the metabolic syndrome to sudden death risk in asymptomatic men: The Paris Prospective Study I. *Eur. Heart J.* **2007**, *28*, 1149–1154. [CrossRef] [PubMed]
32. Hess, P.L.; Al-Khalidi, H.R.; Friedman, D.J.; Mulder, H.; Kucharska-Newton, A.; Rosamond, W.R.; Lopes, R.D.; Gersh, B.J.; Mark, D.B.; Curtis, L.H.; et al. The Metabolic Syndrome and Risk of Sudden Cardiac Death: The Atherosclerosis Risk in Communities Study. *J. Am. Heart Assoc.* **2017**, *6*, e006103. [CrossRef] [PubMed]
33. Perry, J.R.; Voight, B.F.; Yengo, L.; Amin, N.; Dupuis, J.; Ganser, M.; Grallert, H.; Navarro, P.; Li, M.; Qi, L. Stratifying type 2 diabetes cases by BMI identifies genetic risk variants in LAMA1 and enrichment for risk variants in lean compared to obese cases. *PLoS Genet.* **2012**, *8*, e1002741. [CrossRef]

Disclaimer/Publisher's Note: The statements, opinions and data contained in all publications are solely those of the individual author(s) and contributor(s) and not of MDPI and/or the editor(s). MDPI and/or the editor(s) disclaim responsibility for any injury to people or property resulting from any ideas, methods, instructions or products referred to in the content.

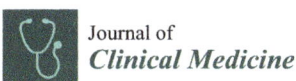

Article

Obesity Is Indirectly Associated with Sudden Cardiac Arrest through Various Risk Factors

Yun Gi Kim [1,†], Joo Hee Jeong [1,†], Seung-Young Roh [2], Kyung-Do Han [3], Yun Young Choi [1], Kyongjin Min [4], Jaemin Shim [1], Jong-Il Choi [1,*] and Young-Hoon Kim [1]

1. Division of Cardiology, Department of Internal Medicine, Korea University College of Medicine, Korea University Anam Hospital, Seoul 02841, Republic of Korea
2. Division of Cardiology, Department of Internal Medicine, Korea University College of Medicine, Korea University Guro Hospital, Seoul 08308, Republic of Korea
3. Department of Statistics and Actuarial Science, Soongsil University, Seoul 06978, Republic of Korea
4. Division of Cardiology, Sanggye Paik Hospital, Inje University College of Medicine, Seoul 01757, Republic of Korea
* Correspondence: jongilchoi@korea.ac.kr; Tel.: +82-2-920-5445; Fax: +82-2-927-1478
† These authors contributed equally to this work.

Abstract: Although obesity is a well-established risk factor of cardiovascular event, the linkage between obesity and sudden cardiac arrest (SCA) is not fully understood. Based on a nationwide health insurance database, this study investigated the impact of body weight status, measured by body-mass index (BMI) and waist circumference, on the SCA risk. A total of 4,234,341 participants who underwent medical check-ups in 2009 were included, and the influence of risk factors (age, sex, social habits, and metabolic disorders) was analyzed. For 33,345,378 person-years follow-up, SCA occurred in 16,352 cases. The BMI resulted in a J-shaped association with SCA risk, in which the obese group (BMI $\geq$ 30) had a 20.8% increased risk of SCA compared with the normal body weight group (18.5 $\leq$ BMI < 23.0) ($p < 0.001$). Waist circumference showed a linear association with the risk of SCA, with a 2.69-fold increased risk of SCA in the highest waist circumference group compared with the lowest waist circumference group ($p < 0.001$). However, after adjustment of risk factors, neither BMI nor waist circumference was associated with the SCA risk. In conclusion, obesity is not independently associated with SCA risk based on the consideration of various confounders. Rather than confining the findings to obesity itself, comprehensive consideration of metabolic disorders as well as demographics and social habits might provide better understanding and prevention of SCA.

Keywords: sudden cardiac arrest; body-mass index; waist circumference; central obesity

1. Introduction

Obesity, which is associated with various medical diseases such as hypertension, diabetes mellitus, dyslipidemia, and coronary artery disease, is a major health concern in developed countries [1–4]. The association between obesity and coronary artery disease is of concern since it can lead to myocardial infarction or sudden cardiac arrest (SCA) [5–8]. A prospective cohort study involving 1 million adults in the United States revealed that the risk of all-cause death and cardiovascular death was significantly increased in obese people [8]. Another study with 2.3 million adolescents from Israel with 40 years of follow-up demonstrated that obesity during adolescence was associated with significantly increased all-cause and cardiovascular mortality in adults [7]. A study from the Republic of Korea also found a significant association between obesity and all-cause mortality [9]. In these studies, body weight status such as normal weight, overweight, and obesity was defined using body-mass index (BMI) criteria, an indicator of general obesity [7–9].

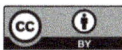

Using BMI can have several limitations [10]. It cannot divide (i) lean body mass from fat and (ii) abdominal fat from the fat of other body sites [10,11]. Furthermore, abdominal obesity, which is not fully reflected in BMI, can have a better predictive value for medical diseases such as diabetes mellitus and myocardial infarction compared with general obesity [12,13].

Sudden cardiac arrest is a medical emergency that imposes a significant burden on both the victim and the society [14–16]. Although both high BMI and waist circumference are known to be associated with the increased risk of cardiovascular death, whether this association is a direct effect of obesity or the result of metabolic comorbidities frequently associated with obesity, such as hypertension, diabetes mellitus, and dyslipidemia, is debated. In addition, prior studies only adjusted a limited number of covariates such as age, sex, height, smoking status, alcohol consumed, educational level, and level of physical exercise, and the influence of other important covariates such as blood pressure, fasting blood glucose, dyslipidemia, and estimated glomerular filtration rate (eGFR) were not taken into account [7,8,17]. We aimed to evaluate the association between obesity measured as BMI and waist circumference and the risk of SCA under adjustment of various metabolic comorbidities using a large prospective cohort from the Korean National Health Insurance Service (K-NHIS) database.

2. Materials and Methods

2.1. K-NHIS Database

This study is a retrospective analysis based on the K-NHIS database, which represents the entire population of South Korea. The K-NHIS is the single and exclusive medical insurance system managed by the government which mandates virtually the entire Korean population to subscribe to. The system is paid for by a nationwide tax system; it also covers those who are not able to afford it, and guarantees basic health care services (citizens are all registered in the system and, therefore, there is less chance of selection bias). The K-NHIS database offers a prospective cohort of subscribed citizens with medical records and various medical measurements during national health check-ups. Therefore, medical data derived from the K-NHIS database are a valuable source for a range of medical research.

If the protocols of the study are approved by both the institutional review board and the official review committee of the K-NHIS (https://nhiss.nhis.or.kr/, accessed on 21 January 2022), researchers are permitted to utilize the K-NHIS database to perform medical research. The Institutional Review Board of Korea University Medicine Anam Hospital and official review committee of the K-NHIS approved this specific study (IRB No.: 2021AN0185). The requirement for written informed consent was waived by the Institutional Review Board of Korea University Medicine Anam Hospital. This study complied with the Declaration of Helsinki and the legal regulations of South Korea.

The K-NHIS provides a regular, biennial, nationwide health check-up to its subscribers. The national health check-up is free of charge for the subscribers as it is covered by the government tax system. During the health check-up, various medical measurements are taken that include height, body weight, waist circumference, blood pressure, serum creatinine, liver function tests, fasting blood glucose (FBG), lipid profile, smoking and alcohol habits, level of income, and physical activity. In the K-NHIS database, various diagnostic codes of the International Classification of Disease, 10th revision (ICD-10) such as hypertension, diabetes mellitus, or heart failure, and prescription history of drugs are recorded. The capability of utilizing these covariates is a distinguished feature of medical research studies based on the K-NHIS database [18,19].

2.2. Participants

In 2009, 66% of people who were meant to undergo the nationwide health check-up actually underwent the check-up. Among adult citizens who underwent nationwide health check-ups in 2009, 40% were randomly sampled and enrolled in this study. Exclusion criteria were participants who were younger than 20 years or those with a diagnosis of SCA prior to enrollment (day of 2009 health check-up). Data obtained from 1 January 2002 to 31 December 2008 were used to identify baseline demographics such as presence of hypertension and diabetes mellitus. Medical follow-up duration was between the day of the 2009 health check-up of each participant and 31 December 2018. No follow-up losses were present except for emigrations.

2.3. Primary Outcome

The primary outcome is the occurrence of SCA during the follow-up period (the day of the 2009 health check-up of each patient and 31 December 2018). The incidence of SCA was defined as event numbers per 1000 person-years of follow-up. Identification of SCA events was based on claims of the following ICD-10 codes: I46.0 (cardiac arrest with successful resuscitation); I46.1 (sudden cardiac arrest); I46.9 (cardiac arrest, cause unspecified); I49.0 (ventricular fibrillation and flutter); R96.0 (instantaneous death); and R96.1 (death occurring less than 24 h from onset of symptoms). According to the definition of SCA, only claims that occurred at emergency department visit were identified as SCA event, and claims during in-hospital admission were excluded.

In order to conform to the definition of SCA, any possible non-cardiac causes of sudden arrest were excluded from the primary outcome [20]. If participants had a prior diagnosis of cerebral hemorrhage, ischemic stroke, asphyxia, suffocation, drowning, gastrointestinal bleeding, sepsis, anaphylaxis, major trauma, hit by lightning, electric shock, or burn within six months of the diagnosis of SCA, the event was not counted as a primary outcome.

2.4. Definitions

The influence of waist circumference and BMI on risk of SCA was evaluated. Waist circumference was measured as the mid-point between the rib cage and the iliac crest. Waist circumference was classified into six stages: waist circumference < 80.0 (cm), $80.0 \leq$ waist circumference < 85.0, $85.0 \leq$ waist circumference < 90.0, $90.0 \leq$ waist circumference < 95.0, $95.0 \leq$ waist circumference < 100.0, and waist circumference ≥ 100.0 for males, and waist circumference < 75.0, $75.0 \leq$ waist circumference < 80.0, $80.0 \leq$ waist circumference < 85.0, $85.0 \leq$ waist circumference < 90.0, $90.0 \leq$ waist circumference < 95.0, and waist circumference ≥ 95.0 for females. Body-mass index was classified into five groups: low body weight (BMI < 18.5 [kg/m^2]); normal body weight ($18.5 \leq$ BMI < 23.0); pre-obesity ($23.0 \leq$ BMI < 25.0); obesity class I (or mild obesity, $25.0 \leq$ BMI < 30.0); and obesity class II-III (or moderate to severe obesity, BMI ≥ 30.0) [21,22].

Alcohol consumption status was defined as follows: (i) non-drinker, 0 g of alcohol per week; (ii) mild to moderate drinker, <210 g of alcohol per week; and (iii) heavy drinker, $\geq$210 g of alcohol per week.

For smoking status: (i) current smokers were defined as those who smoked ≥ 100 cigarettes in their lifetime and continued smoking within one month of the 2009 nationwide health check-up; (ii) ex-smokers were those who smoked ≥ 100 cigarettes in their lifetime, but had not smoked within one month of the 2009 nationwide health check-up; and (iii) never-smokers were those who smoked < 100 cigarettes in their lifetime.

Diabetes mellitus and hypertension were classified into three stages each: (i) non-diabetic (FBG < 100 mg/dL); (ii) impaired fasting glucose (IFG) (FBG 100–125 mg/dL); and (iii) diabetes mellitus (FBG ≥ 126 mg/dL or a prior claim of ICD-10 codes for diabetes mellitus) for diabetes mellitus, and (i) non-hypertension (systolic blood pressure [SBP] < 120 [mmHg] and diastolic blood pressure [DBP] < 80); (ii) pre-hypertension (either $120 \leq$ SBP < 140 or $80 \leq$ DBP < 90); and (iii) hypertension (either SBP ≥ 140, DBP ≥ 90, or a prior claim of ICD-10 codes for hypertension) for hypertension.

Estimated glomerular filtration rate (eGFR) was calculated based on measured creatinine level during the 2009 health check-up, and chronic kidney disease (CKD) was defined as eGFR < 60 mL/min/1.73 m^2 based on the Modification of Diet in Renal Disease (MDRD) equation.

Defining regular physical activity was based on a self-questionnaire acquired during the 2009 health check-up: people who had one or more sessions in a week with high (such as running, climbing, intense bicycle activities) or moderate (such as walking fast, tennis, or moderate bicycle activities) physical activity. The quality of physical measurement and laboratory tests are guaranteed and legally certified by K-NHIS, and the robustness of the aforementioned definitions was validated in our prior studies [19,23–27].

2.5. Statistical Analysis

The categorical variables are presented as number and percentage, and the continuous variables are presented as mean and standard deviation, or median value with interquartile range. The Student's t-test was used for comparison of continuous variables, and the Chi-square test or Fisher's exact test was used for comparison of the categorical variables as indicated. The Cox proportional hazards model was used to calculate unadjusted and adjusted hazard ratios (HR) and 95% confidence intervals (CI). In addition to the un-adjusted model, five multivariate models were adopted: (i) multivariate model 1: adjusted for age and sex; (ii) multivariate model 2: adjusted for model 1 plus smoking, alcohol, regular exercise, and income; (iii) multivariate model 3: adjusted for model 2 plus hypertension, diabetes mellitus, and dyslipidemia; (iv) multivariate model 4: adjusted for model 2 plus hypertension, diabetes mellitus, dyslipidemia, and chronic kidney disease; and (v) multivariate model 5: adjusted for model 4 plus γ-GTP. All tests were two-tailed, and statistical significance was defined as p values ≤ 0.05. All statistical analyses were performed with SAS version 9.2 (SAS Institute, Cary, NC, USA).

3. Results

3.1. Study Population

A total of 4,234,341 participants were randomly sampled from participants that underwent 2009 nationwide health screening (Figure 1). People with prior diagnosis of SCA (n = 491) and with missing data (n = 177,427) were excluded from the study and 4,056,423 people were followed until December 2018. Sudden cardiac arrest occurred in 16,352 subjects among 33,345,378 person-years of follow-up, with an incidence of 0.490 (per 1000 person-years). The flow of the study is summarized in Figure 1. Significant differences in the baseline demographics between people who did and did not experience SCA are summarized in Supplementary Table S1: people with SCA were older and had higher prevalence of male sex, current smokers, hypertension, diabetes mellitus, dyslipidemia, and CKD [25]. The baseline demographics according to BMI status demonstrated a significant difference across all parameters such as age, sex, smoking and alcohol consumption status, regular exercise, income level, hypertension, diabetes mellitus, dyslipidemia, CKD, and γ-glutamyl transferase (γ-GTP) (Table 1). A similar pattern of difference in the baseline demographics was observed according to waist circumference, which is described in Table 2.

Table 1. Baseline demographics according to BMI.

	BMI					
	BMI < 18.5	18.5 ≤ BMI < 23	23 ≤ BMI < 25	25 ≤ BMI < 30	30 ≤ BMI	p-Value
	148,460	1,579,653	1,001,394	1,182,398	144,518	
Male	49,452 (33.3%)	750,152 (47.5%)	602,974 (60.2%)	749,493 (63.4%)	81,460 (56.4%)	<0.001
Age (years)	40.5 ± 16.6	45.2 ± 14.4	48.6 ± 13.4	49.1 ± 13.3	46.2 ± 13.9	<0.001
Age group						<0.001
20–29	52,975 (35.7%)	262,941 (16.7%)	85,034 (8.5%)	83,743 (7.1%)	16,923 (11.7%)	
30–39	33,026 (22.3%)	315,592 (20.0%)	175,039 (17.5%)	219,742 (18.6%)	35,411 (24.5%)	
40–49	23,966 (16.1%)	424,880 (26.9%)	272,812 (27.2%)	309,454 (26.2%)	34,747 (24.0%)	
50–59	13,701 (9.2%)	293,562 (18.6%)	241,153 (24.1%)	284,426 (24.1%)	28,106 (19.5%)	
60–69	10,819 (7.3%)	171,096 (10.8%)	151,983 (15.2%)	194,509 (16.5%)	20,081 (13.9%)	
70–79	10,593 (7.1%)	93,783 (5.9%)	66,893 (6.7%)	81,888 (6.9%)	8526 (5.9%)	
80–	3380 (2.3%)	17,799 (1.1%)	8480 (0.9%)	8636 (0.7%)	724 (0.5%)	
Waist circumference (cm)	66.2 ± 6.1	74.3 ± 6.8	81.2 ± 6.5	87.2 ± 6.5	96.8 ± 8.5	<0.001
Smoking						<0.001
Never-smoker	104,399 (70.3%)	1,009,981 (63.9%)	569,292 (56.9%)	641,966 (54.3%)	81,957 (56.7%)	
Ex-smoker	10,274 (6.9%)	176,612 (11.2%)	166,249 (16.6%)	211,763 (17.9%)	19,715 (13.6%)	
Current-smoker	33,787 (22.8%)	393,060 (24.9%)	265,853 (26.6%)	328,669 (27.8%)	42,846 (29.7%)	
Alcohol consumption						<0.001
Non-drinker	84,650 (57.0%)	844,228 (53.4%)	502,676 (50.2%)	580,170 (49.1%)	74,863 (51.8%)	
Mild-drinker	57,034 (38.4%)	635,906 (40.3%)	415,595 (41.5%)	483,904 (40.9%)	54,251 (37.5%)	
Heavy-drinker	6776 (4.6%)	99,519 (6.3%)	83,123 (8.3%)	118,324 (10.0%)	15,404 (10.7%)	
Regular exercise	14,083 (9.5%)	260,130 (16.5%)	201,750 (20.2%)	235,736 (19.9%)	25,058 (17.3%)	<0.001
Income (lowest 20%)	26,986 (18.2%)	285,175 (18.1%)	170,960 (17.1%)	198,438 (16.8%)	26,103 (18.1%)	<0.001
Diabetes mellitus	5032 (3.4%)	88,229 (5.6%)	89,877 (9.0%)	145,104 (12.3%)	25,156 (17.4%)	<0.001
Diabetes mellitus stage						<0.001
Non-diabetic	123,405 (83.1%)	1,201,431 (76.1%)	672,234 (67.1%)	710,909 (60.1%)	76,152 (52.7%)	
Impaired fasting glucose	20,023 (13.5%)	289,993 (18.4%)	239,283 (23.9%)	326,385 (27.6%)	43,210 (30.0%)	
New onset diabetes	2145 (1.4%)	30,453 (1.9%)	29,509 (3.0%)	49,482 (4.2%)	8994 (6.2%)	
Diabetic < 5 years	1339 (0.9%)	25,901 (1.6%)	29,589 (3.0%)	52,562 (4.5%)	10,096 (7.0%)	
Diabetic ≥ 5 years	1548 (1.0%)	31,875 (2.0%)	30,779 (3.1%)	43,060 (3.6%)	6066 (4.2%)	
Glucose (mg/dL)	90.9 ± 20.9	94.0 ± 21.3	97.9 ± 23.8	100.9 ± 25.7	104.9 ± 30.2	<0.001
Hypertension	14,751 (9.9%)	271,106 (17.2%)	280,148 (28.0%)	451,800 (38.2%)	73,908 (51.1%)	<0.001
Hypertension stage						<0.001
Non-hypertensive	91,041 (61.3%)	725,291 (45.9%)	307,165 (30.7%)	245,829 (20.8%)	16,651 (11.5%)	
Pre-hypertension	42,668 (28.7%)	583,256 (36.9%)	414,081 (41.4%)	484,769 (41.0%)	53,959 (37.3%)	
Hypertension	5325 (3.6%)	90,481 (5.7%)	84,145 (8.4%)	131,823 (11.2%)	24,305 (16.8%)	
Hypertension with medication	9426 (6.4%)	180,625 (11.4%)	196,003 (19.6%)	319,977 (27.1%)	49,603 (34.3%)	
Systolic blood pressure (mmHg)	113.7 ± 14.1	118.6 ± 14.4	123.4 ± 14.4	126.8 ± 14.5	131.2 ± 15.2	<0.001
Diastolic blood pressure (mmHg)	71.3 ± 9.3	74.0 ± 9.6	76.8 ± 9.7	79.0 ± 9.8	82.0 ± 10.5	<0.001
Dyslipidemia	8133 (5.5%)	187,002 (11.8%)	196,442 (19.6%)	300,990 (25.5%)	45,026 (31.2%)	<0.001
Dyslipidemia stage						<0.001
Total cholesterol < 240 (mg/dL)	140,327 (94.5%)	1,392,651 (88.2%)	804,952 (80.4%)	881,408 (74.5%)	99,492 (68.8%)	
Total cholesterol ≥ 240	4679 (3.2%)	95,287 (6.0%)	92,427 (9.2%)	136,280 (11.5%)	19,999 (13.8%)	
Total cholesterol ≥ 240 with medication	3454 (2.3%)	91,715 (5.8%)	104,015 (10.4%)	164,710 (13.9%)	25,027 (17.3%)	
Cholesterol (mg/dL)	177.8 ± 35.1	188.8 ± 39.1	197.9 ± 41.4	202.6 ± 42.1	206.3 ± 42.1	<0.001
High-density lipoprotein (mg/dL)	64.3 ± 37.7	59.7 ± 34.3	55.2 ± 30.4	53.0 ± 32.3	51.7 ± 29.6	<0.001
Low-density lipoprotein (mg/dL)	115.8 ± 351.8	119.1 ± 252.9	122.3 ± 181.8	123.3 ± 158.1	124.6 ± 152.8	<0.001
Chronic kidney disease	8198 (5.5%)	95,435 (6.0%)	71,342 (7.1%)	92,362 (7.8%)	11,257 (7.8%)	<0.001
eGFR (mL/min/1.73 m^2)	93.1 ± 47.9	89.2 ± 44.7	86.5 ± 44.8	85.6 ± 44.6	87.0 ± 45.3	<0.001
γ-GTP *	18.7 (18.7–18.8)	21.3 (21.3–21.4)	27.4 (27.4–27.4)	33.8 (33.7–33.8)	40.5 (40.3–40.6)	<0.001

* expressed as median (interquartile range); BMI: body-mass index; eGFR: estimated glomerular filtration rate; γ-GTP: γ-glutamyl transferase.

Table 2. Baseline demographics according to waist circumference.

	Waist Circumference (Male/Female; cm)						p-Value
	WC < 80/75	80/75 ≤ WC < 85/80	85/80 ≤ WC < 90/85	90/85 ≤ WC < 95/90	95/90 ≤ WC < 100/95	100/95 ≤ WC	
	1,490,892	965,616	803,708	471,183	209,692	115,332	
Male	660,775 (44.3%)	598,889 (62.0%)	499,969 (62.2%)	293,667 (62.3%)	120,066 (57.3%)	60,165 (52.2%)	<0.001
Age (years)	42.4 ± 13.6	47.6 ± 13.2	50.2 ± 13.4	51.8 ± 13.6	52.7 ± 14.2	52.0 ± 15.3	<0.001
Age group							<0.001
20–29	318,255 (21.4%)	88,707 (9.2%)	49,348 (6.1%)	24,681 (5.2%)	11,448 (5.5%)	9177 (8.0%)	
30–39	335,158 (22.5%)	187,253 (19.4%)	133,262 (16.6%)	72,134 (15.3%)	31,459 (15.0%)	19,544 (17.0%)	
40–49	415,596 (27.9%)	272,408 (28.2%)	206,013 (25.6%)	108,027 (22.9%)	42,727 (20.4%)	21,088 (18.3%)	
50–59	242,128 (16.2%)	225,760 (23.4%)	202,887 (25.2%)	117,630 (25.0%)	48,855 (23.3%)	23,688 (20.5%)	
60–69	113,085 (7.6%)	128,347 (13.3%)	140,559 (17.5%)	95,715 (20.3%)	46,428 (22.1%)	24,354 (21.1%)	
70–79	55,993 (3.8%)	55,007 (5.7%)	63,160 (7.9%)	46,864 (10.0%)	25,367 (12.1%)	15,292 (13.3%)	
80–	10,677 (0.7%)	8134 (0.8%)	8479 (1.1%)	6132 (1.3%)	3408 (1.6%)	2189 (1.9%)	
Body mass index (kg/m^2)	21.1 ± 2.1	23.5 ± 1.9	25.0 ± 2.0	26.5 ± 2.2	28.0 ± 2.4	30.7 ± 3.3	<0.001
Smoking							<0.001
Never-smoker	986,822 (66.2%)	532,393 (55.1%)	440,387 (54.8%)	257,592 (54.7%)	120,894 (57.7%)	69,507 (60.3%)	
Ex-smoker	148,357 (10.0%)	156,878 (16.3%)	142,207 (17.7%)	85,813 (18.2%)	35,049 (16.7%)	16,309 (14.1%)	
Current-smoker	355,713 (23.9%)	276,345 (28.6%)	221,114 (27.5%)	127,778 (27.1%)	53,749 (25.6%)	29,516 (25.6%)	
Alcohol consumption							<0.001
Non-drinker	793,738 (53.2%)	470,369 (48.7%)	402,489 (50.1%)	240,337 (51.0%)	113,560 (54.2%)	66,094 (57.3%)	
Mild-drinker	612,902 (41.1%)	412,931 (42.8%)	326,697 (40.7%)	182,237 (38.7%)	74,397 (35.5%)	37,526 (32.5%)	
Heavy-drinker	84,252 (5.7%)	82,316 (8.5%)	74,522 (9.3%)	48,609 (10.3%)	21,735 (10.4%)	11,712 (10.2%)	
Regular exercise	245,521 (16.5%)	190,060 (19.7%)	156,820 (19.5%)	88,629 (18.8%)	37,125 (17.7%)	18,602 (16.1%)	<0.001
Income (lowest 20%)	276,206 (18.5%)	162,310 (16.8%)	133,818 (16.7%)	78,807 (16.7%)	36,187 (17.3%)	20,334 (17.6%)	<0.001
Diabetes mellitus	54,778 (3.7%)	75,069 (7.8%)	89,473 (11.1%)	69,195 (14.7%)	38,400 (18.3%)	26,483 (23.0%)	<0.001
Diabetes mellitus stage							<0.001
Non-diabetic	1,183,986 (79.4%)	665,077 (68.9%)	502,496 (62.5%)	268,100 (56.9%)	109,731 (52.3%)	54,741 (47.5%)	
Impaired fasting glucose	252,128 (16.9%)	225,470 (23.4%)	211,739 (26.4%)	133,888 (28.4%)	61,561 (29.4%)	34,108 (29.6%)	
New onset diabetes	22,574 (1.5%)	27,518 (2.9%)	30,030 (3.7%)	21,671 (4.6%)	11,218 (5.4%)	7572 (6.6%)	
Diabetic < 5 years	15,676 (1.1%)	23,454 (2.4%)	30,162 (3.8%)	24,940 (5.3%)	14,740 (7.0%)	10,515 (9.1%)	
Diabetic ≥ 5 years	16,528 (1.1%)	24,097 (2.5%)	29,281 (3.6%)	22,584 (4.8%)	12,442 (5.9%)	8396 (7.3%)	
Glucose (mg/dL)	92.3 ± 18.7	97.1 ± 23.1	100.0 ± 25.6	102.5 ± 27.5	104.8 ± 29.8	108.0 ± 33.4	<0.001
Hypertension	195,526 (13.1%)	240,734 (24.9%)	276,994 (34.5%)	203,635 (43.2%)	107,014 (51.0%)	67,810 (58.8%)	<0.001
Hypertension stage							<0.001
Non-hypertensive	746,795 (50.1%)	314,141 (32.5%)	196,915 (24.5%)	86,969 (18.5%)	29,483 (14.1%)	11,674 (10.1%)	
Pre-hypertension	548,571 (36.8%)	410,741 (42.5%)	329,799 (41.0%)	180,579 (38.3%)	73,195 (34.9%)	35,848 (31.1%)	
Hypertension	75,002 (5.0%)	80,335 (8.3%)	81,614 (10.2%)	54,905 (11.7%)	26,803 (12.8%)	17,420 (15.1%)	
Hypertension with medication	120,524 (8.1%)	160,399 (16.6%)	195,380 (24.3%)	148,730 (31.6%)	80,211 (38.3%)	50,390 (43.7%)	
Systolic blood pressure (mmHg)	117.3 ± 13.9	122.7 ± 14.3	125.4 ± 14.5	127.6 ± 14.8	129.5 ± 15.1	131.8 ± 15.7	<0.001
Diastolic blood pressure (mmHg)	73.3 ± 9.5	76.5 ± 9.7	78.1 ± 9.8	79.3 ± 10.0	80.3 ± 10.2	81.7 ± 10.7	<0.001
Dyslipidemia	142,044 (9.5%)	170,261 (17.6%)	187,884 (23.4%)	130,610 (27.7%)	66,440 (31.7%)	40,354 (35.0%)	<0.001
Dyslipidemia stage							<0.001
Total cholesterol < 240 (mg/dL)	1,348,848 (90.5%)	795,355 (82.4%)	615,824 (76.6%)	340,573 (72.3%)	143,252 (68.3%)	74,978 (65.0%)	
Total cholesterol ≥ 240	80,387 (5.4%)	85,808 (8.9%)	85,795 (10.7%)	54,982 (11.7%)	26,340 (12.6%)	15,360 (13.3%)	
Total cholesterol ≥ 240 with medication	61,657 (4.1%)	84,453 (8.8%)	102,089 (12.7%)	75,628 (16.1%)	40,100 (19.1%)	24,994 (21.7%)	
Cholesterol (mg/dL)	186.6 ± 37.4	196.6 ± 40.8	201.1 ± 42.8	203.2 ± 43.3	204.9 ± 43.3	206.2 ± 44.2	<0.001
High-density lipoprotein (mg/dL)	60.6 ± 33.7	55.8 ± 32.6	53.9 ± 31.9	52.6 ± 31.9	52.3 ± 31.9	52.2 ± 32.1	<0.001
Low-density lipoprotein (mg/dL)	120.3 ± 292.0	120.6 ± 167.8	122.0 ± 142.0	122.5 ± 143.4	122.8 ± 132.4	123.2 ± 117.3	<0.001
Chronic kidney disease	77,727 (5.2%)	65,384 (6.8%)	62,037 (7.7%)	40,381 (8.6%)	20,738 (9.9%)	12,327 (10.7%)	<0.001
eGFR (mL/min/1.73 m^2)	90.1 ± 45.0	86.9 ± 43.9	86.0 ± 46.3	85.2 ± 44.6	84.7 ± 43.4	85.4 ± 44.8	<0.001
γ-GTP *	20.1 (20.1–20.1)	27.1 (27.1–27.2)	31.2 (31.1–31.2)	34.8 (34.7–34.9)	36.6 (36.5–36.7)	38.9 (38.7–39.0)	<0.001

* expressed as median (interquartile range); WC: waist circumference; BMI: body-mass index; eGFR: estimated glomerular filtration rate; γ-GTP: γ-glutamyl transferase.

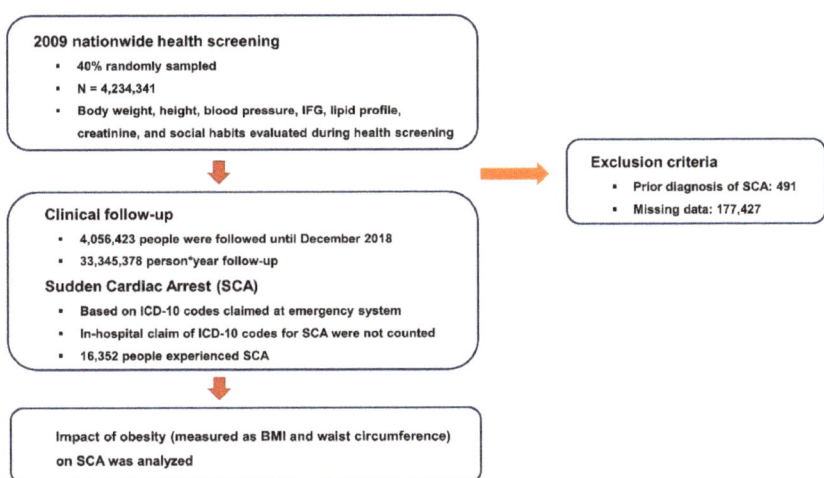

Figure 1. Study flow. BMI: body-mass index; ICD-10: International Classification of Disease, 10th revision; IFG: impaired fasting glucose; SCA: sudden cardiac arrest.

3.2. BMI and SCA

Body weight status measured by BMI was significantly associated with the risk of SCA for both men and women (Table 3, Figure 2a). Moderate to severe obesity (BMI ≥ 30) had 20.8% increased rate of SCA compared with normal weight (18.5 ≤ BMI < 23) (95% CI = 1.12–1.31; $p < 0.001$: Table 3). After adjustment of the influence of age and sex, the increased rate of SCA in moderate to severe obese people was elevated to 35.5% from 20.8% (95% CI = 1.25–1.47; $p < 0.001$: Table 3). The relative risk of SCA in moderate to severe obese people was 38.8% higher after further adjusting for smoking and alcohol consumption status, regular exercise, and income level (95% CI = 1.28–1.50; $p < 0.001$: Table 3). However, the association between BMI and the risk of SCA was lost after adjusting for the influence of hypertension, diabetes mellitus, dyslipidemia, and CKD (HR = 1.05; 95% CI = 0.96–1.13; $p = 0.286$: Table 3, Figure 2a). Furthermore, people with pre-obesity (23 ≤ BMI < 25) and mild obesity (25 ≤ BMI < 30) showed significantly lower risk of SCA compared with people with normal body weight (18.5 ≤ BMI < 23) after multivariate adjustment (HR = 0.80 and 0.79, respectively; $p < 0.001$ for both: Table 3). The multivariate model further adjusting for γ-GTP showed similar results, reflecting no association between obesity and risk of SCA (HR = 0.94; 95% CI = 0.87–1.02; $p = 0.130$: Table 3, Figure 2a) and decreased risk of SCA in the pre-obesity and mild obesity groups (HR = 0.78 and 0.74, respectively; $p < 0.001$ for both: Table 3, Figure 2a).

3.3. Waist Circumference and SCA

Participants were classified into six groups according to waist circumference measured during their health check-up. Without adjustment of covariates, waist circumference showed a significant linear association with the risk of SCA with higher waist circumference associated with increased risk of SCA for both men and women (Table 3, Figure 2b). However, such association was significantly weakened after adjusting age, sex, smoking, alcohol, regular exercise, and income (Table 3, Figure 2b). After further adjusting the influence of metabolic disorders (hypertension, diabetes mellitus, dyslipidemia, and CKD), the highest waist circumference group no longer showed an increased rate of SCA (HR = 1.04; 95% CI = 0.96–1.12; $p = 0.346$). Compared with the reference group (<80 cm and 75 cm for men and women, respectively), middle-level waist circumference (between 80 cm and 100 cm for men, and 75 cm and 95 cm for women) was associated with lower risk of SCA (Table 3). Adjustment of γ-GTP further affected the association between waist circumference and the risk of SCA, with all other groups showing lower risk of SCA compared with the reference group (Table 3).

Table 3. Impact of BMI and waist circumference on SCA.

	n	SCA	Follow-Up Duration (Person-Years)	Incidence	Univariate	Multivariate 1	Multivariate 2	Multivariate 3	Multivariate 4	Multivariate 5
					BMI					
BMI < 18.5	148,460	830	1,196,986	0.69	1.50 (1.40–1.61)	1.70 (1.58–1.83)	1.61 (1.49–1.73)	1.78 (1.65–1.91)	1.79 (1.66–1.92)	1.79 (1.66–1.92)
18.5 ≤ BMI < 23	1,579,653	6016	12,966,752	0.46	1 (reference)	1 (reference)	1 (reference)	1 (reference)	1 (reference)	1 (reference)
23 ≤ BMI < 25	1,001,394	3924	8,249,250	0.48	1.02 (0.98–1.07)	0.85 (0.81–0.88)	0.87 (0.84–0.91)	0.80 (0.77–0.84)	0.80 (0.77–0.83)	0.78 (0.75–0.81)
25 ≤ BMI < 30	1,182,398	4915	9,743,125	0.50	1.09 (1.05–1.13)	0.90 (0.86–0.93)	0.93 (0.90–0.97)	0.80 (0.76–0.83)	0.79 (0.76–0.82)	0.74 (0.71–0.77)
30 ≤ BMI	144,518	667	1,189,264	0.56	1.21 (1.12–1.31)	1.36 (1.25–1.47)	1.39 (1.28–1.50)	1.06 (0.97–1.14)	1.05 (0.96–1.13)	0.94 (0.87–1.02)
					Waist circumference (male/female; cm)					
<80/75	1,490,892	4286	12,283,975	0.35	1 (reference)	1 (reference)	1 (reference)	1 (reference)	1 (reference)	1 (reference)
–85/80	965,616	3665	7,945,666	0.46	1.32 (1.26–1.38)	0.88 (0.84–0.92)	0.90 (0.86–0.94)	0.83 (0.79–0.87)	0.83 (0.79–0.87)	0.80 (0.76–0.83)
–90/85	803,708	3690	6,603,475	0.56	1.60 (1.53–1.67)	0.91 (0.87–0.95)	0.93 (0.89–0.97)	0.81 (0.78–0.85)	0.81 (0.77–0.85)	0.76 (0.73–0.80)
–95/90	471,183	2520	3,859,942	0.65	1.87 (1.78–1.96)	0.94 (0.90–0.99)	0.97 (0.92–1.02)	0.81 (0.77–0.85)	0.80 (0.76–0.84)	0.74 (0.70–0.77)
–100/95	209,692	1310	1,714,019	0.76	2.19 (2.06–2.33)	1.07 (1.00–1.14)	1.10 (1.03–1.17)	0.87 (0.82–0.93)	0.86 (0.81–0.92)	0.78 (0.73–0.83)
≥100/95	115,332	881	938,301	0.94	2.69 (2.50–2.89)	1.39 (1.29–1.50)	1.42 (1.32–1.53)	1.05 (0.98–1.14)	1.04 (0.96–1.12)	0.92 (0.86–0.99)

Incidence is per 1000 person-years follow-up. BMI: body-mass-index; SCA: sudden cardiac arrest; γ-GTP: gamma-glutamyl transferase. Multivariate model 1: adjusted for age and sex. Multivariate model 2: adjusted for model 1 plus smoking, alcohol, regular exercise, and income. Multivariate model 3: adjusted for model 2 plus hypertension, diabetes mellitus, and dyslipidemia. Multivariate model 4: adjusted for model 2 plus hypertension, diabetes mellitus, dyslipidemia, and chronic kidney disease. Multivariate model 5: adjusted for model 4 plus γ-GTP.

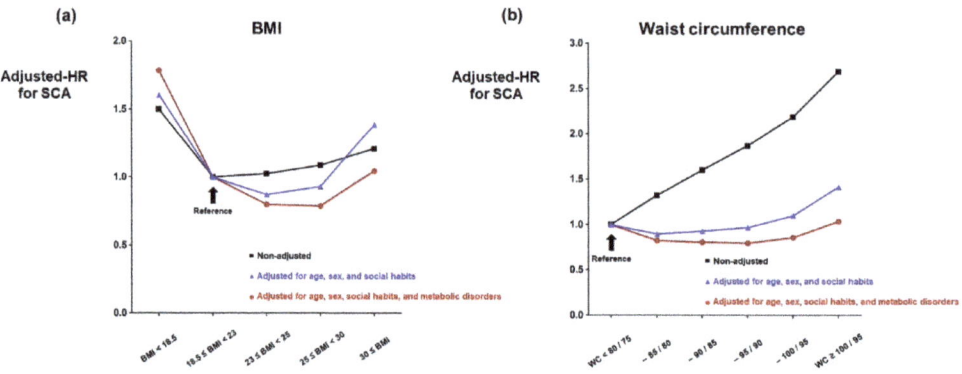

Figure 2. Impact of covariate adjustment. (**a**) The association between obesity (BMI ≥ 30) and SCA was lost when the impact of metabolic disorders (hypertension, diabetes mellitus, dyslipidemia, and CKD) was adjusted. (**b**) Waist circumference showed no association with SCA when various covariates including metabolic disorders were adjusted. BMI: body-mass index; CKD: chronic kidney disease; HR: hazard ratio; SCA: sudden cardiac arrest; WC: waist circumference. Waist circumference is expressed as centimeters. Social habits represent alcohol consumption, smoking status, regular exercise, and income. Metabolic disorders represent hypertension, diabetes mellitus, dyslipidemia, and CKD.

3.4. Obesity, Metabolic Syndrome and SCA

The association of obesity and SCA was further analyzed according to the presence of the classic metabolic syndromes—hypertension, diabetes mellitus, and dyslipidemia.

Participants were divided into (i) those who had the three metabolic syndromes triad (hypertension, diabetes mellitus, and dyslipidemia) and (ii) those who had only one or two, or none of the metabolic syndrome triad Supplementary Table S2. Participants with the metabolic syndrome triad revealed a higher incidence of SCA across all subgroups. After adjusting covariates, participants with the metabolic syndrome triad did not show any significant association between obesity (measured with either BMI or waist circumference) and increased risk of SCA.

3.5. Multivariate Model

In a multivariate Cox-proportional-hazards model, age, sex, smoking status, alcohol consumption, regular exercise, low income, hypertension, diabetes mellitus, dyslipidemia, CKD, and γ-GTP were independently associated with SCA risk (Table 4). Influence on SCA based on the degree of hazard ratio was most prominent in age, sex, smoking, hypertension, diabetes mellitus, and CKD. Waist circumference also showed an independent association with the risk of SCA, but the association was a negative correlation with a 0.6% lower rate of SCA per 1 cm increase in waist circumference (Table 4).

Table 4. Multivariate model for SCA prediction.

	Hazard Ratio with 95% Confidence Interval	p-Value
Age (year)	1.08 (1.08–1.08)	<0.001
Sex		<0.001
Male	2.35 (2.25–2.46)	
Female	1 (reference)	
Smoking status		<0.001
Non-smoker	1 (reference)	
Ex-smoker	1.14 (1.09–1.20)	
Current-smoker	1.81 (1.74–1.89)	
Alcohol consumption		<0.001
Non-drinker	1 (reference)	
Mild-drinker	0.77 (0.74–0.80)	
Heavy-drinker	0.75 (0.71–0.79)	
Regular exercise		<0.001
No	1 (reference)	
Yes	0.89 (0.86–0.93)	
Income		<0.001
High	1 (reference)	
Low	1.09 (1.05–1.14)	
Hypertension		<0.001
Non-hypertension	1 (reference)	
Pre-hypertension	1.16 (1.11–1.21)	
Hypertension	1.51 (1.44–1.59)	
Diabetes mellitus		<0.001
Non-DM	1 (reference)	
IFG	1.06 (1.02–1.10)	
DM	1.74 (1.67–1.81)	
Dyslipidemia		<0.001
Total cholesterol < 240 (mg/dL)	1 (reference)	
Total cholesterol ≥ 240	1.09 (1.03–1.15)	
Total cholesterol ≥ 240 with medication	0.97 (0.93–1.01)	
Chronic kidney disease	1.47 (1.41–1.53)	<0.001
Waist circumference (cm; continuous)	0.99 (0.99–1.00)	<0.001
γ-GTP (unit; continuous)	1.00 (1.00–1.00)	<0.001

DM: diabetes mellitus; γ-GTP: gamma-glutamyl transferase; IFG: impaired fasting glucose; SCA: sudden cardiac arrest.

4. Discussion

This study investigated the association of SCA with obesity, which is represented as BMI and waist circumference, based on a nationwide health insurance cohort of South

Korea. Before consideration of the mediating risk factors, both general and central obesity were positively associated with risk of SCA. General obesity measured as BMI resulted in a J-shaped association with SCA, with highest SCA risk in the low body weight group (BMI < 18.5) followed by the obesity class II-III group (30.0 ≤ BMI), and the lowest SCA risk in the normal body weight group (18.5 ≤ BMI < 23). In contrast, central obesity measured as waist circumference reflected a linear association with SCA risk, resulting in a 2.6-fold increased risk of SCA in the highest waist circumference subgroup (100/95 cm ≤ waist circumference) compared with the reference group (waist circumference < 80/75 cm). However, the association between obesity and SCA risk was lost after adjustment of the covariates of metabolic disease and its surrogate marker (γ-GTP). In other words, a positive association of obesity and SCA was not present after adjustment of the covariates, which accentuates the mediating effect of metabolic disease and sociodemographic factors on SCA rather than the effect of obesity itself. Our study features discriminative strength through assessing the single exclusive nationwide health insurance system, comprising approximately 4.2 million participants, which is the largest population study assessing the association between obesity and SCA. Although the overall incidence of SCA was not high (<0.5%), sufficient cases of SCA (n = 16,352) were analyzed.

4.1. Obesity and SCA

Obesity is a well-established risk factor for mortality as well as atherosclerotic cardiovascular disease, which is represented as BMI, waist circumference, or waist-to-hip ratio. A J-shaped association between BMI and all-cause mortality is shown in prior studies [8,9]. Furthermore, central obesity assessed as waist circumference or waist-to-hip ratio reflected a robust association with mortality after adjustment of BMI, which led to a more comprehensive understanding of the linkage between obesity and mortality by evaluating both general obesity and central obesity [17]. However, both general and central obesity are strongly associated with various metabolic disorders such as hypertension, diabetes mellitus, dyslipidemia, and CKD, as shown in this study. It was unclear whether obesity itself or an associated metabolic disorder is the culprit risk factor for SCA.

Our study found a J-shaped association of SCA with BMI before adjustment of the covariates. Waist circumference also showed a linear association with SCA before covariate adjustment, which is a finding that is consistent with previous studies. However, the association of obesity and SCA was no longer present after adjustment for demographic factors (age and sex) and social habits, which was weakened even more after further consideration of the metabolic conditions and its surrogate marker, γ-GTP. Waist circumference showed a negative association with SCA after covariate adjustment (0.6% decreased risk of SCA per 1 cm increase in waist circumference: Table 4). Our findings suggest that obesity itself is not an independent risk factor for SCA, but is a surrogate marker of metabolic disorders and people demographics. Therefore, not only reducing body weight and waist circumference but also gaining a comprehensive understanding of the metabolic risk factors as a whole in each individual, and the successful management of metabolic disorders, may be important for primary prevention of SCA.

Obesity holds a strong correlation with metabolic disease as well as cardiovascular disease including coronary artery disease, heart failure, and cardiac arrhythmia. However, decreased risk of adverse cardiovascular outcomes in obese patients had been observed in various cardiovascular diseases, known as the obesity paradox [28,29]. The obesity paradox partly explains this loss of association of obesity and SCA. The exact mechanisms of the obesity paradox are yet to be established, but several hypotheses support the obesity paradox. Increased obesity alters hormonal and lipid mediators and cytokines—increased lipoproteins have a protective effect on inflammatory response, such as binding to endotoxin and increase of lymphocytes [30,31]. A decrease of adiponectin level and catecholamine response in obese patients also supports better clinical outcomes [32,33]. In addition, tumor necrosis factor-α I and II receptors produced by adipose tissue may promote an anti-arrhythmic environment, which may lead to decreased lethal arrhythmic events [34,35]. Furthermore, excessive fat and serum cholesterol in obese patients may serve as a reserve for acute inflammatory stress conditions that may provoke SCA [36]. Nonetheless, the use of BMI for measuring obesity should be interpreted with caution since BMI does not accurately reflect different components of body composition such as muscle mass and visceral fat. For instance, a previous study on cancer patients revealed that the obesity paradox was present when it was measured as BMI, but not in sarcopenic obesity patients [37]. It should also be acknowledged that most of the previous studies on the obesity paradox had focused on BMI as an assessment tool of obesity [38]. Therefore, to clarify the obesity paradox, further investigations that utilize more accurate methods to assess body composition and nutritional status are needed.

4.2. Prevention of SCA

Although the consequences of SCA events are highly dependent on the geographical accessibility of emergency medical services and the degree of training of citizens, the majority of SCA events impose considerable socioeconomic costs on their victims and family members [14]. In addition, even after the return of spontaneous circulation, neurologically complete recovery is challenging. Primary prevention of SCA with recognition of the underlying risk factors represents a key strategy in reducing the socioeconomic burden of SCA on public health.

Increased adiposity not only aggravates cardiovascular hemodynamics and leads to structural change of myocardium but also accelerates metabolic condition by the dysregulation of lipid metabolism, elevation of blood pressure, increased insulin resistance, and pro-inflammatory response [39,40]. Our study demonstrated a clear association between obesity (both by BMI and waist circumference) and various metabolic disorders. The increase of BMI and waist circumference was associated with an increased prevalence of metabolic disorders, including diabetes mellitus, hypertension, dyslipidemia, and chronic kidney disease. Clarifying whether obesity is independently associated with SCA or is indirectly associated with SCA through the influence of metabolic disorders is important for the prevention of SCA. If coexisting metabolic disorders are the culprit risk factor for SCA, weight reduction itself may not be sufficient to effectively prevent SCA, and concomitant management of metabolic disorders such as hypertension and diabetes may be more important.

4.3. Limitations

There are several limitations in this study. First, obesity defined through BMI and waist circumference was measured at the time of enrollment (2009), and temporal change of the parameters was not considered. Certain populations with systemic conditions such as malignancy or tuberculosis might have experienced acute change of body weight. The results of the current study cannot demonstrate cause and effect relationships. Consequently, further analysis of temporal change of BMI and waist circumference may provide more valuable clinical implications. In a similar vein, although obesity was quantified as BMI and waist circumference, it was not further analyzed specifically, such as analysis of fat mass and proportion of visceral fat. Second, since the outcome was restricted to out-of-hospital cardiac arrests, this study might have underestimated the actual incidence of SCA. Due to heterogenous etiologies of in-hospital cardiac arrests, it is difficult to distinguish the predisposing condition of in-hospital cardiac arrest by ICD-10 codes—whether it was a sudden, unexplained cardiac arrest or a hemodynamic collapse due to non-cardiac underlying conditions. Moreover, the major reason for excluding in-hospital cardiac arrest is due to its different clinical characteristics compared with out-of-hospital cardiac arrest [41]. Patients with in-hospital cardiac arrests are reported to have older age, higher proportion of non-shockable rhythm, and also a higher proportion of chronic illness such as infection, malignancy, or chronic respiratory disease [42]. Therefore, we restricted the analysis to out-of-hospital cardiac arrest to decrease heterogeneity and reduce other possible confounding factors. Last, our cohort exclusively consisted of an East Asian population and extrapolation to other ethnic groups should be undertaken with caution.

5. Conclusions

Obesity assessed as BMI and waist circumference did not show an independent association with SCA risk after adjustment of mediating risk factors. In conclusion, rather than focusing on obesity per se, an integrated approach with consideration of pre-existing metabolic disorders as well as people demographics and social habits might provide a better understanding and prevention of SCA.

Supplementary Materials: The following supporting information can be downloaded at: https://www.mdpi.com/article/10.3390/jcm12052068/s1. Table S1: Baseline characteristics of patients with and without SCA; Table S2: Impact of BMI and waist circumference on SCA according to metabolic syndrome.

Author Contributions: J.-I.C. had full access to all data in this study and takes responsibility for data integrity and analytical accuracy. The concept and design of the study were developed by Y.G.K., J.H.J., S.-Y.R., Y.Y.C., K.-D.H., J.-I.C. and Y.-H.K. Data analysis and interpretation were performed by Y.G.K., S.-Y.R., Y.Y.C., K.-D.H., J.H.J., K.M. and J.-I.C. The manuscript was drafted by Y.G.K., J.H.J., K.-D.H. and J.-I.C. Statistical analysis was performed by Y.G.K., J.H.J., K.-D.H. and J.-I.C. Data collection was performed by Y.G.K., K.-D.H., J.S. and J.-I.C. All authors have read and agreed to the published version of the manuscript.

Funding: This work was supported by a Korea University grant (J.-I.C.), a grant from Korea University Anam Hospital, Seoul, Republic of Korea (J.-I.C.), and in part by a National Research Foundation of Korea (NRF) grant funded by the Korean government (MIST, Ministry of Science and ICT) (No. 2021R1A2C2011325 to J.-I.C.). The funders had no role in data collection, analysis, or interpretation; trial design; patient recruitment; or any other aspect pertinent to the study.

Institutional Review Board Statement: The current study was approved by the Institutional Review Board of Korea University Medicine Anam Hospital and official review committee of the K-NHIS. The ethical guidelines of the 2013 Declaration of Helsinki and legal medical regulations of Republic of Korea were strictly undertaken throughout the study.

Informed Consent Statement: The requirement for written informed consent was waived by the Institutional Review Board of Korea University Medicine Anam Hospital.

Data Availability Statement: The data underlying this article are available in the article.

Conflicts of Interest: The authors have no conflict of interest and no relationships with industry.

Abbreviations

BMI: body mass index; CI: confidence interval; CKD: chronic kidney disease; DBP: diastolic blood pressure; DM: diabetes mellitus; eGFR: estimated glomerular filtration rate; FBG: fasting blood glucose; γ-GTP: gamma-glutamyl transferase; HTN: hypertension; HR: hazard ratio; ICD: International Classification of Disease; IFG: impaired fasting glucose; K-NHIS: Korean National Health Insurance Service; SBP: systolic blood pressure; SCA: sudden cardiac arrest.

References

1. Heymsfield, S.B.; Wadden, T.A. Mechanisms, Pathophysiology, and Management of Obesity. *N. Engl. J. Med.* **2017**, *376*, 254–266. [CrossRef]
2. Hall, J.E.; da Silva, A.A.; do Carmo, J.M.; Dubinion, J.; Hamza, S.; Munusamy, S.; Smith, G.; Stec, D.E. Obesity-induced hypertension: Role of sympathetic nervous system, leptin, and melanocortins. *J. Biol. Chem.* **2010**, *285*, 17271–17276. [CrossRef] [PubMed]
3. Knowler, W.C.; Fowler, S.E.; Hamman, R.F.; Christophi, C.A.; Hoffman, H.J.; Brenneman, A.T.; Brown-Friday, J.O.; Goldberg, R.; Venditti, E.; Nathan, D.M. 10-year follow-up of diabetes incidence and weight loss in the Diabetes Prevention Program Outcomes Study. *Lancet* **2009**, *374*, 1677–1686. [CrossRef] [PubMed]
4. Stecker, T.; Sparks, S. Prevalence of obese patients in a primary care setting. *Obesity* **2006**, *14*, 373–376. [CrossRef] [PubMed]

5. Flint, A.J.; Rexrode, K.M.; Hu, F.B.; Glynn, R.J.; Caspard, H.; Manson, J.E.; Willett, W.C.; Rimm, E.B. Body mass index, waist circumference, and risk of coronary heart disease: A prospective study among men and women. *Obes. Res. Clin. Pract.* **2010**, *4*, e171–e181. [CrossRef]
6. Wilson, P.W.; D'Agostino, R.B.; Sullivan, L.; Parise, H.; Kannel, W.B. Overweight and obesity as determinants of cardiovascular risk: The Framingham experience. *Arch. Intern. Med.* **2002**, *162*, 1867–1872. [CrossRef]
7. Twig, G.; Yaniv, G.; Levine, H.; Leiba, A.; Goldberger, N.; Derazne, E.; Ben-Ami Shor, D.; Tzur, D.; Afek, A.; Shamiss, A.; et al. Body-Mass Index in 2.3 Million Adolescents and Cardiovascular Death in Adulthood. *N. Engl. J. Med.* **2016**, *374*, 2430–2440. [CrossRef]
8. Calle, E.E.; Thun, M.J.; Petrelli, J.M.; Rodriguez, C.; Heath, C.W., Jr. Body-mass index and mortality in a prospective cohort of U.S. adults. *N. Engl. J. Med.* **1999**, *341*, 1097–1105. [CrossRef]
9. Jee, S.H.; Sull, J.W.; Park, J.; Lee, S.Y.; Ohrr, H.; Guallar, E.; Samet, J.M. Body-mass index and mortality in Korean men and women. *N. Engl. J. Med.* **2006**, *355*, 779–787. [CrossRef]
10. Cerhan, J.R.; Moore, S.C.; Jacobs, E.J.; Kitahara, C.M.; Rosenberg, P.S.; Adami, H.O.; Ebbert, J.O.; English, D.R.; Gapstur, S.M.; Giles, G.G.; et al. A pooled analysis of waist circumference and mortality in 650,000 adults. *Mayo Clin. Proc.* **2014**, *89*, 335–345. [CrossRef]
11. Snijder, M.B.; van Dam, R.M.; Visser, M.; Seidell, J.C. What aspects of body fat are particularly hazardous and how do we measure them? *Int. J. Epidemiol.* **2006**, *35*, 83–92. [CrossRef] [PubMed]
12. Wang, Y.; Rimm, E.B.; Stampfer, M.J.; Willett, W.C.; Hu, F.B. Comparison of abdominal adiposity and overall obesity in predicting risk of type 2 diabetes among men. *Am. J. Clin. Nutr.* **2005**, *81*, 555–563. [CrossRef]
13. Yusuf, S.; Hawken, S.; Ounpuu, S.; Bautista, L.; Franzosi, M.G.; Commerford, P.; Lang, C.C.; Rumboldt, Z.; Onen, C.L.; Lisheng, L.; et al. Obesity and the risk of myocardial infarction in 27,000 participants from 52 countries: A case-control study. *Lancet* **2005**, *366*, 1640–1649. [CrossRef]
14. Myat, A.; Song, K.J.; Rea, T. Out-of-hospital cardiac arrest: Current concepts. *Lancet* **2018**, *391*, 970–979. [CrossRef]
15. Cummins, R.O.; Ornato, J.P.; Thies, W.H.; Pepe, P.E. Improving survival from sudden cardiac arrest: The "chain of survival" concept. A statement for health professionals from the Advanced Cardiac Life Support Subcommittee and the Emergency Cardiac Care Committee, American Heart Association. *Circulation* **1991**, *83*, 1832–1847. [CrossRef]
16. Ong, M.E.H.; Perkins, G.D.; Cariou, A. Out-of-hospital cardiac arrest: Prehospital management. *Lancet* **2018**, *391*, 980–988. [CrossRef] [PubMed]
17. Pischon, T.; Boeing, H.; Hoffmann, K.; Bergmann, M.; Schulze, M.B.; Overvad, K.; van der Schouw, Y.T.; Spencer, E.; Moons, K.G.; Tjonneland, A.; et al. General and abdominal adiposity and risk of death in Europe. *N. Engl. J. Med.* **2008**, *359*, 2105–2120. [CrossRef] [PubMed]
18. Kim, Y.G.; Han, K.D.; Kim, D.Y.; Choi, Y.Y.; Choi, H.Y.; Roh, S.Y.; Shim, J.; Kim, J.S.; Choi, J.I.; Kim, Y.H. Different Influence of Blood Pressure on New-Onset Atrial Fibrillation in Pre- and Postmenopausal Women: A Nationwide Population-Based Study. *Hypertension* **2021**, *77*, 1500–1509. [CrossRef]
19. Kim, Y.G.; Han, K.-D.; Choi, J.-I.; Choi, Y.Y.; Choi, H.Y.; Boo, K.Y.; Kim, D.Y.; Lee, K.-N.; Shim, J.; Kim, J.-S. Non-genetic risk factors for atrial fibrillation are equally important in both young and old age: A nationwide population-based study. *Eur. J. Prev. Cardiol.* **2021**, *28*, 666–676. [CrossRef]
20. Al-Khatib, S.M.; Stevenson, W.G.; Ackerman, M.J.; Bryant, W.J.; Callans, D.J.; Curtis, A.B.; Deal, B.J.; Dickfeld, T.; Field, M.E.; Fonarow, G.C.; et al. 2017 AHA/ACC/HRS Guideline for Management of Patients With Ventricular Arrhythmias and the Prevention of Sudden Cardiac Death: Executive Summary: A Report of the American College of Cardiology/American Heart Association Task Force on Clinical Practice Guidelines and the Heart Rhythm Society. *J. Am. Coll. Cardiol.* **2018**, *72*, 1677–1749. [CrossRef]
21. World Health Organization; Regional Office for the Western Pacific; the International Association for the Study of Obesity; the International Obesity Task Force. *The Asia-Pacific Perspective: Redefining Obesity and Its Treatment*; World Health Organization: Geneva, Switzerland, 2002; 56p.
22. Seo, M.H.; Lee, W.Y.; Kim, S.S.; Kang, J.H.; Kang, J.H.; Kim, K.K.; Kim, B.Y.; Kim, Y.H.; Kim, W.J.; Kim, E.M.; et al. 2018 Korean Society for the Study of Obesity Guideline for the Management of Obesity in Korea. *J. Obes. Metab. Syndr.* **2019**, *28*, 40–45. [CrossRef] [PubMed]
23. Kim, Y.G.; Oh, S.K.; Choi, H.Y.; Choi, J.I. Inherited arrhythmia syndrome predisposing to sudden cardiac death. *Korean J. Intern. Med.* **2021**, *36*, 527–538. [CrossRef] [PubMed]
24. Roh, S.-Y.; Choi, J.-I.; Park, S.H.; Kim, Y.G.; Shim, J.; Kim, J.-S.; Do Han, K.; Kim, Y.-H. The 10-year trend of out-of-hospital cardiac arrests: A Korean nationwide population-based study. *Korean Circ. J.* **2021**, *51*, 866–874. [CrossRef]
25. Kim, Y.G.; Han, K.; Jeong, J.H.; Roh, S.-Y.; Choi, Y.Y.; Min, K.; Shim, J.; Choi, J.-I.; Kim, Y.-H. Metabolic Syndrome, Gamma-Glutamyl Transferase, and Risk of Sudden Cardiac Death. *J. Clin. Med.* **2022**, *11*, 1781. [CrossRef]
26. Kim, Y.G.; Roh, S.Y.; Han, K.-D.; Jeong, J.H.; Choi, Y.Y.; Min, K.; Shim, J.; Choi, J.-I.; Kim, Y.-H. Hypertension and diabetes including their earlier stage are associated with increased risk of sudden cardiac arrest. *Sci. Rep.* **2022**, *12*, 12307. [CrossRef] [PubMed]
27. Lee, J.; Lee, J.S.; Park, S.H.; Shin, S.A.; Kim, K. Cohort Profile: The National Health Insurance Service-National Sample Cohort (NHIS-NSC), South Korea. *Int. J. Epidemiol.* **2017**, *46*, e15. [CrossRef] [PubMed]

28. Lavie, C.J.; McAuley, P.A.; Church, T.S.; Milani, R.V.; Blair, S.N. Obesity and cardiovascular diseases: Implications regarding fitness, fatness, and severity in the obesity paradox. *J. Am. Coll. Cardiol.* **2014**, *63*, 1345–1354. [CrossRef]
29. Zeller, M.; Steg, P.G.; Ravisy, J.; Lorgis, L.; Laurent, Y.; Sicard, P.; Janin-Manificat, L.; Beer, J.-C.; Makki, H.; Lagrost, A.-C.c. Relation between body mass index, waist circumference, and death after acute myocardial infarction. *Circulation* **2008**, *118*, 482–490. [CrossRef]
30. Ravnskov, U. High cholesterol may protect against infections and atherosclerosis. *Int. J. Med.* **2003**, *96*, 927–934. [CrossRef]
31. Cavaillon, J.; Fitting, C.; Haeffner-Cavaillon, N.; Kirsch, S.; Warren, H.S. Cytokine response by monocytes and macrophages to free and lipoprotein-bound lipopolysaccharide. *Infect. Immun.* **1990**, *58*, 2375–2382. [CrossRef]
32. Kistorp, C.; Faber, J.; Galatius, S.; Gustafsson, F.; Frystyk, J.; Flyvbjerg, A.; Hildebrandt, P. Plasma adiponectin, body mass index, and mortality in patients with chronic heart failure. *Circulation* **2005**, *112*, 1756–1762. [CrossRef] [PubMed]
33. Csige, I.; Ujvárosy, D.; Szabó, Z.; Lőrincz, I.; Paragh, G.; Harangi, M.; Somodi, S. The impact of obesity on the cardiovascular system. *J. Diabetes Res.* **2018**, *2018*, 3407306. [CrossRef]
34. Lee, S.-H.; Chen, Y.-C.; Chen, Y.-J.; Chang, S.-L.; Tai, C.-T.; Wongcharoen, W.; Yeh, H.-I.; Lin, C.-I.; Chen, S.-A. Tumor necrosis factor-α alters calcium handling and increases arrhythmogenesis of pulmonary vein cardiomyocytes. *Life Sci.* **2007**, *80*, 1806–1815. [CrossRef] [PubMed]
35. Mohamed-Ali, V.; Goodrick, S.; Bulmer, K.; Holly, J.M.; Yudkin, J.S.; Coppack, S.W. Production of soluble tumor necrosis factor receptors by human subcutaneous adipose tissue in vivo. *Am. J. Physiol. -Endocrinol. Metab.* **1999**, *277*, E971–E975. [CrossRef] [PubMed]
36. Goossens, C.; Marques, M.B.; Derde, S.; Vander Perre, S.; Dufour, T.; Thiessen, S.E.; Güiza, F.; Janssens, T.; Hermans, G.; Vanhorebeek, I.; et al. Premorbid obesity, but not nutrition, prevents critical illness-induced muscle wasting and weakness. *J. Cachexia Sarcopenia Muscle* **2017**, *8*, 89–101. [CrossRef] [PubMed]
37. Gonzalez, M.C.; Pastore, C.A.; Orlandi, S.P.; Heymsfield, S.B. Obesity paradox in cancer: New insights provided by body composition. *Am. J. Clin. Nutr.* **2014**, *99*, 999–1005. [CrossRef]
38. Prado, C.M.; Gonzalez, M.C.; Heymsfield, S.B. Body composition phenotypes and obesity paradox. *Curr. Opin. Clin. Nutr.* **2015**, *18*, 535–551. [CrossRef]
39. Bastien, M.; Poirier, P.; Lemieux, I.; Despres, J.P. Overview of epidemiology and contribution of obesity to cardiovascular disease. *Prog. Cardiovasc. Dis.* **2014**, *56*, 369–381. [CrossRef]
40. Parto, P.; Lavie, C.J. Obesity and Cardiovascular Diseases. *Curr. Prob. Cardiol.* **2017**, *42*, 376–394. [CrossRef]
41. Penketh, J.; Nolan, J.P. In-hospital cardiac arrest: The state of the art. *Crit. Care* **2022**, *26*, 376. [CrossRef]
42. Andersson, A.; Arctaedius, I.; Cronberg, T.; Levin, H.; Nielsen, N.; Friberg, H.; Lybeck, A. In-hospital versus out-of-hospital cardiac arrest: Characteristics and outcomes in patients admitted to intensive care after return of spontaneous circulation. *Resuscitation* **2022**, *176*, 1–8. [CrossRef] [PubMed]

Disclaimer/Publisher's Note: The statements, opinions and data contained in all publications are solely those of the individual author(s) and contributor(s) and not of MDPI and/or the editor(s). MDPI and/or the editor(s) disclaim responsibility for any injury to people or property resulting from any ideas, methods, instructions or products referred to in the content.

MDPI
St. Alban-Anlage 66
4052 Basel
Switzerland
www.mdpi.com

Journal of Clinical Medicine Editorial Office
E-mail: jcm@mdpi.com
www.mdpi.com/journal/jcm

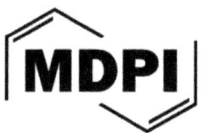

Disclaimer/Publisher's Note: The statements, opinions and data contained in all publications are solely those of the individual author(s) and contributor(s) and not of MDPI and/or the editor(s). MDPI and/or the editor(s) disclaim responsibility for any injury to people or property resulting from any ideas, methods, instructions or products referred to in the content.

www.ingramcontent.com/pod-product-compliance
Lightning Source LLC
LaVergne TN
LVHW070401100526
838202LV00014B/1364